THE AWAKENING WEST

THE AWAKENING WEST

CONVERSATIONS *with* TODAY'S NEW WESTERN SPIRITUAL LEADERS

Lynn Marie Lumiere & John Lumiere-Wins

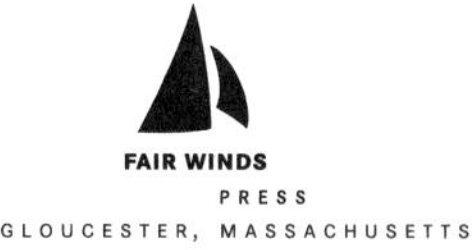

FAIR WINDS
PRESS
GLOUCESTER, MASSACHUSETTS

First revised edition published in the U.S.A. by
Fair Winds Press
33 Commercial Street
Gloucester, Massachusetts 01930-5089

Library of Congress Cataloging-in-Publication Data available

ISBN 1-59233-010-x

10 9 8 7 6 5 4 3 2 1

Cover design by: Peter King & Company
Book design by: Peter King & Company
Photo of ShantiMayi on page 255 by: Gyani Speyer

Printed and bound in Canada

DEDICATION

To all those who have been our teachers
and to the awakening of all beings

May all beings remain free from suffering
May all beings have happiness
May all beings be free

ACKNOWLEDGMENTS

Special thanks to Joolz Haugen and Sheila Hancock-Sheridan for editing.

And thanks to our Spiritual Community who has supported this project since its inception.

"BUDDHA, JESUS, AND OTHERS WERE RARE FLOWERS, THE FIRST FEW FLOWERS. AND NOW WE ARE ABOUT TO EXPERIENCE A COLLECTIVE FLOWERING OF HUMAN CONSCIOUSNESS...IT'S A COMPLETELY NEW DIMENSION OF CONSCIOUSNESS ARISING. IT REALLY IS LIKE THE BIRTH OF A NEW SPECIES OUT OF THE OLD."

Eckhart Tolle

CONTENTS

INTRODUCTION

Within the past ten years, we have noticed a wave rising steadily in the sea of human consciousness. And it continues to swell in strength and size. We noticed something unanticipated and unheard of quickening within our community of spiritual seekers and humanitarian servers. We saw ordinary people like ourselves having what had previously been considered to be extraordinary experiences of freedom and enlightenment. What we are talking about here can be called by many names: awakening, enlightenment, freedom, liberation, self-realization, etc., and has long been considered something that occurs for only the rarest few. And those rare few have primarily been found in the Eastern world.

With this book we are acknowledging and, in a series of conversations, beginning to document and explore an awakening in human consciousness on a scale that seems to us wholly unprecedented in Western civilization. Surprising though it may seem, as we proceeded with the research for this book, we discovered that the growing number of awakened Westerners now stretches far beyond the limits of a single volume. The number included here is only a small fraction of the many we have encountered and heard about, not to mention those in other areas and countries, of whom we have not yet heard. We expect that the examples in this book will stimulate you to explore this nascent phenomenon for yourself.

This is a beginning, a dawning of a shift in the evolution of Consciousness. As with all beginnings, there is so much more to learn and discover. We are learning to speak a new language of being that is just now forming in the Western world. This process has its own beauty and seems to be self-correcting and unfolding naturally. The depth of understanding about who we are is considerably more expanded than it was ten years ago. And it will have expanded even more ten years from now. We feel blessed to be a part of this expansion.

Although many more are now having experiences of awakening and glimpses of freedom, it is still rather rare for this to blossom into the full embodiment of Truth—where the awakening becomes a lived experience moment to moment and is expressed through a person's humanness in everyday life. There appears to be a spectrum of awakening from initial glimpses to fully embodied liberation. It seems to us that the people included in this book were in various places along this continuum at the time we spoke with them.

We chose to speak to spiritual teachers because they are eyewitnesses to the awakening that we are documenting here. Many of these teachers are traveling around the world and so have considerable exposure to this phenomenon. Our own observation is that many others who have had an awakening do not adopt the formal role of teacher.

For the most part, we asked the same questions of each person. We chose to do this in order to show the various flavors of the responses as well as the sameness. Each person is saying essentially the same thing in his or her own unique way. (Unfamiliar terms and names can be found in the Glossary.) Also, except for the last six interviews, we kept them in the order in which they took place, which shows some development in our own process and understanding over the period of four years that we worked on the book. In this second edition, we have added six interviews that were not included in the first edition.

So, what does all this have to do with you? It has something to do with you if your heart is quickened by what you read. It has to do with you if, when you look at the world we have created for ourselves and, seeing how far it has gotten out of balance, you feel compelled to do something to right it. Perhaps you don't know what to do. Or if you do know, you might prefer to do it with love in your heart rather than with resentment and anger.

If this book resonates with you, then explore these things for yourself. Test this. Look for yourself. Drop all preconceived notions and look. Really, what is experiencing your experience of your senses, your body, your mind and your world? See for yourself what, if anything, you find and begin to rest as that. Is there any separation between you and that? Or is that really who you are?

We invite you to join with us in this most magnificent of discoveries. In sharing these messages we pray that this book may be of service in the rapid and easy awakening of our world. May each and every one of us enjoy ease and peace and well being; may we all recognize our inextricable, innate interconnectedness with all of life in all its immediacy and diversity. May we all complete this spiritual journey together.

THE TIME IS NOW

Throughout human history there have been a handful of individuals whose awakening to Truth and the meaning of life has been the source of the great religious and spiritual traditions of the world: the anonymous Vedic sages, Lao Tzu, Buddha, Moses and the prophets, Jesus, and Muhammad. Each of these traditions has spawned saints and sages in each century who are acknowledged to have realized the same absolute Truth.

This is the awakening from the dream of separation and impermanence into the recognition that we are in reality the very consciousness that is the permanent and immanent substance of everything that appears within itself. Even our material bodies, which appear so separate, exist enmeshed within the living web of elements that compose and continually recreate them and all of life. Today, despite appearances to the contrary, contemporary science is demonstrating that nothing is disconnected from anything else: the entire universe is all one system composed of interlocking, interpenetrating, and mutually sustaining subsystems. And we humans are conscious participants within this wholeness.

This awakening can be described as a shift in perception and identity. This is a shift from a separate, personal "I" living in a world among "others," to the realization that this "I" does not fundamentally exist, except as a conceptual construct and a social convention. This awakening is about realizing that we actually are the impersonal and ever-present Awareness in which our "I" and its apparent world are arising, existing and disappearing, moment by moment.

As all sages from all traditions throughout time have asserted, that which we actually are cannot be truly captured in words. We can only be it. It cannot be fully described nor can it even be known through the mind, which is merely a part of it. Nevertheless, it is what we always have been and cannot not be. We can and have overlooked it however, in our conditioned and socially sanctioned identifications with our mind, our body, and our personal stories about who we are and what life is all about.

This dawning of awakened consciousness appears to be calling all of us in these times of increasing turmoil, greed, violence, and environmental destruction; and we are just beginning to discover how available and "contagious" this awakening actually is. It seems that for humans as a species, now is the time! Unless there is a widespread and profound shift in our confusion and fear, our ignorance, greed, rage, and polarization, we humans may soon end life as we know it on our planet.

As a species, we humans—especially in the West—have been living in a disconnected, media-driven, conceptual culture. We have been unaware of our natural role within the web of life. We have been disconnected from one another, from the Earth, from the feminine, and most painfully, we have been disconnected from our own essential Being. This is even apparent in most Western churches and temples which have lost touch with the living spirit that infused their roots and have largely become dogmatic and spiritually dry.

Over the last thirty years many Westerners, finding our own traditions lacking, have turned toward the more experiential traditions of the East—Hinduism, Buddhism, Taoism and Sufis—as well as to indigenous peoples' traditions, which recognize and honor the ecological dynamics of all our relations. These experiential approaches have significantly influenced the development of humanistic and transpersonal psychology. These movements have grown tremendously since the consciousness expansion of the 1960s, which was largely stimulated by the use of mind-expanding drugs. During those heady times, thousands if not millions of us, glimpsed another vision of what it means to be human—a vision that was kinder, more conscious, more cooperative, and humane. We believe that the awakening we are referring to in this book is the next wave of consciousness expansion and is already having far-reaching effects.

The Eastern practices promised a way to realize what was glimpsed on psychedelics, and new forms of psychotherapy offered increased awareness and improved functioning in one's life. Since those early days, a growing number of Western seekers, ourselves included, became sincerely involved in Eastern spiritual practices and in healing our past childhood trauma and conditioning. As it turned out, for most of us, it has been very slow going. We have been struggling to change our entrenched, conditioned patterns without the realization of That which is already free of these patterns.

Contributing further to this search for something more is the disillusionment with materialism that many in the West experience. Not only has it failed to bring the fulfillment it advertises, but worse, it seems to be destroying our planet's ecosystem. In the face of the current global marketing of material consumption, and near total corporate control of democratic processes around the world, there is a growing concern for ecological and human values. Dissatisfaction with life as we have known it, as well as the ominous feeling that things have gotten way beyond our personal control, has contributed to a search for authentic meaning and connectedness. As Isaac Shapiro says, "Now we are at a place and time where we are ready for a mass awakening on this planet." And, as the great Indian sage Ramana Maharshi once said, "When there is a nightmare, everybody wants to wake up."

Yet in the midst of this increased interest in personal growth and spirituality, there is at the same time an increasing disenchantment with psychology, religion, and spiritual practice. They have failed to fulfill their promise for all but the rare few. In fact, after twenty or more years of effort, many spiritual practitioners are now recognizing that practice itself can be a potential obstacle to awakening. Spiritual practice tends to perpetuate the belief that true fulfillment is not here and now, but has to be attained at some time in the future through effort. The problem with the future is that it is always in the future.

Many people are thirsty for a true and lasting fulfillment which is practical and accessible, not something that takes forty years of meditation practice or happens only after you die, if you're good enough. As Lama Surya Das says, "People are getting more sophisticated, more subtle and deeper, and less fascinated with the side effects and the special effects of spiritual life, and more interested in the heart of the matter."

There is a tremendous surge of interest in the United States and throughout the Western world in what is known as the direct or immediate paths: the non-dual teachings such as Advaita Vedanta and the Tibetan Buddhist, Dzogchen. These approaches teach that what we most essentially are is already, always, immediately available to be directly experienced right here, right now. In this book you will notice the repeated pointing to immediacy in each person's message. None of these people are directing us to a path of long, arduous spiritual practice; instead, each is asking us to notice something so simple that we tend to discount it. It is so present and near at hand that we tend to look right past it in our determined effort to find lasting peace and happiness in the future by becoming different or "better."

The Truth of who we are is a direct experience, available at all times, but it also seems that we must be ready to hear that. We can't say what led us personally to that readiness. But we do know that sitting with people such as those presented here in this book has been extremely helpful and inspiring. Being in their presence can inspire both the recognition that this present awareness is what we truly are and the deepening of this recognition into the ground from which we live, moment to moment.

We have the deepest gratitude for those who have been our teachers —most of whom are included in this book. Although in an absolute sense, it can be said that we don't need any help because we already are what we seek, paradoxically most of us need to be in the presence of one who is awake in order to awaken ourselves. Otherwise, our restless sleep of delusion continues uninterrupted, and others who are asleep only support it.

For us, this book is in part an honoring and a sharing of our teachers. Most of all, we want this book to communicate that now is the time that we can all awaken from our dream of separation; the suffering and dissatisfaction we have so long endured and struggled with can end. This awakening is not limited to an exceptional few. Since it involves realizing what we already actually are, it is available to everyone who sincerely wants it. Beyond that, we anticipate that encountering the individuals in this book will help to break up many of the myths people have about enlightenment and the "awakened ones." We hope to dispel the myth that they must have had special or extraordinary lives, or that they only became enlightened through various rigorous practices or a particular creed.

In fact, the people you will meet here are from many different walks of life. Some come from ancient spiritual traditions and are the contemporary lineage holders of direct transmissions handed down through many centuries; others are from no particular tradition. Some have done a great deal of spiritual practice, some very little or none at all. Some have teachers or gurus; others do not.

An important principle that this book illustrates is that despite the diversity of their gender, race, class, and religious backgrounds, these people agree that there is only one Truth and each and every one of us is That. The difference in the flavors of its expression is particularly rich and distinct among these Westerners. Perhaps that is because our awakenings are not as influenced by ancient cultural traditions with long established patterns of what constitutes "enlightened" behavior. We find a fresh uniqueness in the ways that Truth is expressed here. Each one is a radiant facet of one luminous gem. Each offers their unique wisdom and understanding of the same one Truth.

Ultimately, it appears that everyone is seeking happiness through something: power, pleasure, self-improvement, spiritual attainment or simply the acquisition of more and better things. The recognition that what we seek is what we, essentially, already are is a radical, evolutionary shift in perspective, now dawning among a rapidly widening circle of people. Behind all of our striving is an unquestioned belief that there is something missing. The time has come to stop searching for what we think is missing and discover what has never been lost. The resulting peace and ease of being influences every facet of our lives, and infuses all our relations with kindness, compassion, and love.

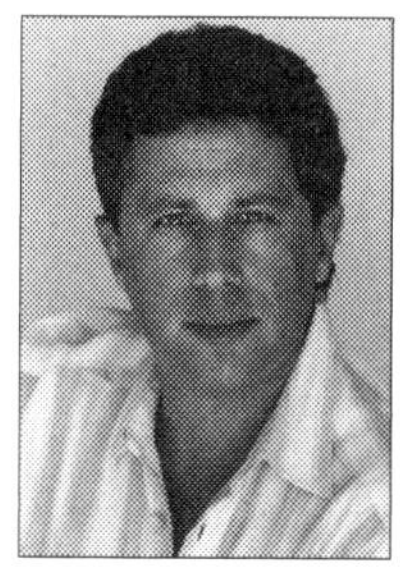

ROBERT RABBIN

"WE DON'T NEED TO SEEK: WE HAVE ALREADY FOUND.
WE DON'T NEED TO LEARN: WE ALREADY KNOW.
WE DON'T HAVE TO BECOME: WE ALREADY ARE.
SEE THIS AND BE FREE."

from The Sacred Hub

While browsing a magazine, John came across a couple of quotes from a book, *The Sacred Hub*, by Robert Rabbin. Upon reading them, he recognized that this man had had an awakening and contacted him in southern California by phone. This was the first contact made after the idea for this book was born.

When Robert came to the Bay Area a month later, we were able to attend one of his evening talks. The silence in his presence was palpable and Robert's responses to questions were thorough and often revealed an unusual perspective and a very creative vision. During a conversation after the class, Robert agreed to do an interview with John, and so the book began. At this point, Lynn Marie had not yet joined the interviewing process.

Initially Robert seemed to be profoundly unpredictable which was somewhat unnerving. This quickly passed, however, as a warm relatedness and our common interest took its place. Robert's interest in the spontaneous, original expression of Truth was complemented by John's genuine appreciation of the immediate potency and beauty of his words.

Robert now lectures and leads seminars around the country and is consulted by individuals as well as corporate and community leaders on a broad range of personal and professional issues. He has authored several books in addition to *The Sacred Hub*, and his articles and columns are published internationally in magazines and newspapers. Robert is a frequent speaker to groups in the business, academic, and spiritual communities.

Robert has had a lifelong interest in the nature of the human mind and consciousness. He studied with Swami Muktananda in India, and subsequently, his spiritual inquiry has been profoundly influenced by Ramana Maharishi and Nisargadatta Maharaj.

CONVERSATION *with* ROBERT RABBIN

JLW *Who are you?*

ROBERT There are several levels at which that can be answered. However, whatever one says, however precise and comprehensive one's self definition is, the deepest truth of who one is only begins to be revealed in silence. An old Chinese poet once remarked, "99.9 percent of everything you do and of everything you think is for the sake of your self. And you don't have one."

We are all, in our essence, the dynamic eternal awareness in which the secondary definitions that include one's role in life, one's personal history and personality and character particulars are not very important. They shouldn't be taken too seriously. We ought to have disclaimers attached to our personal histories similar to the ones used by psychic hotlines: For entertainment purposes only.

JLW *What is enlightenment, realization, awakening?*
ROBERT They are merely words, and as with all words they must be defined within a particular context. With respect to the thrust of our conversation, these words point beyond themselves. We must not get caught in what they might mean conceptually. They refer to something beyond conceptual knowing.

JLW *Do they refer to something for you? What would you say?*
ROBERT Of the terms you mentioned, the one that has the most relevance is awakening. Awakening is an interesting word. It feels alive to me. The way we use it in common language is to say that I have awakened from sleep or that I have awakened from a dream or from a nightmare or from some kind of delusion. The awakening we're talking about here is very similar to the experience of waking up from sleep, from dreams, from a nightmare, to the waking state. But in this "awakening" we awaken from the waking state into the awakened state, or reality. This kind of awakening is an experience not unfamiliar to most of us, though we experience it briefly and are conditioned to turn away from it quickly. You mentioned this the other night when you described your own glimpses into reality.

Many people have experienced this sudden stab of love in the heart and the effortless expansion beyond doubt. In this awakening we find ourselves in love and struck by beauty such that we become silent. In that silence we realize our oneness with that awareness in which everything occurs.

I think that what awakening refers to is to the experience of being truly alive, aware and free from the distortions imposed by the limitations of our senses and the patterns within our mind. And this awakening certainly liberates us from the accumulation of false identities through which our memory creates and sustains a sense of separateness from the whole.

Of course, the practical memory remains. You'll still be able to program your VCR.

JLW *So awakening refers to the awareness of that in which all things may or may not be occurring. Is that what you mean?*

ROBERT I do mean that, but it isn't enough to be able to just say it. It is necessary to have the direct experience, because what you just said, while I don't disagree, is still conceptual. We should remember what Rumi said, "No matter how you think it is, it's different than that!"

The actual experience is always different from the words used to describe the experience, and in this case so radically different that there is no correlation between saying it and experiencing it.

It's very important to use concepts, especially ones built upon the words of others, carefully. We ought to remain suspicious of our own comfort with conceptual knowing because in the matters of which we are speaking, it is the difference between the menu and the meal. It's so important that we learn to see the ease with which we quickly develop a conceptual representation of that which is utterly beyond representation, and then think it's the same thing. The mind is such a gossip and busybody and loves to pretend to know what it cannot know.

Rather than developing our reliance on concepts and the words of others, we ought to develop an original form of self-expression that demonstrates the experience of our oneness with that awareness. I think we become lazy because of our habitual borrowing of expressions from Lao Tzu, or the Buddha, or this teacher or that scripture. It's much more exciting and alive and fun to speak with originality about one's direct experience.

As we practice articulating in an original way the subtle facets of our being, we will live in the evocative climate of that awareness. We will be able to see for ourselves how ever-present the awakened state is. And we will know, through experience, reflection, and expression that it is much greater than the phrasing "the awareness in which everything occurs."

JLW *So, how did this awakening occur for you?*

ROBERT Actually, there isn't an awakening, even though we speak as though there is. The awakening refers to an original, uncorrupted presence. It isn't a state of mind or being because anything we can say will not be true enough to approximate what the word "awakening" points to.

Even if the awakening did occur, it wouldn't occur to anyone because that is the price of admission, so to speak. Whoever one thinks one is, that disappears in the awakening. This awakening doesn't belong to anyone and it doesn't occur to anyone. It is eternally present and apparent; so it can never be more revealed than it is right now. It can never be more present than it is right now. It is never lost. It is never achieved. The clarity and freedom inherent in what we are calling awakening begins to shine through when an individual becomes transparent enough.

So really one doesn't awaken. One stops pretending to be other than what they are. It has more to do with either taking off the various costumes, or keeping the costume on but knowing it is a costume and taking great delight in the costume.

I did spend a lot of time and energy investigating myself; I explored my attachment to various costumes, various forms of make-believe and pretense. And then, in the course of these investigations and explorations, there was a kind of passing away of the dense constellation of elements that we take to be the personal self. I'm trying to remember what actually happened, but it is beyond my recollection because it was not really a particular experience or singular event. It seems that it was more like a piece of ice melting. At some point, there was only water: fluid, flowing, expansive.

It's more like one day, your self-interest and self-concern just drifts out to sea and you stop recycling the reactivity gathered from past experiences. What remains when the preoccupation with "self" disappears is a different kind of person, one in whom suffering and confusion and doubt don't stick. The sense of being an individual remains, but it remains within a much larger context of awareness. It is as though the individual self is a cloud in a vast sky. The cloud is suspended within the sky, changing shape according to situations.

JLW *Do you have any suggestions or recommendations for others who are experiencing a desire for awakening to the truth?*

ROBERT I would say to those people who have an interest in awakening that they become very close to that urge within them which is inciting them to investigate the truth of things. That will be their guide. And, being their guide, it may take them to India, Japan, Korea, or South America. It may take them to Berkeley or Redwood City or St. Louis or

Los Angeles. It may take them into the presence of a teacher or not. It may take them into the presence of a structured path or not.

Trust that. Learn to discern its effect in your life. And when it takes you someplace, then give yourself to where it has taken you fully and without reservation. If it takes you into the presence of a teacher, then for as long as you are there, become the absolute best student you can be. If it takes you to a hatha yoga studio, then become the absolute best yogi you can be. If it takes you into a job at the post office, then do your work with absolute clear-eyed integrity, open-hearted compassion, and skill. In that way, know that the energy which is urging you, the pressure within you that is moving you towards the awakening is the awakening itself. And follow that.

For those people who are tired of pursuing and want to end the whole game in a hurry, just investigate who you are as an experiencer, as a perceiver, as an individual. See who you are through merciless self-inquiry. Awakening occurs naturally as we release our hold on conceptual thinking, as we develop our ability to listen deeply, to see beyond appearances. The state of clarity exists within us, fully developed, ripe and ready for eating. This clarity becomes self-evident in silence.

I am also tempted to say that people should meditate, by which I mean to turn one's attention inward so as to be able to observe the nature and function of mind directly. In this way, one can easily see the ways in which we block the light of our innate clarity. This seeing occurs in silence. It is spontaneous and beyond words. That with which we observe the nature of the mind from a place of silence and openness is awareness itself.

JLW *Thank you... It seems that more and more people are awakening to the truth of their being in the Western world. Does it seem so to you, and if so, what does it signify?*

ROBERT I would say that the nature of people's beliefs is expanding to include non-conventional realities, and because their beliefs are expanding, the range of their perceptions and experiences is expanding. But new beliefs do not equate to clarity, which is the hallmark of awakening. Awakening is a fireball that engulfs the fantasies of the mind. The awakening has a scorched earth policy. Everything that was is reduced to silence, and then from that silence a new life emerges. But there must be the silence first; the furnace must do its work.

Certainly, there is a widespread interest in spirituality, in awakening. One can see Deepak Chopra or Marianne Williamson on Larry King. One can see Gary Zukav on Oprah. We can see the influence of the Dalai Lama or Thich Nhat Hanh within political and business circles. Ram Dass has been to the White House.

If there is a great awakening going on, we should be able to see more and more people expressing that clarity and freedom in their lives, not just in their conversations. As Chogyam Trungpa said, "There is no enlightenment. There is only enlightened activity."

JLW *What do you see as the source of suffering in the world, and what, if anything can or should be done about it?*

ROBERT Suffering in the world is not different from suffering in one's own self. There is no suffering in the world that doesn't originate within one's own consciousness. It is my view that suffering originates from alienation from the truth, from the despair, the loneliness, the tension, and the fear of misperceiving who one is. In the moment of awakening, suffering ends, regardless of the subsequent conditions or circumstances in a person's life. And when the suffering ends within oneself, one is no longer capable of inflicting suffering on others and therefore does not contribute to the suffering in the world.

So, if suffering is to end in the world, suffering must end within ourselves. For suffering to end within ourselves, we must come to know who we are. In knowing who we are, all forms of unnecessary violence and chaos and oppression disappear because there is no longer any motivation for them. The motivation for those acts of terrorism dissolves in the awakening. After that, suffering and violence can't occur.

JLW *Awakening ends the sense of a personal "I." Without operating out of a personal "I", how do you make decisions and get things done?*

ROBERT I think this is the most frequently-asked question. It is the question of greatest concern for people. "Well if I don't do it, how will it get done and what will happen to me?" Things will happen as they have always happened. As the limited sense of "I" becomes submerged in the expanse of clarity, we begin to see how things have always happened. I think it was Nisargadatta Maharaj who said that anything that happens is a result of everything that happens. It is only our egocentric perspective that likes to take sole ownership for what happens.

Of course, from this perspective, we can believe that through one's own efforts particular results occur. And this is true, but it is true within the relativity of this limited self. From this egocentric perspective, we can indeed make a relationship between "our" intention and effort and a particular result. From this perspective, cause and effect are linear. From another perspective, this is not true.

When one awakens, the solidity of oneself dissipates, and thus it is more difficult to draw precise lines between this effort and that result, because it is more difficult to locate a starting point of intention or effort. As long as we are embodied, we will be compelled to participate, to act, to be involved in producing outcomes. But we do so from within a larger context than our own "personal" effort.

In that greater context than the personal, in that awakened state, things happen of their own accord, in such a way that the mind can never understand because a mind cannot fathom that reality. To say that things happen of their own accord does not mean that we are not involved in the happening.

The greater problem here is that it is our mind that wants to know, definitively, how things happen. The mind can never know. It is too limited a means: it cannot recognize how things occur outside of time and location and effort and intention. It wants to remain the center of things, one way or another. It wants a degree of certainty, and thus control, to mitigate the fear that lurks within its own center.

I would like to say in passing that when we awaken, the "outcomes" we seek are much different than before. We do not work against life, seeking something only for the sake of the limited self. Our concern for the limited self is not our motivating force. We begin to live happily in the larger unfolding of life, with all of its mystery and spontaneity.

JLW *Beautiful... Rob, without operating out of a personal "I," from the perspective you have been describing, how do you experience relationships with others?*

ROBERT Relationships are created according to the quality that I bring to my encounter with each moment. So it is always a new event, moment to moment, according to the qualities that I bring to my encounters with others. If I'm open, if I'm grasping, if I'm not. If I'm ambitious, if I'm lustful. All of these qualities determine the nature of a relationship.

Relationships are a very powerful mirror for how we are being. It is a wonderful practice field to see whether or not our clarity is expressing itself in action, or whether the many hands of our mind and ego are grabbing, pulling, and tearing.

JLW *As you know, Westerners are very much into self-improvement. Does involvement in the various therapies and spiritual practices assist in awakening?*

ROBERT Anything can be a catalyst for the awakening. But there is no exact formula that will be effective for all people all the time. For example, if in reading your particular Enneagram model something strikes you and you have a revelation of Self, we could say the Enneagram was useful for you in your awakening. I think it would then be a mistake for you to go out and insist that all of your friends take up the study of the Enneagram. It would be a mistake to think that the Enneagram has any particular value in terms of its ability to awaken. It was a part of the whole moment. Every moment, because it lives in awakening, is an expression of the awakened state. Everything—a cat, a flower, the Enneagram, a seminar, a guru's touch, reading a book, a Fritos commercial on TV—can in some way facilitate the awakening. Remember, what we are calling awakening is a pre-existing fact of existence. Clarity can burst forth any moment, with or without discernible cause, because everything grows out of the soil of that clarity.

JLW *Is there anything else you would like to add?*

ROBERT I would add that silence is the greatest teacher. I know that we want to be able to "know" how things happen and who we are. We can know these things, but only within the sphere of the mind. There comes a moment when one no longer needs explanations and definitions.

There comes a moment when simplicity is enough, when clarity in each moment is enough, when spontaneous action is enough. A great peace and contentment exists within us, perfectly formed, and that is enough. Within silence, all is known, silently. Whatever is said about that silence is too noisy and complex. Ramana Maharshi said, "When you know yourself, all else will be known." This is my experience. We know ourselves in silence, and it is from this silence that a life of freedom, clarity, and joy emerges effortlessly.

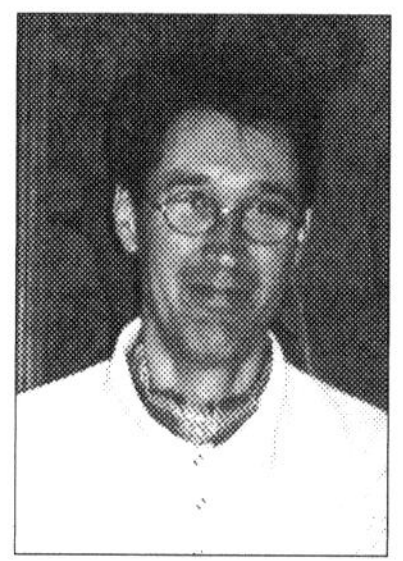

FRANCIS LUCILLE

"ACCEPT THE POSSIBILITY THAT YOU ARE ALREADY PERFECTLY OKAY. YOU ARE ALREADY FULLY ENLIGHTENED, COMPLETELY FREE. YOU HAVE TO BE OPEN TO THAT POSSIBILITY, AND IF YOU ARE OPEN TO THAT POSSIBILITY, THEN IT BECOMES REALITY."

We first met Francis over four years ago while attending one of his dialogues in the Bay Area. Since then we have had the pleasant opportunity of being with him many times. His presentation is quiet, soft, and gentle. At the same time, he expresses a sharp clarity and precise insight. With Francis there is a simple welcoming of all that arises which is noticeable in the aroma of his presence.

Through his presence, as well as through the method of dialogue, Francis points to our timeless essence, awareness, as the real substance of our body and the world, thus showing a way to end fear and suffering. Francis also teaches a form of body work, or "body-sensing," which helps one to experience their "body of awareness" which is at the root of the sensing of the static body. Through this method, the energies that were tied up in the somatic structure are set free and an expansion of consciousness free from the limitations of the ego becomes a living experience.

Francis Lucille was born in France in 1944. He is a graduate of École Polytechnique in Paris, where he was trained as a mathematician and physicist. In 1973, he began his spiritual search after encountering Vedanta and Zen scriptures. His deep thirst for the Truth of life took over and all other pursuits were lost. This search found its resolution through meeting his teacher, Jean Klien, in 1975.

Besides working as a scientist and diplomat, Francis has held dialogues, workshops, and retreats in Europe, Canada and the United States over the past twenty years. He is now retired from employment and works full time sharing his understanding with truth seekers. He is also the author of *Eternity Now, Dialogues on Awareness* and has made available a series of tapes of recorded dialogues which are focused on themes such as happiness, relationships, and our natural state.

CONVERSATION *with* FRANCIS LUCILLE

JLW: *Who are you?*

FRANCIS: I am awareness. I am the same as you are, the same awareness.

JLW: *What is enlightenment, realization, awakening?*

FRANCIS: I don't know, what does that mean to you?

JLW: *To me it means the recognition of just what you are saying, that at the very ground there is awareness, that's the fundamental ground of being, and everything occurs in that. Awakening means the realization of that. Somehow I think it means the permanent and final realization of that rather than just a glimpse. Would you change or add to what I am saying?*
FRANCIS: Are you implying that the glimpse of awareness is not enlightenment?

JLW: *It seems so. The glimpse seems to be an enlightenment, a realization experience, but if it is repeatedly getting covered over or obscured, then maybe there is a process in which one becomes stabilized in that knowledge or recognition, I don't know... I thought I was asking you!*
FRANCIS: I think that Truth-seekers may put too much emphasis on awakening and not enough on awareness. Awareness is the substance of awakening and what is important is the substance. Awakening is often construed as an event in space and time. Although there are events which are very important, and it certainly is an important event, whether it's a glimpse or a magnitude-eight earthquake, the important element is not the awakening but it is That to which one awakens. So, if the important thing is That to which one awakens, then the glimpse of it is very important... and creating an idea of a person who has had the glimpse is already falling from it.

JLW: *Yes, and how did this awakening come about for you?*
FRANCIS: I don't like to tell personal stories because they have the drawback of being personal.

JLW: *I think in this case it might be advantageous because...*
FRANCIS: I'm not trying to dodge the question, but the main drawback is that people may try to identify with the specific succession of events that I present and conclude, "It has not happened for me this way, so there must be something wrong." There are as many paths as there are Truth-lovers and seekers and this has to be said before we can go into a personal story.

I think that the quest for Truth starts with dissatisfaction. As long as we are happy with the state of things, we feel no need to look for anything. We begin the search when we feel deep dissatisfaction or the recognition of failure in our life. In my case, I was not happy despite having obtained a good education, a good job, marriage, children, and so on. There was a deep sense of failure in my life. It was a sense of urgency that brought me to the quest.

The quest began with a serendipitous circumstance in a Parisian bookstore during which I came across a book by J. Krishnamurti. I sat in a bistro and read this book which was something completely new for me. I had read thousands of books in my life, but it was the first book that interested me in this way. I went back to the bookstore and purchased all the books I could find by Krishnamurti. Then, I flew back home and started talking about him to my friends. I was disappointed when I discovered that they did not share my deep interest.

At this time there was an abrupt and dramatic change in my life focus. I stopped doing almost everything else in order to read and meditate. After a while, the desire arose to find someone who would be an embodiment of living free from fear, someone who could birth this in me. I began looking and met a few interesting people and at some point I met my teacher.

JLW: *Thank you... do you have any suggestions or recommendations for others who are experiencing a desire for awakening?*
FRANCIS: Follow your desire for the Truth. It may lead you to strange people or places, but in the end you'll be fine!

JLW: *I'd like to step back a little... after two years you met your teacher. At some point you realized what he represented and was endeavoring to communicate to you. How did this happen?*
FRANCIS: You see, it was a two-step process because there was a delay between the actual experience of awakening, which came first, and the recognition that he was my teacher. After having met him, in a way I can say, his presence was still within me... his silence, his listening, and his welcoming. Through his presence somehow he taught me welcoming—through his welcoming.

After I met him I thought, "What a nice man, I would like him to be my friend. I would like to spend more time with him." It did not occur to me that at last I had found my teacher even though at the time I was looking for a teacher. It was with this goal in mind that I had met him, and yet all that came to me after the meeting was the thought, "Maybe he is the one you are looking for." Nothing in his behavior nor in what happened told me he was not, so I was open to that possibility; that's all.

During the following days and weeks, I would quite often think about him. I was spending a lot of time with a disciple of his, who had become a good friend of mine. One day we were meditating at my place and toward the end of the meditation, unexpectedly, my friend started chanting the Gayatri Mantra. When I listened to the sound and felt the beauty and sacredness of the first Aum, I felt mysteriously attracted toward this beauty, toward this sacredness. At the same time I had the distinct impression that something was preventing me from surrendering, from being one with this sound. Since I was experiencing the welcoming attitude I had learned from my teacher, I let come up whatever it was that was preventing me from being one with the sound.

As I welcomed this obstacle, it soon grew into a very intense panic and fear of dying. At that point, I was so committed to the search that I was simply willing to die. I can remember knowingly making the decision to die if necessary. I thought, "So what! Let it be so if it must."

The moment I accepted that possibility, the fear almost instantaneously became purely a bodily sensation; it was completely seen. The structure of the fear at the level of thinking was also being completely witnessed. I could see both the top of the structure at the level of thinking and the bottom at the level of feeling. I could see this vanishing from both ends, only the single trunk of the tree remained, and this was the "I" thought. I could see the "I" thought vacillating like the flame of a candle just before it is extinguished. Then it just vanished. All of this was happening during the first Aum of the incantation, to give you a temporal frame of reference.

JLW: *What a sacred moment!*

FRANCIS: Yes. And what occurred after that could not be expressed in words. Even if I say that it was beauty, immortality, absolute love, absolute understanding, I am ashamed to use these words.

Putting things in perspective, what this event accomplished, almost instantaneously, were two things: First, because it gave me the certainty of my immortality, it permanently "cured" me from fear. Second, it gave me a bliss that was absolute. It was unlike any happiness I had known up until that point, which had been relative, meaning I could always expect something more—this was absolute. With it came the knowledge, "This is it; there is nothing which could be greater because this is beyond measure." The experience of this bliss cured me from desire. So I was cured from both fear and desire.

It does not mean, by the way, that fear and desire instantaneously stopped, because for a while the old habits kept reoccurring. But that which was fueling them was no longer alive, and so there was nothing to fuel them any longer.

JLW: *Yes, I've heard that reoccurring old habits continue like a fan that has been turned off but is continuing to spin out its momentum.*

FRANCIS: Right. Although the mind was struck by something that was beyond its comprehension, from the vantage point of the mind at that moment, it was an event in space and time. This was a misinterpretation of the mind. I remember going to my teacher a few days later, being overwhelmed by that which I couldn't put into any box with a label on it. I described the experience and I asked him, was this the experience you are talking about? And he said, with a smile, "If I understand you correctly, it had a beginning in time and an end in time?" At that moment I said, "Yes." And then he said, "Well, then it is not the experience I am talking about," And then he added, with a smile, "No matter what it was or wasn't, just keep the perfume of it; live with the perfume of it."

It is very important to never acknowledge an experience because you have to find it by yourself; it has to find itself in you. It reminds me of the Zen story of the student who had an experience of satori. He came to see his teacher and said, "I had this experience, Master, was it satori?" The master says, "No, it is not satori; it is just no big deal." So the guy goes back to his room but still this powerful experience is with him that his mind cannot digest. He has no place he can put it within his mind. There is a freedom within him and this beauty and power. A few days or months later he comes back to his teacher and asks him again, "Are you really sure that this experience I told you about is not the satori?" Then the teacher tells him, "Of course I am sure." Then the student tells him, "Okay. In this case you keep your satori; I will keep this experience." And then the teacher says, "That is satori!"

JLW: *So, initially your mind was interpreting it as an event in space and time, but obviously you have since recognized that although there was an event, it was a revelation of* *something that was transcendental, that was beyond space and time. How did that come about?*

FRANCIS: It is something that came about thanks to my teacher. In my case, I had a longstanding relationship with my teacher after the initial awakening. I had a lot of baggage intellectually and in my body that I had to get rid of. My teacher was instrumental in helping me put things in the correct perspective. He also helped to transpose this understanding not only intellectually, but also at the level of feeling in the body. He helped to bring it into the level of daily life. It was wonderful just to live with him, to spend long vacations together and see how he would do his shopping, how he would cook his food, or how he would interact with others and so on. There was a kind of silent teaching that went on.

JLW: *It was a living of the understanding or a living of the revelation.*

FRANCIS: Yes. They were very wonderful vacations I had with him. The teaching goes on all the time. The teaching does not stop the moment you have this revelation. In fact, the teaching never stops.

JLW: *Can you say a little bit more about that? Is there an ongoing deepening or a further revelation that you notice or experience?*

FRANCIS: Every moment is a revelation; this moment is a revelation. The perfect teacher is in fact the perfect student; there is no difference. The perfect student is totally open, eager to learn, open to the unknown from moment to moment. That is also what the perfect teacher is. In a way, you are a disciple of Truth for life. It's just that two things disappear—fear and desire. That is the only difference.

JLW: *And, as you said earlier, the "I" thought disappeared as well.*

FRANCIS: Yes. Prior to the revelation I am referring to, I had glimpses and ecstatic experiences of beauty and harmony. The difference with this revelation was that I witnessed the disappearance of the ego, of the "I" thought and its train of fears and desires. At that precise moment when it disappeared, I knew my Self, and I remained as That.

JLW: *When you say that there was intellectual and physical baggage, what are you referring to?*

FRANCIS: The baggage is made out of memories, repetitions, patterns, habits, both at the level of thinking and at the level of bodily perceptions and tensions. These old patterns originated from the inner core "I" thought, and in a moment I directly saw this inner core disappear and be replaced first by the immensity and then within this immensity, a beauty, absolute love, splendor, and immortality. Having seen that, there is no possible identification even if the old "I" thought reappears as a matter of habit. Once there has been this recognition, you don't go for the ride. It is just not possible. It is seen for what it is. If it appears you say, "Oh, the clown and the monkey are showing up again." It is almost laughable.

I had a period of about two years when it was very intense. The first year was an especially difficult adjustment, but there is a grace in this. The difficulty happened when I was not in the physical presence of my teacher. At that point I still did not know that he was my teacher. For a while I kept seeing other teachers; I kept looking. I spent the next summer with my teacher as a friend. I was invited to his place, and we would do some meditation, some body work in the morning, and I would ask him questions all day long. Still my life was chaotic somehow. I had pain about my relationships with women and the old habits were still powerful. Approximately one year later, during one of his public dialogues, I knew he was my teacher. I knew it because it came from the same source; it was unmistakable. From that moment on, it was a one-to-one relationship; I didn't see any other teacher; I just focused on his teachings.

JLW: *Regarding the old habits, do they just play themselves out and then cease because there is no one engaging in them?*

FRANCIS: Yes. For example, I used to smoke. After the awakening, I almost instantaneously went down from twenty cigarettes a day to two cigarettes a day and kept smoking one or two cigarettes a day for ten years. Then I just suddenly stopped altogether. It was effortless.

I also noticed a big change in my sleeping patterns. I used to sleep for eight or nine hours; now I sleep for only five hours. There is an awareness present during sleep that was not there before. You could say that something was never sleeping in me. I go into dreaming and remain aware during the transition, completely aware.

JLW: *I'd like to ask what you see as the source of suffering in this world, and what you think can be done about it?*

FRANCIS: The source of suffering is to think of oneself as a person, as a separate entity. The body is going to die; it is going to suffer. As long as you are identified with the body, its physical pain and the dying process, you are the agony and the psychological suffering. The moment you are not someone in this world, but this world is in you, the picture changes completely—you are free. You then see the beauty of things, of the leaves that come out in the spring, of the flower that takes its full expansion, then fades away and a new flower comes. The cycles of life, the seasons of life and death, there is a great beauty to that. You don't see that beauty with the narrow, obstructing prism of the personal entity.

JLW: *Without having a personal identity, how do you make decisions, how do things get done?*
FRANCIS: Things get done. Decisions get made. Nobody makes them. Nobody does anything. This has always been the case in fact. Even from the vantage point of a so-called ignorant person... the ignorance is just a presumption that he or she does anything, good or bad.

JLW: *So things get done and then there's an afterthought claiming ownership of the doing, but there is no individual doer?*
FRANCIS: Right, exactly.

JLW: *How do you experience relationships with others?*
FRANCIS: There are no others. There appear to be others, but you move directly beyond the appearance and you contact the other where we are one. I am not a limited body, but rather space. The so-called "other," already as a physical entity, is not distant. It is welcomed within this space. The "other" is already me. When I look into your eyes, I see only That which is beyond—and That is what I am.

JLW: *Westerners are very much into self-improvement. Does psychotherapy assist in awakening?*
FRANCIS: I would say that it depends on the therapist. If the therapist is free, he or she will make you free no matter what is said or done. The really important factor is the inherent freedom in the therapist.

JLW: *Are there some people who are relatively free, or is it like a light switch that's either on or off?*
FRANCIS: That which we all are is freedom, awareness; in this sense you cannot say that someone is not free. We are all awareness, and awareness is free. However, this freedom expresses itself in different ways depending

on the individual. There are people, for example, who are free from the notion of being a person, but somehow don't have a feeling for beauty. They are more sensitive to the truth and understanding aspect of it and less to the beauty aspect of it, like there are all kinds of flowers.

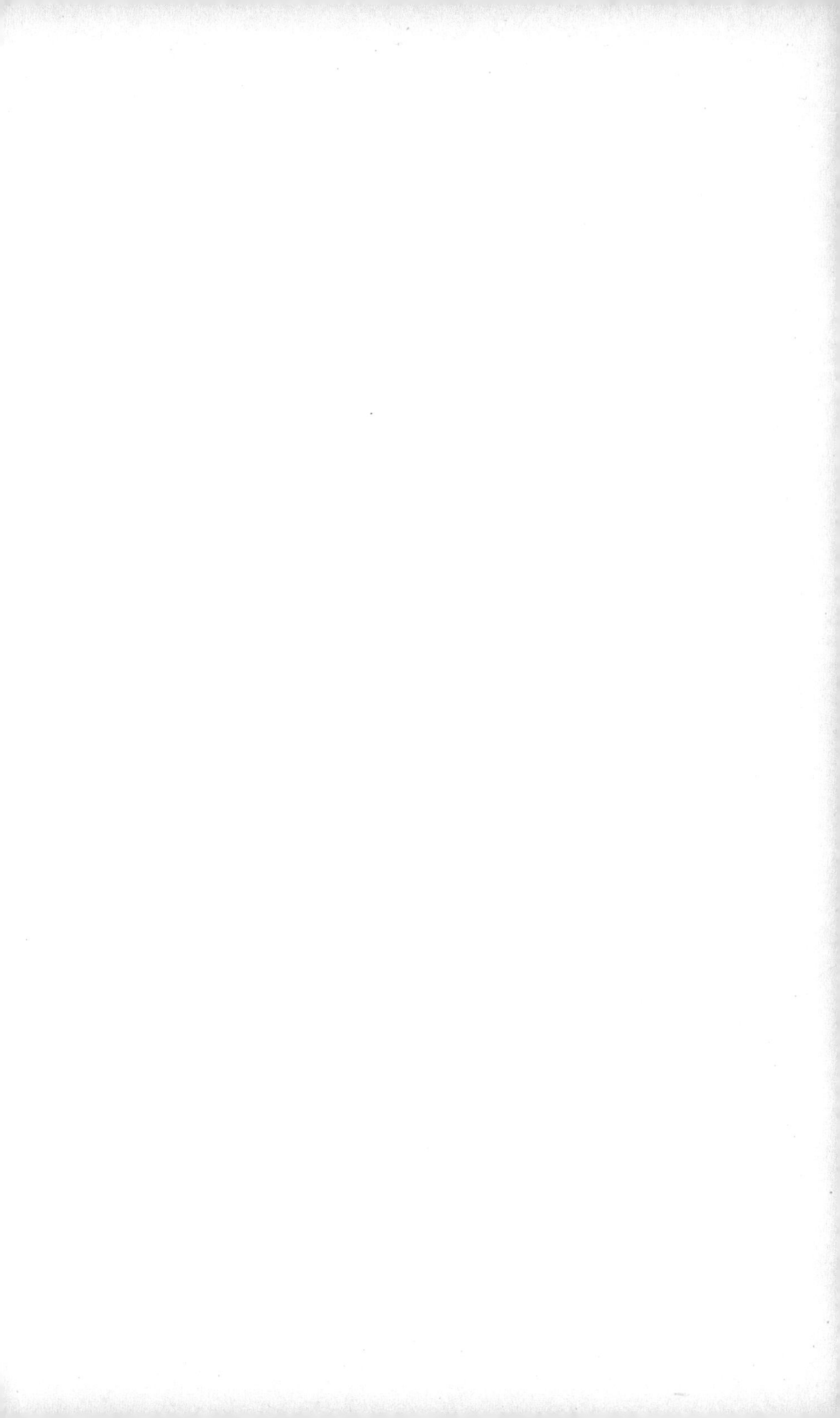

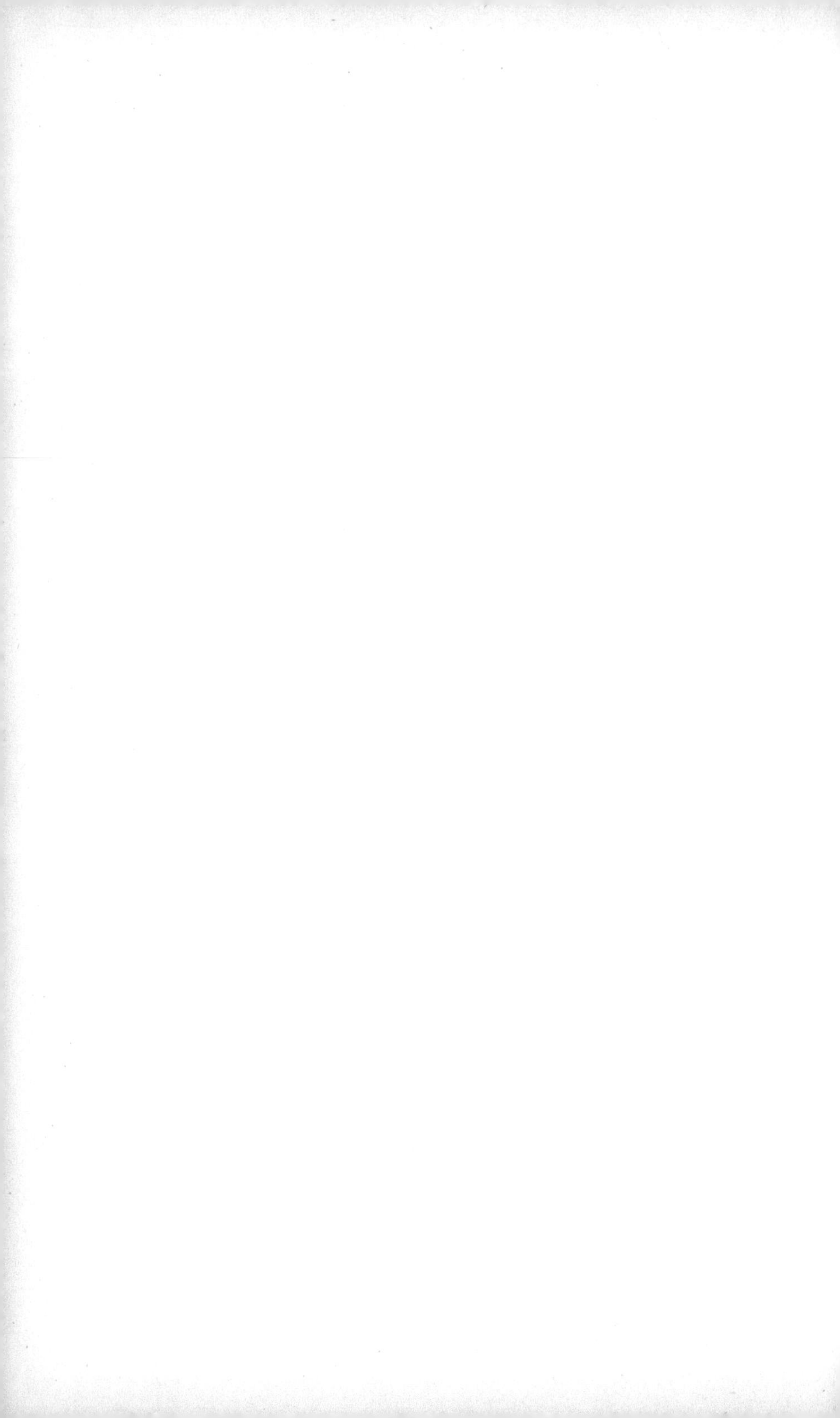

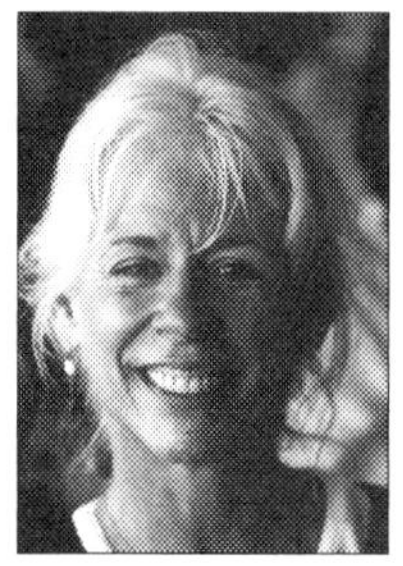

GANGAJI

"YOU WILL NEVER BE SATISFIED UNTIL YOU REALIZE WHO YOU ARE. THE TIME IS NOW. NOW IS THE TIME TO RECOGNIZE THE CORE OF PEACE THAT EXISTS WITHIN YOURSELF. YOU ARE THAT! YES, NOW IS THE TIME."

from You Are That!

Gangaji was born Antoinette Varner and raised in the southern United States. Toni, as she was called, has been a schoolteacher, workshop leader with her husband, Eli Jaxon-Bear, and an acupuncturist. She practiced Zen, Vipassana, and Tibetan Buddhist meditations. Although her search and longing for the Truth was deep, she has expressed that she had no interest in traveling to India or in having a guru. Yet, in 1990 she found herself on the banks of the Ganges River where she met and awakened with her Master, Poonjaji. He named her Gangaji and declared that, "the river Ganga would flow in the West." Poonjaji asked her to go "door to door" sharing the Truth she had realized. This request resulted in the many satsangs Gangaji has given throughout the world. She now devotes herself fulltime to spreading Truth.

Gangaji has been a powerful catalyst for both of us. It was Gangaji who first gave us the experience of hearing the Truth spoken in Western vernacular. And since Gangaji has lived in the Bay Area and been a part of some of the same political, psychological, and spiritual movements as we have, our response was immediate. Not only was she a Westerner, but from such a similar background as well. This is what led us to see that awakening to the Truth of our Being was possible for us. Seeing Gangaji brought it too close to home for us to deny.

We have found Gangaji to be articulate, clear, and absolutely unwavering. Her message is consistent, and her presence is powerful. At times she can be ruthless, even fierce, in her pointing to the Truth. At other times she is lovingly playful and joyous in her delight in seeing others recognize who they are.

Gangaji is a private person who is not easily accessible outside of her public satsangs, except through correspondence. Unfortunately, we did not have the opportunity to interview her in person. At her request, we sent her questions and she typed out answers for us. Although the interview is not interactive, we feel that it expresses the qualities of this excellent teacher. The emphasis on certain words was added by Gangaji.

WRITTEN INTERVIEW *with* GANGAJI

Q: *Who are you?*

GANGAJI: Nothing that can be defined—before everything and present in everything and after everything. Not a person yet present in every person. Not anything and not separate from anything. I is in all forms, after all forms. I is—I is not. I am present in formulations of I is and formulations of I is not and yet untouched by either!

Q: *What is enlightenment, realization, awakening?*

GANGAJI: The certainty of realizing boundlessness as one's true nature.

Q: *How did this occur for you?*

GANGAJI: In fact, it does not occur. It is realized to be. With a shock (Poonjaji's gaze, the grace of his presence) that which has always been present in its boundlessness was revealed to be. In the experience of this mind-stream, the lightening began in his presence, under his guidance, and at a certain point—back in California a few weeks after leaving India—a thunderbolt split open the clenched fist of the doubting mind. This thunderbolt appeared by surprise. Self-evident Truth of all one Self is continually revealed, even as conditioned existence forms, dies, and reforms.

Q: *Do you have any suggestions or recommendations for others who are experiencing a desire for awakening? Are there any things one can do or refrain from doing to experience this?*

GANGAJI: Honor the desire. Fall into it headfirst. Let the desire for awakening direct the choices of life. This desire is the Sat Guru (true revealer of light). It can and will use every opportunity to strike your Self-denial with its force of purity, if it is honored—respected—listened to. Let the Sat Guru do its work.

Q: *It appears as though more human beings are awakening to the Truth of their Being in the Western world at this time. Does this seem so to you, and if so, what does it signify to you?*

GANGAJI: Yes, it does seem so. Perhaps the human being is waking up to how Self-denial only results in egoic indulgence and hence, enormous suffering (greed, hatred, war).

Q: *What is the source of suffering in the world, and what can be done about it?*

GANGAJI: The root of suffering is ignorance of the truth of who one is. This root is fed and nourished by believing and tending the idea of who one is. The root is simple, but obviously, the repercussions of this deadly root are extremely complex, and the forms of suffering manifested by eating this root startling in their horror.

When you recognize yourself to be—in truth—all of the known and unknown, the desire for others to be held back so that you may get ahead is recognized as an outgrowth of the root of ignorance. When this root is not nourished, the outgrowth cannot continue. This root is extinguished by realizing all thoughts and emotions and actions relating to rejecting or clinging to other (in whatever form) are formed from the ignorance of Reality.

You are other. Discover who both you and other is, and you recognize there is no need to cling or reject. Then when tendencies arise to keep or keep away, they can be met in Truth and freed.

Q: *Without operating out of a personal "I," how do you make decisions and get things done?*

GANGAJI: Decisions appear naturally. Things get done (or not done) naturally. The concept of personal "I" is just a concept. It is not the reality of I. A concept doesn't decide! It is simply a concept about the one deciding. Discover who decides, and you discover yourself as consciousness. Is a limit or a boundary discovered there? No. Is a person discovered there? Only as an object in consciousness—appearing and disappearing.

Q: *From the perspective of no personal "I," how do you experience relationships with others?*

GANGAJI: Mysterious and deep. Relationships are always an opportunity to more clearly experience the endlessness of who I am with the grace of Truth. This includes all relationships, unpleasant as well as pleasant.

Q: *Westerners are very much into self-improvement. Does involvement in the various therapies and spiritual practices assist in awakening?*

GANGAJI: It depends. If the goal is the deepening of client and therapist into the endless mystery of Truth, then yes, of course it is helpful, as relationship is helpful. If the goal is to shore up an image of oneself, it may be helpful in the short run, but only as propellant for the recognition that your image of who you are is only an image, and therefore, all images are limited. There may be a transition from bad image to good image which calms the mind enough so that no image is embraced. However, usually the pleasure experienced with good image is a strong temptation to continually make your image better and better, leading of course, to megalomania. In our culture, megalomania is often given adulation as the ideal. True Self-acceptance is the recognition that no image fits! All images are really only the constructs of mind to avoid surrendering to Truth of Self.

Q: *Are there any questions you are often asked that should be included here?*
GANGAJI: A question I'm often asked is, "What to do with negative emotions?" Simply put, I say meet everything fully and completely as it is. A true meeting can only occur when there are no expectations or agenda for what the meeting will deliver. In other words, there is stillness of mind— no story about the meaning of the emotions, the history, the categorization, the conclusion, the analysis. All of this mind activity is fine, and even entertaining, but in the moment of meeting, it becomes a distraction.

Meet fully whatever arises without following the dictate of mental strategies to flee or hide or fix or get rid of. The activity of mind that follows (rather than leads) true meeting is fresh and insightful naturally. It is quite a surprising meeting!

Q: *What does this mean for the world?*
GANGAJI: That is unknown. We know what following the mind as if it were reality leads to. We can see and read and experience that daily. Let us see what being true to Truth means!

Q: *Are there any others who have had similar awakening, whom you know or know about that you feel should be included in this book?*
GANGAJI: Many others. In fact, anyone reading this who is interested in uncovering true Self already has some echo of a memory of Self, shining in its radiance. I would say for everyone to be true to that (with no image of what being true looks like!) For each of us, immediate, direct experience with enlightenment is already present

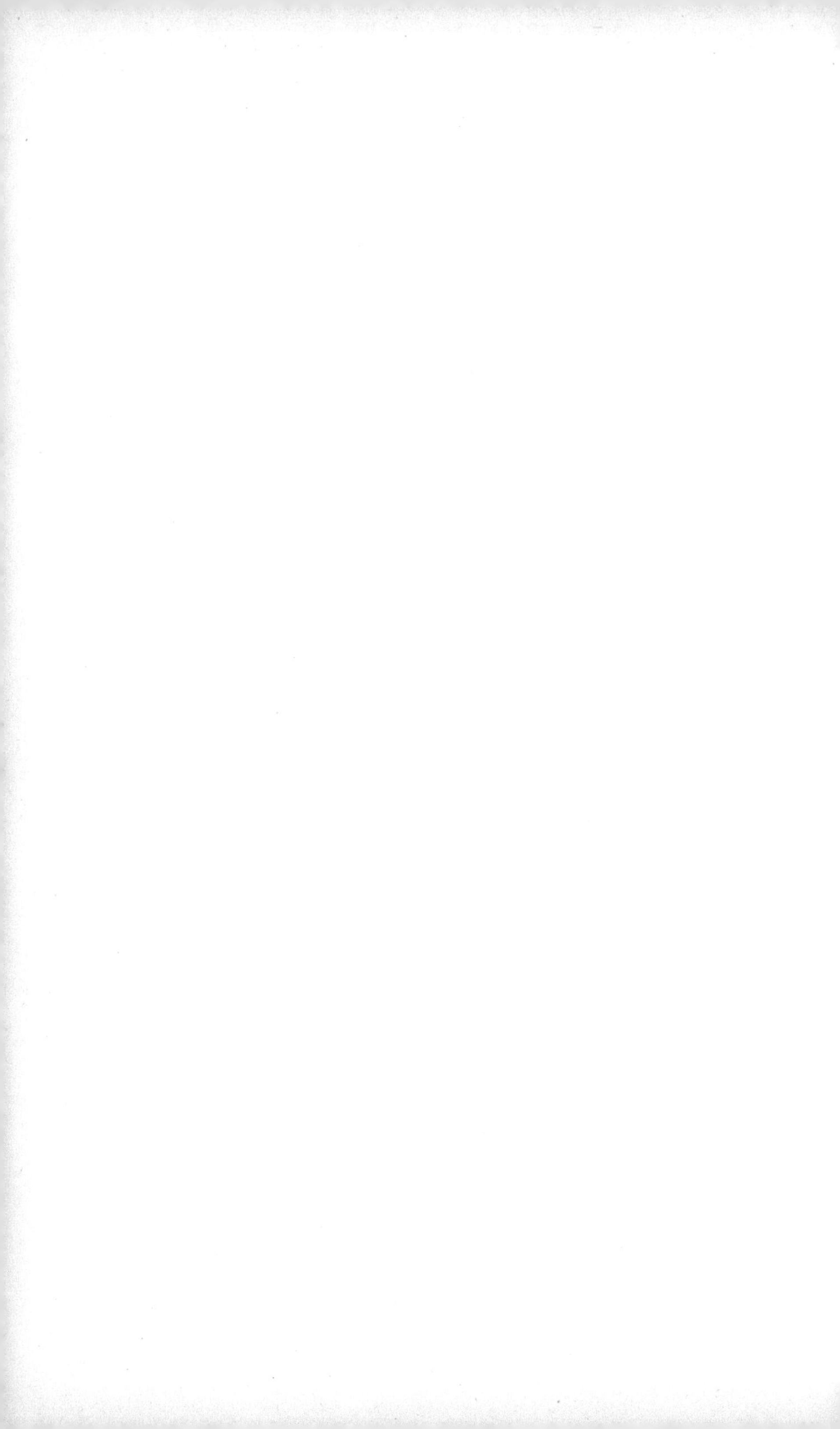

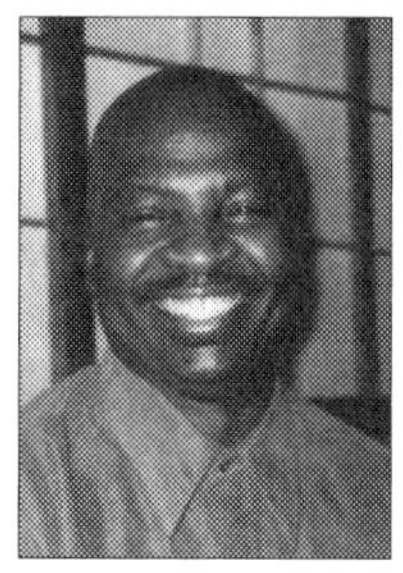

KENNY JOHNSON

"WHEN YOU REALIZE THAT YOU ARE AWARENESS, YOU COME TO KNOW THAT YOU ARE ETERNITY AND WILL NEVER CEASE TO EXIST. ALL YOU HAVE TO DO IS SIMPLY STOP AND LOOK AND YOU UNERRINGLY KNOW THAT YOU HAVE ALWAYS BEEN HERE, NOW AND YOU WILL ALWAYS BE HERE, NOW."

When we asked Gangaji whether she would like to be a part of this project, she recommended others to us whom she thought should be included. One of these is Kenny Johnson. At the time of our first contact, Kenny was in prison.

Kenny's life of crime began at age fifteen he was cheated out of the money he had worked hard for all summer. Devastated, he turned to stealing in order to get the money he needed. From then on he lived as a career criminal, in and out of prison. In 1982, Kenny was sentenced to forty years in the Federal Bureau of Prisons. He was released on parole in December 1996.

It was in jail that his spiritual interest quickened. He would read any spiritual text he could. Open to all paths, he explored many. He was introduced to Eastern spirituality through Siddha Yoga, but felt that his understanding was not complete until meeting his teacher, Gangaji. Kenny says, "I have no regrets when it comes to spending my entire adult life in prison. Never would I have studied so hard and prayed so long for real freedom. My mind would never have turned toward the Truth unless I had been made to sit in one small area and contemplate the meaning of life."

The interview is a composite of responses from Kenny through letters and phone calls. The prison phone calls were limited to ten minutes, but it was enough to give us a sense of him. For us, Kenny's enormous heart is what stands out, so sincere and loving. The simplicity and beauty of his expression moves us deeply, and we are pleased to share it with you.

Now that Kenny is out of prison and living in the Bay Area, we have the pleasure of being able to spend time with him. When we first met with Kenny, we asked if he wanted to redo the interview that was done when he was in prison since so much time had passed. He was pleased to read what he had said at such a difficult time in his life and requested that we use this interview without making any changes. The emphasis on certain words has been added by Kenny.

Kenny is now learning to adjust to the world outside prison after spending most of his life there. This new world has an entirely different set of rules, which has been a major adjustment for him. Kenny was teaching for a while after he got out of prison, but has stopped for now until he completes more of this adjustment period.

INTERVIEW *with* KENNY JOHNSON

Q: *How did an awakening to the Truth of your Being occur for you?*

KENNY: As a thief, cheat, and robber, I chased the American dream through crime. I could never make that big score that criminals talk about, but few gain. However, while in prison, I would read. The Bible became my breakfast; the Holy Koran my lunch; the Gita was my supper. My prayers to Christ were filled with tears and wails for freedom. There were many years of fasting during the holy month of Ramadan, and waiting anxiously for a special blessing from Allah. As a devotee to Krishna, I would eat no meat and chant the holy names of Krishna, day in and day out. Please do not allow me to leave out all those Hatha Yoga practices of standing on my head and the intense breathing exercises.

My quest for the Beloved began in earnest once I came to accept the fact that I needed to meet a guru or teacher. I prayed for a guru or teacher in the year 1990 and the revelation of meeting my teacher came later that year. I was shown in a dream that I would meet my teacher in Colorado, and that she would be a white-haired woman. The catch was that I would have to be released from federal prison in 1992 and go back to prison before this would happen. This dream was so real and uplifting, but horrifying at the same time. You must realize that I was sentenced to forty years in 1982 and would not be eligible for parole until 1992. The thought of going to prison again after a ten-year sentence was not at all acceptable to this man. Needless to say, I got out of prison and was returned to federal prison in 1993 because I violated parole. In the Englewood, Colorado Federal prison I joined a meditation group and started sitting. During one session a video was shown, and I was amazed when I saw this white-haired woman named Gangaji. My heart leaped, but my mind was agitated. I recognized her as the woman I had dreamt about.

Then some more great news came that night. Gangaji would be visiting the prison in the spring of '94. When she came that spring, a fellow brother in the sangha "woke up." I was jealous; I thought I was ready. Her next visit would be in the fall of '94. She came back in September and sat for about twenty minutes. The first words out of her mouth were, "Kenny, I've been thinking about you." What a treat! What a joy! I blurted out these words to Gangaji, "In the Bible it says that we must wait for God's grace to descend upon us." She said, "God's grace is here now!" Then she looked at me and asked me to extend my head towards her and tapped me three times lightly upon my bald head. All things stopped and speeded up at the same time. I had no more questions, but there were a million thoughts racing through this mind. When a person is in such a state, they can only sit and watch.

For the next fifteen months, I was in a state of being "totally pleased." I found myself going to the chapel and just sitting, or watching videos of Gangaji, Papaji, and Ramana Maharshi. When at work, I would slip away from my computer and go to a closet and sit all alone. During my lunch breaks, you could find me walking the track gazing a few feet in front of me absorbed in bliss. In the middle of the night I would get out of bed and ask the officer if I could use one of the rooms to meditate while everyone was asleep. Then there was my Walkman radio—it was always on my head and tuned to some spiritual program or gospel music show. I was completely absorbed in awareness, unable to speak of this awakening.

On December 8, 1995, I was scheduled to be released from prison and to be returned to my home in Kansas City, Missouri. To my utter dismay, the state of Iowa wanted me detained until they could come and pick me up to serve a five-year sentence for them. I was taken to a county jail and placed in a one man cell. For seven days all I did was sit, walk, lie, and stand in meditation. On the seventh day I was released to the authorities who were transporting me back to Iowa.

While lying in a holding cell in some jail in New Mexico with seventeen prisoners, an inmate asked me, "How can you be so calm amidst all this confusion?" My reply to him was that I hear and see nothing but silence. He wanted more information, "How can you see and hear silence?" I told him it was simple, and that he didn't have to become affiliated with any religious group. It didn't matter if he was a Muslim, Christian, Hindu, etc. All that is required was a desire to be free. He said, "Show me." I directed him to look into his own mind and watch the thoughts that arose in the mind. He looked for a minute or so, then I said, "Let the first thought that appeared, go." He did as I asked. Then I asked him what remained? He replied, "Nothing—Emptiness—Void." We looked at each other and laughed. He was free, and he knew it!

Whenever a fellow prisoner "wakes up," I am so pleased and thrilled to be here in jail. For when a person serves this Truth totally, they truly do not care where they are. All that matters is serving the Truth.

Q: *How has this awakening changed the quality of your life?*
KENNY: One's quality of life improves immeasurably. The best part is that you no longer have any question about people, life, God, and so on. Each time a question appears, the answer is right along with it. It is sort of like having this "Wish Fulfilling Tree" inside of you, and there is never a sense of lack. You are always full. Wisdom is your best friend. You are no longer a victim. No game can be played upon you. You no longer play games with people. You value your fellow human and want only the best for him or her.

Before this awakening, there was a distinct feeling of hollowness in all my pursuits. I would buy a new car believing that the car would bring me much joy. But the opposite happened. There was a longing for something else to make me happy. So I would go shopping and buy some new shoes. Again there came the longing for something else to fill this hollowness. After experiencing this awakening, all desires have been quenched. If I get a new pair of shoes, so what. If a new car comes my way, so what. I am full always. Being here now is all that is. Since joy comes from the immaterial awareness, then it is only natural for me to remain in the place where all happiness, all joy, all peace emanates and pervades this universe. When one turns the searchlight of awareness on the field of desire, there is nothing.

Q: *How would you answer the question, "Who are you?"*
KENNY: When someone asks me, "Who are you, Kenny?" I reply, "I am That which was and which is and which will be."

Q: *Could you please elaborate on what you mean by this?*
KENNY: Simply put, this means there never was a time when what you are, eternity, did not exist. When you realize that you are awareness, you come to know that you are eternity and will never cease to exist. All you have to do is simply STOP and LOOK and you unerringly know that you have always been here, now, and you will always be here, now.

Q: *What do the words enlightenment, realization, awakening mean to you?*
KENNY: People always want to know, what is realization, enlightenment, awakening? It is going home — being home, and in your home you have all that you could ever ask for. It is your natural state. You are no longer sleeping the sleep of delusion. You are always worshiping the divine form

of the Beloved. You see Her in the squirrels, the trees, the rocks, and in every human whose eyes you gaze into.

My reward is only a chance to kiss Her, hold Her, embrace Her. She is me and I am Her; you can see that we are One. I have no life as Kenny any more. The Beloved has destroyed the false concepts of "I," "me," and "mine." There is only the spontaneity of just being in the present moment and doing whatever job needs to be done. Just being!

Q: *I notice that you speak in terms of the feminine, "Her." Could you comment on this?*
KENNY: This is coming out of my amazement at how all things spring forth from the earth, nature that is. When you contemplate this miracle of life, you automatically recognize the feminine aspect of God—the causeless cause. When absorbed in Awareness, love continually flows from the heart. Since the Beloved cannot be captured in any manner physically, there is a longing. The Beloved is everywhere and yet nowhere. You see the impossibility of possessing Her, so you just adore Her in all things. We are married in this "no thing."

Q: *You speak in a beautiful, devotional manner. Could you please say something about devotion when there is a realization of non-duality, of no "other?"*
KENNY: For the longest time there was this sense of separateness within my mind and in the way I dealt with people. However after realizing the Self, I became aware of the unity of all things. In this unity I saw the loving hand of the Creator. I saw that everything is perfect. There are truly no problems in a perfect creation. There was no need for schemes or deceit. Everything just takes care of itself marvelously. This revelation made me happy, ecstatic with joy and gratitude. I came to see how nature praises the Creator. How the sun rises and continually submits itself to the will of Father God. Then I would look and see the moon also doing its duty with no complaint. Wherever I look I see everything embracing and submitting to the Self.

So, I became like the sun, each morning embracing the mean guard in my heart, or the angry inmate. At night I would become the moon and embrace the dark moods of the prisoners who longed to be with their loved ones. My heart sent forth torrents of love to them. Even in my dreams I would find myself telling others to let go of all conceptual thoughts and become filled with this love, this bliss. Just by being focused on the Self every hour of the day, the child of devotion was born. My every action became devoted to the Self in all of its manifest form.

Q: *What do you see as the source of suffering in the world?*
KENNY: So many suffer because there is identification with the thoughts that arise in the mind and because of attachment to these thoughts. Prisoners suffer a great deal because they are attached to loved ones on the outside who they can't be with. Whenever I ask someone to simply inquire into their mind and find the source of a thought, they find nothing and instantly realize that all thoughts are empty and have no power but the power we give them. A question I ask others is, "Where does the thought come from and where does it go or return to?" A lot of the brothers say, "Wow!" They can't believe it is so easy to be free and yet be able to live a productive life. They come to realize that if they are sweeping the floor, they are here. If they are shoveling snow, they are here. There is no place where they are not here. When in a group of people, there is the Beloved! Laughing, talking, lifting weights, or jogging.

Q: *It seems to us that more Westerners are waking up then ever before. Can you comment on this?*
KENNY: It is the perfect season for Westerners to "wake up." "When the fruit is ripe it shall be harvested!" We Westerners have inundated ourselves with material things, which has left us hollow inside. The drugs get us high for a while and then we pursue sex, which leaves us drained. Then after years and years of searching for permanency in impermanent things, feelings, relationships, we are ready! We come to know that all created things can only give us temporary thrills. It is the perfect time for Westerners to experience this awakening. We have prepared ourselves well with all the suffering that we have inflicted upon ourselves.

Q: *Is the awakening for everyone or just a rare few?*
KENNY: It is my experience that anyone can "wake up." No one is excluded. They must simply desire to be free. The Beloved is patient and has eternity to wait, so all can and will be free. No one will be lost—for how can the Beloved ever lose Herself?

Q: *Do you see spiritual practices as necessary in order to wake up?*
KENNY: As I stated earlier there is no requirement to being free. However

so many ask, "Do I need a practice?" After experiencing this awakening, some say that they need a practice. I ask them, "When are you not doing the practice? Who is doing the practice? If you sat on the meditation cushion and meditated all day, what would be gained or lost? If you worked hard at your job and you were aware of your True Self, what would be gained or what would be lost?" They say, "Nothing." "So, please tell me when are you not in meditation?" And always, they stop. They realize that it is the ego-mind still fighting to stay alive. There comes an understanding that thoughts are not able to stick to the mind, when in Truth, there is no mind.

Q: *How do decisions get made and things get done without identification with the ego, a separate "I?"*
KENNY: All duties, all performances, are done spontaneously. There is no conscious planning on my part. There's no looking for reward. While working, there is only the consciousness of being here. There is only serving the Guru in all activities. When one has submitted to the Guru, there develops a single purpose. That purpose leads one to work unselfishly and contentedly. You come to know that pleasing the Guru is in essence the best service. In Truth there is no work, no Guru, and no one doing the work. You are continually established in the present Now, Totally Aware. Totally Pleased. Totally Rewarded. Totally Devoted to this Love.

Q: *When you say the word "guru" to whom or what are you referring?*
KENNY: The Guru is not a person you are submitting to. People fear submitting to another person or institution, simply because they fear abuse, misuse or mind control. There's the fear of having their freedom to think and be themselves limited. But once you submit to the True Guru, the Sat Guru, you are in reality submitting to your True Self, what you truly are. You are the Guru. God, in His/Her infinite mercy and wisdom gave everyone their own Guru. He/She is in you as the Guru. So you are able to experience all the blessing of the universe. You possess your own magic lamp and every wish is fulfilled the moment you think the thought—behold, a gift from you to you. Even before you can formulate a wish—behold, it is there. Do not waste another second of your life looking outside of yourself for your Self.

Q: *How do you experience relationships with others since this awakening?*

KENNY: When dealing with others, one sees each person as himself. One wishes true enlightenment for each person. If a person speaks about life being unfair, instantly there comes the realization that they are in suffering. But how can there ever be suffering when there is nothing but Love everywhere? Love is the cry of the baby for food. Love is the cry of the grownup for better wages to feed his family. Love is the essence that causes the baby to cry, the grownup to cry, and Love is the satisfier of all those who cry. From Love comes the cry and from Love comes the response to the cry.

We are continuously reaching with our minds for something other than the present moment of Now. We reach into the past for those good old days. We project our mind into the future for visions of happiness in some event. For example: "Remember the 60s when everyone was getting a real salary, and everything was cheap?" Or, "Honey, next year we will take the kids to Disney World, and we will have a great time." Whenever we perform such mental gymnastics we are always doing them now! So, my brother, my sister, Be Here Now!

Q: *Anything else you would like to add?*

KENNY: As a lover of the scriptures, I read the word and could only gain a little solace from what was being conveyed by Jesus, Muhammad, Krishna, and Buddha. There seemed to be a missing element that evaded my grasping mind. I would go to the churches, the mosques, to hear the preacher preach on these sacred texts; still there was no rest for the weary mind. Then came the awakening! The mind was slain. Awareness was revealed. Now, each book only confirms the inner awakening; each word, each verse points to this spiritual experience. You come to know that the books come from the very same source that is you. The book, the Source is you, no difference.

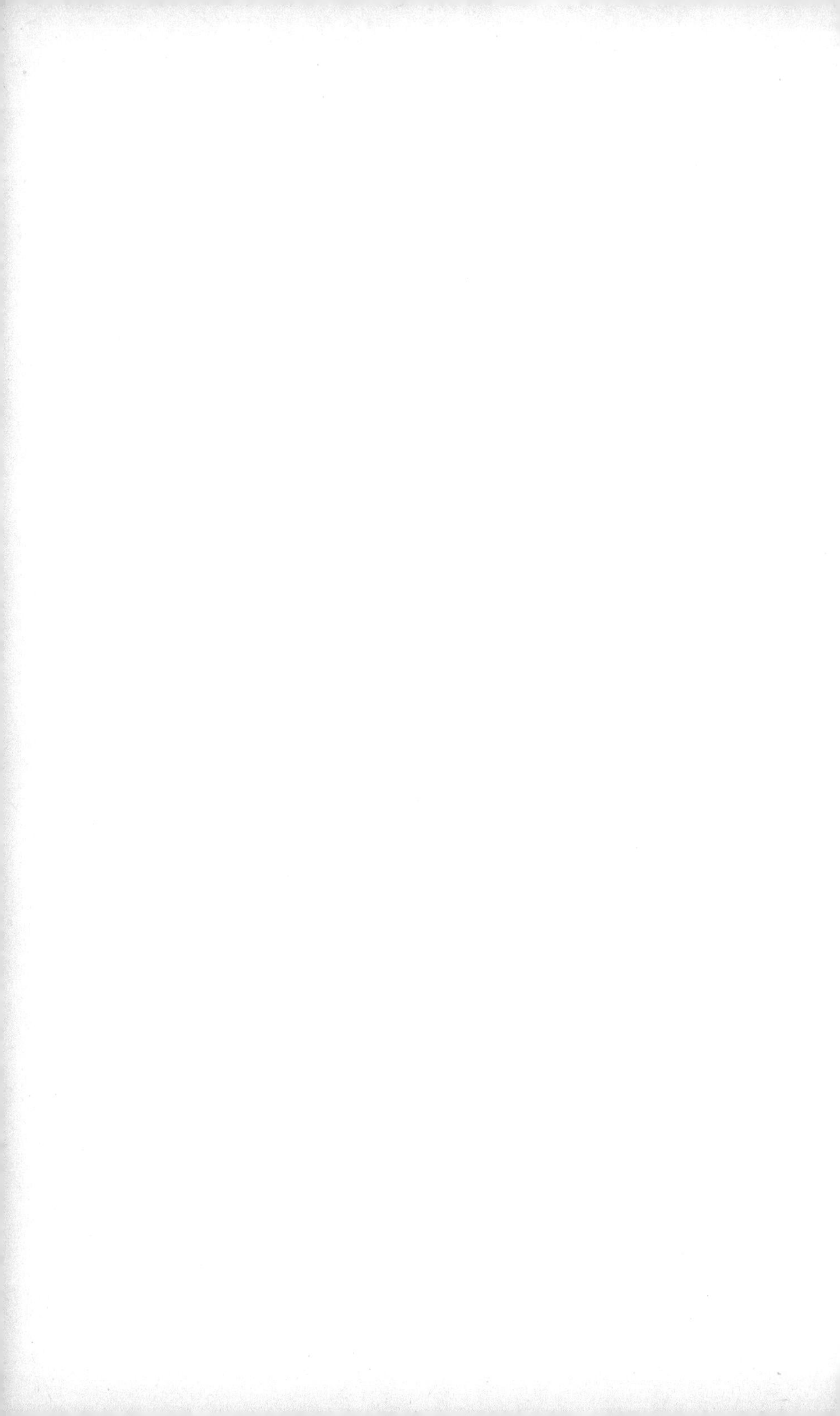

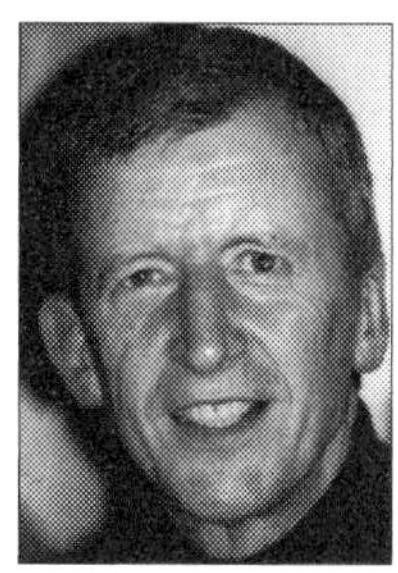

CHRISTOPHER TITMUSS

"THERE IS NOW A SENSE THAT THE MOST PROFOUND ELEMENTS OF SPIRITUAL TEACHINGS — FINDING THE TRUTH, LIBERATION — ARE ACCESSIBLE. IT IS AVAILABLE IN THE HERE AND NOW AND PEOPLE ARE WILLING TO PUT UP WITH THE SWEAT OF EXISTENCE TO DISCOVER FREEDOM."

Before meeting Christopher, we had been told by someone who knows him that there had never been a time in Christopher's life when he imagined he was not awake to who he truly is. Intrigued, we attended several of his Dharma talks during a weeklong Meditation retreat he was holding in the Bay Area. What convinced us to pursue this interview was his emphatic declaration of the immediacy of the presence of Truth.

Christopher is considered by some to be a challenging teacher. He tends to turn questions back on the questioner and probes for what's behind what they're asking. He pulls people away from the intellectual realm into the depths of their question, going right to the heart of the matter. He points students toward their own direct experience and insight. Christopher is a blatant radical, both politically and spiritually. He adheres strictly to the Truth itself and its immediate availability rather than filtering it through any doctrine or idea of what is appropriate to say or do.

We met in a backyard in Albany, California on a warm summer afternoon. In the far corner of the yard, dwarfing our little gathering, was an enormous, ancient redwood tree. Sheltered within a natural arch in the thick bark of the tree was a stone Buddha. Christopher, a well-respected Buddhist teacher, is a humble being who is delightfully warm, friendly, jovial, and gracious. It was a pleasure to spend time with him and hear his story as the three of us looked up at that enormous, ancient tree and all the space around it.

Christopher is a former Buddhist monk who teaches spiritual awakening and Insight Meditation retreats worldwide. A poet and writer, he is the author of several books including his most recent work, *An Awakened Life—Uncommon Wisdom from Everyday Experience*. He is the co-founder of Gaia House in Devon, England which is an international retreat center. He lives there when he is in England with his teenage daughter who attends the local school. Christopher is also a founding member of the international advisory board of the Buddhist Peace Fellowship.

CONVERSATION *with* CHRISTOPHER TITMUSS

LML: *You are a teacher of Vipassana Meditation...*
CHRISTOPHER: [Interrupting] I am a Dharma teacher. I don't use the word Vipassana. I prefer to call it Insight Meditation. Insight Meditation is essentially a meditation which establishes awareness for the purpose of insight and liberation, that's its primary function. In its relative, practical expression, it's a sitting place of existence, a walking place of existence and that's the core theme that runs through the sit, walk form. It is a supportive method and technique for realization.

JLW: *What do you mean by realization?*
CHRISTOPHER: Realization means the realization of the Truth, which is one, without a second. The essential realization is that one is a free and liberated human being and the clear indication of that is when the problems of life have gone out of existence.

JLW: *This is your experience?*
CHRISTOPHER: Oh yes!

LML: *Do you have a story of how this realization came about for you?*
CHRISTOPHER: No, I don't have a story. There was no before or after in my life.

JLW: *In other words, this has always been so for you?*
CHRISTOPHER: Yes. The usual story, as you know and probably have confirmed through the contact and association with the others that you are meeting and speaking with for this book, is generally that there is a very distinctive moment in time where a tremendous transition occurs. That is a situation for a small number of people. Then, there are other people who simply cannot point to a before or after event, yet they recognize through the duration of their life that through practice, path, commitment, and love of the discovery they found that they realized their freedom. But they could never say it happened in this meditation or listening to this teacher, or in this event, or when I was in nature or whatever. Then there are others who have no sense of movement in any way, either dramatic, which you are speaking about, or gradual, which I was just speaking of. They don't have a thinking that moves along those lines whatsoever, and in fact never had.

LML: *Is the latter description true for you?*

CHRISTOPHER: I am speaking of the latter, yes. Some people will say, "I was just living my life, then there was an explosion, and this had tremendous repercussions in my life." The person then may ascribe with their thought and language, words to that experience: "... found God, ... realized no-self, ... discovered the vastness, ... touched Buddha nature, ... no words to describe, or whatever." The influence of that has had a continuity in the person's life—sometimes joyfully, sometimes with quite some degree of struggle to comprehend what has happened.

There are those who don't have that explosion have no specific reference point, yet, are free. There is a genuine sense and knowing that for years, I was like this and this and this and then it transformed. This transforming was not located in a specific time and place but over a period of time. The outcome is not determined by whether it was dramatic or over a period of time; what is important is whether one is liberated. It is only that which really matters.

Throughout my life I have had a wide variety of spiritual and religious experiences. I have never heard an experience from somebody else which I haven't had, and I have been in religious circles my entire life. I spent ten years in the East, six years as a Buddhist monk, lived in a cave, lived in a monastery, etc. But I don't have a thought which has in it, before and after or during. Therefore, I can't think in sudden or gradual terms.

LML: *So, you just don't perceive things in those terms.*

CHRISTOPHER: Never did. Never could. And never will.

LML: *One question I have, Christopher, is, if you can't perceive things in terms of sudden or gradual, can you say something about being a teacher of a gradual path? Many people perceive Insight Meditation as a gradual path.*

CHRISTOPHER: Well, some people see it in gradual terms, that mirroring of the path of the Dharma. "The path" is a useful metaphor, it is a reminder to people in terms of the Eightfold Path, to genuinely examine each and every area of our human existence, and to leave no stone unturned. So, some in the Insight Meditation community do like, appreciate, and enjoy the benefit of the metaphor of "the path." Sometimes, when it is useful, I will make appropriate gestures toward that. But it is not a focus of my way of teaching.

As an Insight Meditation teacher, I am pointing to immediacy. So, if there is any leaning in my teaching, it is that freedom is discoverable right here and now. There is no better opportunity in the field of existence than what this moment offers. In this sense, "path" has a mild feeling of postponement. I think there is a practical aspect of that for some people in certain situations; and therefore, the language of the path is a skillful means for some. But in general, as an Insight Meditation teacher, I am striking for immediate discovery. That is the focus. Some may say that in comparison it is a bit more rare but not as rare as some people in the tradition would like to think.

LML: *Do you have a sense that this immediate discovery is occurring more frequently for Westerners at this time?*
CHRISTOPHER: I have no sense of it increasing or decreasing, nor staying the same. I honestly don't have a measuring thought.

JLW: *It seems though that you would have a good perspective on what is going on around the globe.*
CHRISTOPHER: Yes, I have a very good sample in so far as each year I am in three or four continents and work most days of the week with people who are exploring the spiritual life and the spiritual experience in it. That is what I do. So, in my various visits to these various continents, I hear all of that. But again, I would not think in the language of there is now more or less, or staying the same. Only because I would have had to have been around in previous years and generations. My experience as a teacher is confined to twenty years from the mid-1970s through this time.

What one can generally say is that there are a growing number of teachings taking place in the West, both the shallow and those with depth. There are a growing number of teachers flowering and coming through, but I think that is the result of a number of people's tremendous love, dedication, and commitment.

That is giving more confidence for people who are having these sudden experiences, totally out of the blue, without any relationship to anything that they have known, to actually come forward and say, "This is happening to me; it is not an emotional problem; it is not a psychological state of mental ill health. It is of a different order and dimension."

Those people now are finding comfort and understanding in the Eastern traditions that they didn't before because one healthy aspect of the Eastern traditions is that they aren't demanding loyalty. Sometimes, as I have heard regularly enough, people will go to other religions—Middle Eastern or Western religions or elsewhere—and be spoken to in a very unimaginative and deprecating language of being "possessed by the devil" or "you need a psychiatrist"or "you need to be saved," or whatever.

JLW: *It is not popular in Christian or Muslim communities, for example, to say, "I am God."*
CHRISTOPHER: Yes, exactly. It just sends alarm signals through certain circles. But I do have to say that any "I am" with an appendix to it such as "God" sends signals from the standpoint of insight, the world of Dharma and the Buddhist tradition as well. "I am" of itself is a conceit. To put "I am" and then load a charged word on the end… be watchful of "I" and clinging and grasping, "I am this, or that" and "I" identifying with anything. One can use the language but with caution and care. It could be a signal of imprisonment as much as liberation.

LML: *In terms of "I am," how would you answer the question, who are you?*
CHRISTOPHER: Well, you might get a little frustrated with Christopher here. The inner life doesn't conceive and move in those ways. So, any response wouldn't be fair. One can just go along with the conventional—just a human being sitting in this chair, and we are communicating. That is more than enough really, too much actually.

LML: *Do you experience life from a personal "I," a personal reference point?*
CHRISTOPHER: The personal reference would be just for you and I communicating. I am sitting here; that's the personal reference. The "I" is a shorthand for forms of experience. "I" is a shorthand for the bodily life, such as "I" am feeling this—there is feeling going on inside, and so that is a simple way to make communication easy. And that's enough, more than enough.

LML: *So, you are free from identification with a personal self as "I."*
CHRISTOPHER: Totally. Yes, without doubt, without question.

LML: *So, then how do you experience relationship with others?*
CHRISTOPHER: The primary perception that runs out of the heart is that each human being I know and see is fundamentally free. When others do not see this freedom themselves, it shows me that there is just some

movement going on in the inner life, which they believe obscures their free liberation. I don't believe it. But they believe it. So, my job is to make a rather small contribution in assisting the dissolution of their belief. I see freedom first, then the movement of events outwardly called heart, mind, and body, and address it.

LML: *So, most people believe they are not free; they are identified as being a separate self. Do you see that as the source of suffering in the world?*

CHRISTOPHER: I would be reluctant to pinpoint it to identification; some people don't relate to that very well. But identification is an important factor—the movement of the mind, the social conditioning, the old karma, the structures of society, the kind of world that human beings interact with—put all of that together and it is called "dependent arising" in Dharma language. The dependent arising is what generates the suffering.

LML: *Some people reading this may wonder what they can do to be free of their suffering. What do you have to say to them?*

CHRISTOPHER: Having moved extensively in spiritual circles for fifty-two years, I see in the view of some people (which may be reflected in some of the people you are interviewing, because I know a few of them) that there can be a very profound, insightful, liberating experience that takes place, and then they say that it is unconditioned; therefore, there is nothing you can do—nothing whatsoever. It either happens to you, or it doesn't. Then the language of grace comes in.

It's very important to remember that this is a viewpoint. This viewpoint, if identified with, gets an absolute tone to it. The ego identifies with the view that there is nothing you can do, and then this view becomes its own imprisonment through clinging to the viewpoint.

Then there are others who will take the opposite extreme and say that you have to go on a gradual path. They say it is moment by moment gradual practice, and then maybe in this lifetime or in another lifetime surely, you will find liberation. This is another view, another extreme, with easily more clinging there.

So, somewhere is the non-clinging to a position, either gradual or immediate, radical or progressive. One needs to be watchful because the person not only can deceive himself or herself but deceive others as well. Generally speaking in the tradition of Dharma, an attempt to strike the middle way says, "OK you can acknowledge yourself, you can acknowledge the I," if someone wishes to explore these things. But then, look at your life, look at your livelihood, look at your actions, look at your intentions, look at the attitude, meditation, face your existence, get exposure to teachings—these are all a way to show whether something is deeply missing in your life.

If you feel that you are just a product of secularism, which has as its Triple Gem, producing, consuming, and prestige—if one has serious doubts about that as a reason for existence, then they need to initiate some method of exploration and, therefore, a process of waking up. The Dharma teachings make that unambiguous and clear. So, the middle way is no clinging anywhere.

JLW: *You mentioned that you do not operate out of a sense of a separate "I." Sometimes people wonder how you make decisions and get things done with no self?*

CHRISTOPHER: Yes, and people deserve to know this. I do think that teachers of the Dharma who have a privileged position of authority do need to be held accountable, do need to be questioned, and people do deserve answers to those kind of questions. In that respect, both of you have an important task on your hands. You've got to be asking the questions that a guy or women walking down the street would ask like, "Yeah, but how do you get things done if there's no self? Are you just like a vegetable or what?" It's understandable, because the language, insight, and experience can generate confusion for people.

Conversely, we could look at it the other way: how could the "I" get anything done? [Laughter] What is the track record for what the "I," "me" and "my" has done?

LML: *Not very good!*

CHRISTOPHER: Yes. So, turning it around and bringing a doubt to the conventional solidification of "I." Perhaps out of that diffusing of the significance of "I"there can come about a more open and expansive awareness of "I"and its identifications.

There are three major areas of identification: self, family and country—three powerful forms of identification of "I," "me" and "my." The questioning of all of that can genuinely open the field of awareness, the field of the heart, the field of attention and out of that can come an action which was born of awareness and interconnectedness that is not bound up in "I," "me" and "my." The manifestation of this is kindness, warmth, friendship, and deep intimacy with humanity, nature, etc. All of that, in Dharma language, is free from clinging, free from holding, free from "I," "me," and "my," no "I" engaged with existence — full awareness, full love, full of compassion. But all of that is a language itself which others would use to describe it.

So if you were to say, "Christopher I have come here to interview you today because I have so much compassion for a lot of people." I [Laughter] would want to sit back from you! So the language of awareness, compassion, and love — let others use that description and say, "Oh this person has so much light, so much kindness, and so much compassion." But if the "I" thinks "I" have this compassion, etc…

LML: *It just doesn't belong to anyone.*
CHRISTOPHER: Exactly. It doesn't belong to self, to "I," it doesn't belong there. It is a misunderstanding. Love doesn't belong to anyone.

JLW: *Beautiful. Thank you. It is a pleasure to be with you.*

LML: *Is there any description of the experience of freedom that you can share with us?*
CHRISTOPHER: No problem, no suffering. In daily life the essential inner experience is happiness and friendship. That's the norm of day to day life.

LML: *It is a freedom from suffering then?*
CHRISTOPHER: Yes. The suffering is of the inner life, so, it would be a mild limitation on suffering just to associate it with the inner life. Freedom doesn't belong here [gestures toward himself], it's free!

To make a small distinction, with suffering, it has its locality in conventional terms. Human beings suffer; sentient life suffers; etc. and therefore, we put it in time and place. But freedom isn't co-dependent, isn't bound to conditions; it is free! As it were, living proof that freedom is the true nature of things manifested in this immense diversity [gesturing toward the nature in the yard around us]. What could better show freedom than the freedom that permits all of this?

Freedom makes this multiplicity possible. This freedom is the true nature; this freedom therefore, makes this [gestures to indicate his body] possible. It is a kind of a small event, this little thing going on between the head and toes. So, it is freedom in that sense. The manifestation out of this is happiness, joy, no problem in the life living itself like the trees and the flowers. Nothing special.

... I did a couple of books of interviews myself. My interviews were not so concentrated and focused as yours—you are a good pair of interviewers—mine were with a bunch of people who I basically have a lot of love and affection for, and whose contribution to wisdom in the world I enjoy and appreciate.

LML: *Thank you. We'd like to see those books. One of the things we are endeavoring to show here is that it appears as though there is more openness to awakening at this time in the West. Awakening is being seen as a possibility by many, and in fact realized to be immediately available by increasing numbers of us.*

JLW: *In our own experience over the last twenty years we've seen a change from doing spiritual practice to become a happier, better person to actually seeking freedom. In the past this was seen as something that occurred to only a very rare few, and mostly in the Eastern world.*

CHRISTOPHER: I would agree with that. I think the significant development in that respect is that there are teachings getting established which makes a climate of receptivity many, many, many degrees higher. The integrity and authenticity of teachings which emphasize a sound ethical basis, which emphasize depth of meditation and commitment to it, the wisdom of the heart and the potential for a genuine, free life without the pressures, and clinging that can occur in it—there is greater receptivity to that.

As I said, I think that the twofold factors are people coming forward, like some of the people you are interviewing, the determination of people to put themselves deeply into these areas, and the facilities which are nourishing that—whether it's the three month retreat, or the hermitage wing at Gaia House where people are living in solitude, or people going to India, Burma, Thailand, and elsewhere.

There is now a sense that the most profound elements of spiritual teachings—finding the Truth, liberation, whatever the word — are accessible. It is available in the here and now, and people are willing to put up with the sweat of existence to discover freedom.

LML: *We are endeavoring here to document this in some small way.*

CHRISTOPHER: It is an invaluable role. The conveying of this to wider circles is a very important role and task—partly for the insight, partly for the inspiration and partly for the confidence. If, for example, we take the Insight Meditation community, which I know as well as any other human being, both East and West, the past ten years of teaching have been pretty consistent in pointing here and now, and that the non-dual is really immediate and available; it is not far away. There have been some shifts in the Vipassana community in which the view of the "gradual path" as being "that's what we do" and we'll leave it to Zen for sudden, we'll leave it to Dzogchen for sudden, we'll leave it to Advaita and Poonjaji in Lucknow for sudden. That common view both within and without the Vipassana community has undergone, from my observation and listening, a significant shift.

LML: *A shift towards immediacy?*

CHRISTOPHER: Yes, it is a shift towards immediacy, but more importantly, a shift towards the potential that it's closer than we think. I think that is a reflection of people's liberation, people's realization and that finally, being here and now is not a kind of quiet convenient meditative moment-to-moment practice. Being here and now is being here and now because this is where it is at. There ain't nothing else. You either realize it now or it's hopeless. This view is entering into the Vipassana community, and it is reflected in the rigor of the inquiries that go on in the retreats. It's reflected in the requests from many friends who say, "Don't pitch the Dharma low, Christopher. Keep them on the edge rather than giving a teaching that concentrates on the beginners. Rather than going to the beginners, let the beginners come to the cream of the milk in the Dharma, which is freedom, here and now. Let them grow into it." That's what's going on now.

LML: *You say that freedom is immediate and available here and now. People may wonder then, "how can I see this?" "How do I do it?"*

CHRISTOPHER: Of course, it's the mantra of the West, "How do I get it, and how do I do it?" The "how" word is not very helpful. We might say we introduce a little scaffolding which we call meditation method and technique, a little structure to give a little support to consciousness so it gets steady. How? Breathe in and out. How? Be watchful of the body. How? See your thoughts arising. That's a typical Vipassana style.

All that's just to get the consciousness steady. Steady for what? Steady so that we can not be preoccupied with feelings, thoughts and body, to enable us to wake up. See, some people get stuck with just the observing, but the observing is a "how" designed to liberate one from all the effort to have to observe and just let it come naturally. So, rather than the "how," if anything, it's "what." What is liberation; what is bliss? Sometimes it is quite necessary to drop the "how" because it is still thinking, "Here I am and how do I get there? What do I have to do to go from A to B?" Rather than, there's no B, no A to Z, this is it!

LML: *Just asking the "how" question presumes that you are some place other than where freedom is.*

CHRISTOPHER: Exactly. So, it's that kind of emphasis. As I said before, for some, given the degree of pain and stress, unhappiness and confusion, etc., it is important to, out of kindness, provide people with a sense of direction, of practice, of going from A to B and getting them well established on the path. It's a perfectly useful resource to do so.

Woe be to those who dismiss it all at hand and say, "Practice is just striving; it's just ego; it's just desire." To take support away from people in that way shows a lack of wisdom and a lack of kindness and a clinging to a view that there's nothing you can do. That view does have to be watched carefully. It's unfair to people who come with great need and great longing for well being, happiness, and peace in their life, to then be told that there is nothing that they can do. It leaves some people disheartened and despairing.

There are others, of course, who respond to "nothing to do" by questioning any holding and clinging to their form of structure, and become free of it. But I have listened to many voices of those who have been hurt by major charismatic authority figures saying there is nothing you can do. And, one can also be hurt by those who say that it is a long, long, long, hard road.

LML: *Both are extremes.*

CHRISTOPHER: Exactly.

JLW: *In light of what you were saying earlier about the importance of asking questions that "people on the street" might ask, are there any questions of that nature that you would like to include here?*

CHRISTOPHER: In terms of response to your question, there are people who have profound experiences that they can't make sense of. Some people have these experiences but they don't have the insight of what it is about. People can give me tremendous accounts of their experience, and every word that comes out of their mouth is a description of liberation, freedom, joy, cosmic awareness, the inseparable nature of reality, without a whisper of intention to exaggerate or deceive. This happened to a few in the retreat I just did. So, there's experience and apparent understanding or insight.

It may not be quite fair and it may not be quite appropriate on my path of teaching with authority here, but I have to say to the person, "If you can come in a year and a day and say the same to me, the insights have stayed; then it's cohesive." If they haven't, it could be just a wonderful experience, a tremendous brief shift of consciousness, an enormous opening up. But if the outcome of it is that within days or weeks they go back into a kind of normal drudgery, miserable relationships, hating work, worrying about things, etc., then I would just put that into the language of having an experience. No matter what is said; that is not the realization. The realization makes that real; that's what realization is.

LML: *A realization holds no matter what is happening good or bad, no matter where you are at, or what you are doing.*

CHRISTOPHER: Exactly, exactly. Of course, in the period after realization the self can arise. Of course, ego and "I" can arise. Of course, some suffering can arise. But there is this sense that there's a qualitative difference. In making that freedom real it must manifest through the heart. It's the only decent criteria we have. Therefore love, kindness, warmth, and openness become much more a feature of one's life. If it isn't, it's not realization; it is an experience. That difference is something that is vital.

There are people who come, and they say to me, "I've had this experience, but I've never expressed it. No language, nothing fits, nothing feels right in the way I try to put words to it." So there's just silence and a brief comment. The outcome is that their experience does transform, and they never bring in the known to give it a language such as no-self, emptiness, truth, or the buzzword, enlightenment. Yet, their life is transformed. There's realization without interpretation. Realization without language. So, the significance of the experience begins a quest to get the insight into the experience. Generally speaking, that quest forward cannot come through the mind itself. It has to find it through the dynamics of understanding with others.

The risk, and it's a significant risk, is that there is the experience, there is the insight and understanding, but then there is the talking about the experience. In talking about the experience, insidiously, the self can re-emerge and possess it. Then what will show is the person in a dualism of the self talking about "no self." Conflict will arise, suffering will arise.

In the Dharma tradition, let's take monks for example, monks, except with the teacher, are not allowed to speak about their experience. The danger is that it goes the other way and gets a bit enclosed.

JLW: *It can become reified; it can become a "thing."*

CHRISTOPHER: Yes. So, in the monastery where I stayed for three and a half years, you knew. You didn't need someone to come and say "I've realized." One just knew. There is a presence; there's something that goes on that is communicating itself.

LML: *Nonverbally.*

CHRISTOPHER: It is nonverbal. The danger is of the reification of "no self" through self. Some spiritual teachers tend to talk a lot about themselves —"I, me, and mine." One can listen with a lot of interest and appreciation, but after awhile one just gets exhausted in hearing about this person's experience. So, people who are sharing the no-self experience, the realization of emptiness, have to be very watchful. One must be quite cautious not to reify realization in the question, "How did this happen to you?" Nothing happened to me! How could anything happen to me! Me is just a little event going on here. It's important to watch this.

LML: *May I share some of my experience with you?*

CHRISTOPHER: Certainly.

LML: *I've never been trained in Insight Meditation, yet what is occurring naturally seems to be similar—an observing of what arises and falls within the spacious awareness. There has been a progression of sorts into more and more detachment from what arises, less clinging, less relationship with it one way or another—or if there is a relationship that enters, that is seen as well. When I hear Insight Meditation described, it sounds similar.*

CHRISTOPHER: From your description there, you're right. It's a very similar feature, the ability to be conscious of what appears in the bodymind, to see it clearly so what is seen isn't producing something—either fear of the observation projected onto the object, or it appears to be coming from the object, causing "me"suffering. Mindfulness, consciousness, and the quality of attentiveness help one to see that something is not as "bad" as it appears. Things are not what one imagines them to be. Witnessing can dissolve that and show the simple, pure, undiluted, interconnectedness with things and that they are all held together in freedom, Buddha nature.

There is a significance in the observation, the significance of giving attention to the awareness itself rather than the content. The Buddha says in the *Four Foundations of Mindfulness Awareness*, which is a kind of bible of the Vipassana community, that one is aware and mindful to the extent necessary in order to abide independent and free in this life. Sometimes the tradition has gotten too exaggerated in its focus, endeavoring to be mindful, moment to moment, all the time.

So, sometimes people come to me and ask outright, "Are you free?" Which I said before, it's people's right to ask those questions to teachers. One time I asked the person, "What does to be free mean to you?" The person said, "To be free is to be mindful and aware moment to moment." I said, "Then I'm not free," and left it at that. The next day somebody came and asked, "Are you liberated? Are you free?" When I asked this person what it meant to be free he said, "A tremendous sense of expansiveness and not suffering anymore." I said, "Yes."

The key of the observation and mindfulness is "to the extent necessary." If we make a holy cow out of it, we'll constantly be judging ourselves, "I'm mindful," "I'm not mindful." When it's there and it's natural, it's just to the extent necessary. If there are areas in our lives where we need greater vigilance—an example in my own life is that I am a parent—I have a teenage daughter. I love her to bits. There's an extra vigilance that is required "to the extent necessary"—it's not an easy world to be in for teenagers, and for adults as well.

There are risks involved in being in this world—alcohol, drugs, sexual abuse, being on the streets at night—many factors. It requires an extra mindfulness and vigilance to the extent necessary in relation to my daughter. I can't take her for granted. That's beautifully stated in Buddha's text. But if we exaggerate mindfulness; we are always judging. Mindfulness comes naturally, awareness comes naturally, connectedness comes naturally. It is not the work of the self.

LML: *There is a growing sense I have that mindful awareness is naturally occurring all the time and cannot not be.*

CHRISTOPHER: Beautiful, beautiful. That sense and appreciation, it's very freeing. It is the whisper. It is the outcome.

LML: *And then it is seen that there truly is nothing one needs to do.*

CHRISTOPHER: Exactly. Once one knows that, there's not a trace of boredom, apathy, or indifference to existence. There's nothing to do, yet one is actively concerned with life, with the ending of suffering, with justice issues or whatever it might be. Yet, one knows deep down there's nothing to do because it's doing itself. So maybe on that note we can end since it's doing itself! [Laugh]

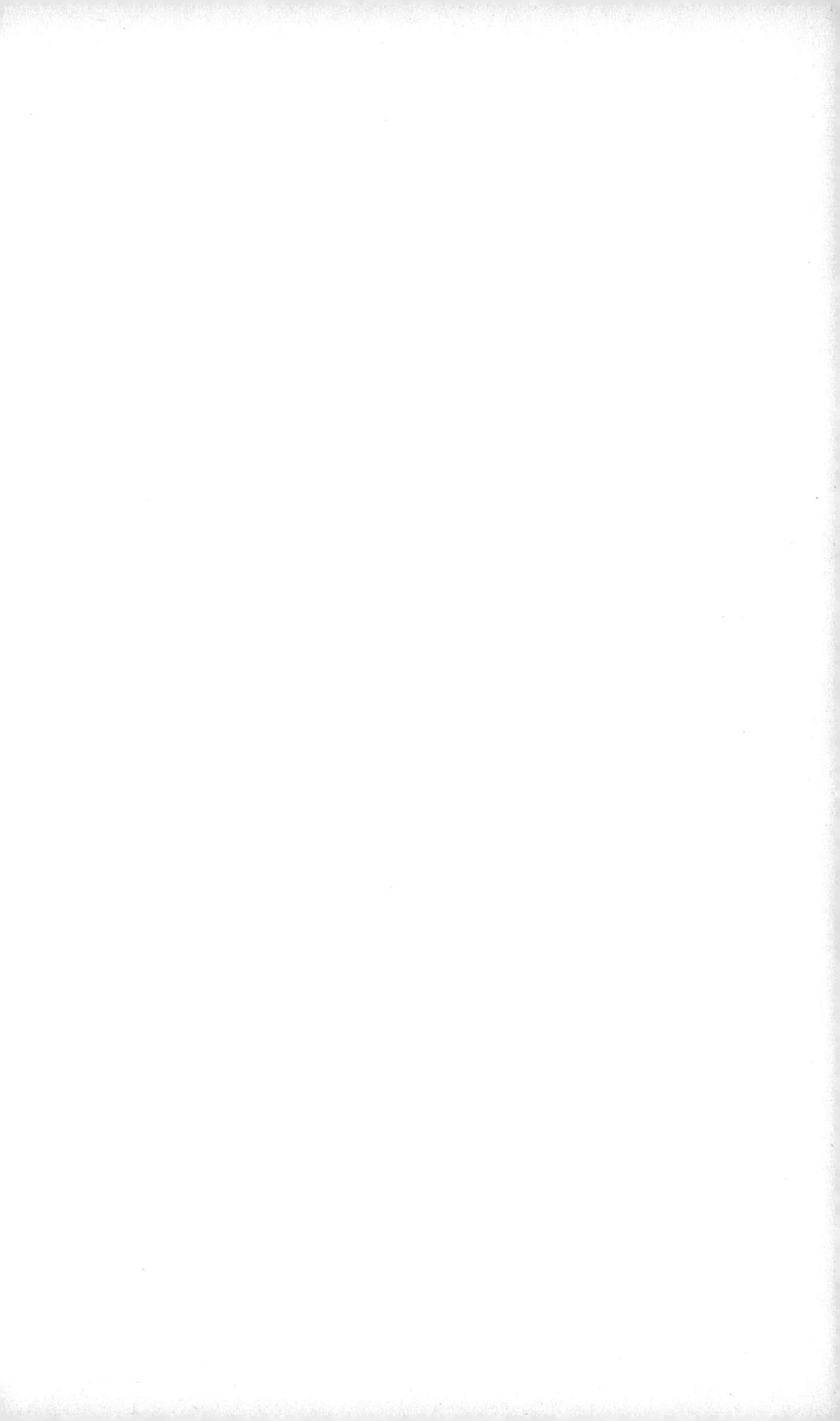

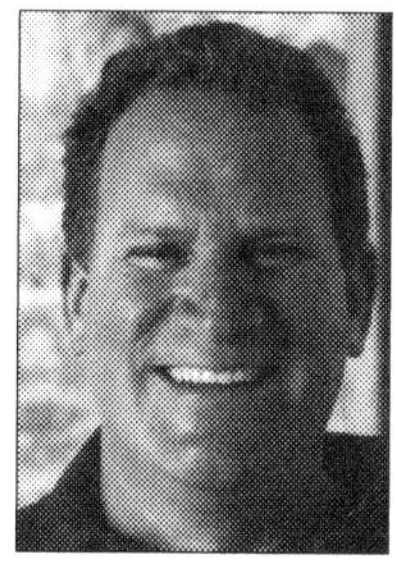

LAMA SURYA DAS

"WHY SHOULD ANY OF US SPEND OUR LIVES AS ONLOOKERS AT THE SEASIDE, NERVOUSLY WADING IN THE SHALLOWS? OTHERS HAVE FOUND FREEDOM, SATISFACTION, AND LIBERATION. YOU CAN DO IT TOO. WE CAN ALL DO IT. TOGETHER. THE TIME HAS COME TO STRIDE IN AND BEGIN SWIMMING IN THE DEEPER WATERS. SURF'S UP!"

from Awakening to the Sacred

Surya Das found time to see us on his day off after completing a six-day retreat in Big Sur, California and before flying back to Massachusetts to teach again. Our first questions initiated a torrential response which continued, virtually without ceasing for several hours. To say his knowledge and understanding of Buddhism in general and Dzogchen in particular is impressive would be quite an understatement. In accord with his traditions, Surya was not interested in talking about his own personal story. But he was forthright when speaking about the Buddhist teachings, the qualities of clarity, compassion, kindness, and wisdom of his teachers, and the lineages and teachings they passed on to him. Surya has a strong, imposing presence that could seem intimidating. But on the inside is a huge, generous, bodhisattva heart that is completely dedicated to serving the Truth.

Born Jeffrey Miller in New York in 1950, he was given his name Surya Das by one of his first teachers, Neem Karoli Baba. Surya is one of the first Westerners to become an authorized lama and teacher of Dzogchen, the consummate teaching of Vajrayana Buddhism. He is a poet and author of several books including the best seller, *Awakening the Buddha Within*.

Surya Das has studied and practiced meditation with the greatest spiritual teachers throughout the Far East and in the Himalayas. The secret Dzogchen teachings were once closely guarded treasures of Tibet, whispered into the ears of only those ethical and accomplished disciples who had successfully completed anywhere from ten to thirty years of preliminary practices. Now for the first time in history, these "mind-nature teachings" are being made available to anyone who wants them. These are the ancient lineages' most powerful teachings for recognizing the mind's essence, understanding emptiness, and living with compassion in our turbulent times.

The Dalai Lama once told Surya: "Dharma in the West is up to you Westerners now. Be creative in adapting the timeless essence of the teachings to your own culture and times." At this time, Surya is the primary Western messenger spreading these great teachings in his clear, understandable, Western vernacular. To help serve this goal, he founded the Dzogchen Foundation of America in 1991, based in Massachusetts, New York, and California. He has taught many Western Buddhist teachers and has initiated and organized the annual Western Buddhist Teacher's Conferences with the Dalai Lama. He also leads regular meditation retreats in twelve different countries around the world.

We found Lama Surya Das to be warm, humorous, and articulate; the treasury of his learned wisdom, insight, anecdotes, and quotes is extremely rich. Although John had been interested in and involved with the Dzogchen teachings for several years, it was through this contact with Surya that Lynn Marie found the Dzogchen teachings come alive and felt them touch her heart deeply. She has been influenced by these teachings ever since. Surya Das is one of John's main teachers.

CONVERSATION *with* LAMA SURYA DAS

JLW: *Dzogchen is a Tibetan Buddhist teaching that is not yet widely known in the Western world. As a teacher of Dzogchen, could you speak about this teaching?*
SURYA: Dzogchen literally means the innate great perfection, the natural great perfection. Many Tibetan lamas and masters these days say that Dzogchen is the teaching for today because it's not culturally based; it's beyond Buddhism. It's not something that depends on dogma, study, rituals, or forms like visualizations on deities, initiations, and so on. It's a naked awareness practice. It's a way of awakening to your American Buddha nature, not your Oriental Buddha nature. It does not depend on becoming oriental and changing your furniture or clothes, but instead to awaken the Buddha within you. Buddha nature is not American or Tibetan. So, this is about something you can directly get to—our own innate wakefulness, our inner Buddha, the sleeping Buddha. Even to call it "Buddha" is to make it too foreign. It is as Western as we are because it is what we are!

So, Dzogchen is called the teaching for today. It's right to the point; it doesn't take a lot of study or memorization. You don't have to convert from anything to anything in order to awaken to who and what you truly are. Dzogchen says we are all Buddhas by nature. Our only task is to awaken to what we truly are. We are not discussing Tibet, India, the Himalayas, or Buddhism twenty-five hundred years ago. To awaken to who and what we truly are is right now. It's always now. It's now or never.

JLW: *You were once connected with Neem Karoli Baba?*
SURYA: Yes, my first guru was Maharaji Neem Karoli Baba. He gave me my name Surya Das in 1972. He always said, "Learn from everyone;

learn from all the sages and saints because they are all one." So in those days I spent a lot of time in ashrams, particularly with Tibetan masters, but also other teachers in Sri Lanka and India, Burma, Thailand, Bhutan, and Japan.

I found that the Dzogchen teaching is sort of a culmination or the luminous heart of the Dharma. That's why I say it's beyond Buddhism. I'm not saying it's the best teaching or the only way; it's just that it's the heart of the matter. It's the mystic principle underlying all the authentic teachings and paths; it's where all teachings converge.

That's why people say, "What's the difference between Dzogchen and non-dual or Advaita Vedanta?" All the innermost, mystical, non-dual traditions are so very similar. They don't depend on external forms that look different—like Asians look different from Westerners and Buddhas look different from Christs and they both look different than Hindu gods, etc. In the inner meaning of the Great Perfection, in the light, what's there to look different? They are the same. It's pure luminosity. So, Dzogchen is the living heart of the Dharma. The Dharma is something do-able today. People always ask me to talk about Dzogchen and teach it in the West and so, I am talking about it and teaching it in the West. It's very complimentary to all other practices. It's an outlook, a bigger view that can enhance any practice that you do. Most spiritual practices we do today can be enhanced by the non-dual understanding, the "view from above," while we practice in a conventional way.

JLW: *Yet, Dzogchen isn't just a view; it's also a set of practices.*

SURYA: Yes, Dzogchen tradition, like Mahamudra, to which it is similar, and the Zen tradition are the so-called highest teachings of Buddhism. "Consummate teachings" may be better than "highest."

Dzogchen is explained according to view, meditation, and action. There is the view of things as they are, the Natural Great Perfection; and there's the meditation of non-meditation, of being, not of doing. It's a naked awareness practice; it's not mental calisthenics, its not bowing or rituals; it is not self-improvement. It's recognizing things as they are. In Buddhism there's no self to improve so that solves that problem. Whereas Socrates says, "Know thyself," in Buddhism it's, "There is no thyself." [Laughter]

So, there's the view, meditation and then, spontaneous action. This is enlightened activity, impeccable activity, selfless action. Dzogchen is a sort of profound non-dual, mystical approach. The general Buddhist path is action to retrain morality, meditation to cultivate wisdom, and the view of things as they are. Dzogchen, however, starts with the view of how things are first. This is why it is called the more advanced or mystical teaching.

With this view, it's like Buddhas practicing Dzogchen because it's our Buddha nature doing it anyway and we recognize that from the beginning. It's not trying to transform an imperfect me into a perfect me. It is recognizing who is doing what around here.

JLW: *It's recognizing the perfection in both the perfect and imperfect.*
SURYA: Exactly. That's why Dzogchen is called not just the Great Perfection, but the great wholeness, the consummate wholeness. One is perfect; the view is perfect. But two is also perfect; dualism is perfect in the Great Perfection. The one and the many are inseparable.

JLW: *It's the perfect display of That.*
SURYA: Yes, it is That. That's why we say that samsara and nirvana are inseparable. The Dzogchen Master Long Chempa said, "Fools who despise samsara and long for nirvana will have a very long road to peace." It is not that nirvana, enlightenment, peace is on the far other shore like you sometimes hear in the general teachings. Nirvana is here, in nature. It is nature; it is the nature of things as they are. It's not many lifetimes and three kalpas in the future; it's now or never. It's always here. That's why the Zen Master Hakuin said, "This very land is the pure land, nirvana, this very body, the body of Buddha." He didn't mean Japan; he didn't mean his "bod." He meant ours, here in America; he meant everywhere, everybody.

LML: *Dzogchen is new to the West, isn't it?*
SURYA: Yes, it's new, but it is also a timeless truth. There must have been many who have realized it before we ever heard of Asia. But Dzogchen is new to the West as a teaching, as a practice, as a Buddhist path. Buddhism is fairly new to the West—the last two hundred years. Dzogchen has come to the West since the Tibetan lamas left Tibet after the Chinese invasion in the 1950s. This Tibetan wisdom was dammed up for two thousand years in Tibet. Then, the dam broke, and it spread all over the world.

Dzogchen is often called the "sacred, secret teaching." In general Zen Buddhism has been more well-known, and then more recently Mahayana Buddhism has become more well-known. In the 1980s and 1990s the Dzogchen teachings have been a little more translated and introduced in the West by Tibetan teachers and now by some senior Western students and authorized Western lamas and teachers.

JLW: *This morning we were just talking about how the awareness is never not present. It's always what we are, but somehow we focus our attention on the display of phenomena and the events of our experience and never notice the context in which it's all occurring.*
SURYA: It's easy to say that and difficult to really live it, and in between is our life.

JLW: *Yes, and that's where I understand the practices come in with Dzogchen. It's one thing to understand, to have the view, and then the practices help you to cultivate the presence of awareness.*
SURYA: We don't say "cultivate" because that implies more of a developmental model, as if there is something to cultivate and improve. The Dzogchen tradition says—I'll just keep quoting Dzogchen texts—"Buddha nature is not improved in nirvana, and it is not ruined or degenerated in samsara."

JLW: *What is the difference between sleeping Buddhas and awakened Buddhas?*
SURYA: The difference is recognition or maturity or wisdom, not just understanding. This is why I started to talk about how this is neither improved by enlightenment nor ruined by delusion. Again, I'm just translating out of Tibetan texts: "It's primordially pure and perfect from the beginningless beginning." So, whether it looks like light or dark, or rainbow colors, or whatever in between, that's just a refraction of itself—like the light that comes to a crystal and makes many colors. It is still one light diffracted, and displayed.

In the Dzogchen tradition we talk about the view of how it is. This is introduced and pointed out. Hopefully, it is experienced. The Dzogchen tradition starts at the point of introduction or recognition. Hopefully, that implies something on the part of the sleeping Buddha, the student.

LML: *So, it begins with the view, the recognition of the natural Great Perfection and the practice comes out of that. The usual way of thinking is the other way around—practice* *is done until recognition occurs. If Dzogchen begins with the view, how then does this recognition occur?*

SURYA: That's a good question. First of all, we all have it. It's the innate wisdom. It's the innate awareness. It's our Buddha nature. It's the light by which we already see. It's not just a light to see. We are just highlighting that it is here. You can find it anywhere. Everything is it. Everything is radiant, everything is light, energy—whatever you want to say. The mystical theists say everything is God, or we are all God's children, similar to the refractions in the crystal.

In Dzogchen this introduction is emphasized first. We're translating the word "nutra." It doesn't just mean introduction it also means identifying and recognizing. It's not just being introduced to something like you, John, introduced me to Lynn Marie. I know it sounds like you have to have a teacher to introduce you to this new thing. Like some people believe you have to have a guru to zap you so you have an awakening or recognition. That is hierarchical and very Oriental.

But there have been millions of people in the world who awoke without a teacher: Ramana Maharshi, Tilopa, wherever you want to look. Satori is an introduction. It's not that someone gave you satori, you broke through, you woke up. Maybe your practice ripened, maybe something fell away. That's why it's a balance between being introduced to something that was already there and recognizing, identifying what was always there. Without that recognition you aren't really doing Dzogchen practice you're doing some kind of mind practice. Dzogchen practice is Rigpa practice, the non-dual, naked awareness practice.

JLW: *Could you explain further what naked awareness is?*

SURYA: Rigpa or pure presence, primordial presence, naked awareness… it's like gnostic awareness; it knows. It's not something you develop by getting more concentrated. It's not something you develop like stages of insight. It is what has insight. It is the nature of the mind. It's not the mind that's developing a stream of thoughts. It is the presence of awareness through which those thoughts stream.

Buddha nature is the nature of all sentient beings, enlightened, unenlightened, and in between. It's called the primordial nature or awareness. The word in Sanskrit is vidya. Vidya is the opposite of avidya, which is ignorance.

LML: *How is it that we can so completely overlook our own primordial nature?*
SURYA: Because it's so close that we overlook it. We are so turned outward that we are looking elsewhere. It's too transparent, so we don't notice it. We see through it. It's too good to be true, so we don't believe it. It's like, "What, I'm the Buddha? No, I'm a sinner. Jesus was the Buddha. I'm a sinner," or whatever our cultural and inner conditioning is that keeps us away from it. So, we turn outward, and we look past our Jesus or Buddha nature. We're looking up on the stage at the guru or the master, or we're looking to the future eons from now to our enlightenment. We're not recognizing how innate Buddha nature is. This is basic Buddhism, but with Dzogchen it's a very profound attack—access, immediate access. Not just developing it through a path in many lifetimes.

JLW: *It's not trying to eliminate, "Oh, I'm a sinner." It's recognizing that prior to sinner/saint, here it is.*
SURYA: You recognize that all beings, everything is Buddha nature, or whatever it is you want to call it, your True Nature. In Dzogchen the awareness we are working with is really innate wakefulness. It's not states of mind developed by concentration, bliss or highs or lows, good, bad; those are relative, dualistic. Which is fine on the conventional, horizontal level, the level of relative truth as it is called in Buddhism.

On the level of Absolute Truth, emptiness, prajna, shunyata, wisdom—that is the nature of things; that is how things actually are, always. In the relative, conventional level, things appear and function in different ways, but from the Absolute perspective, they are all equal. As it says in the sutras, they are characterized by shunyata, they are all equally impermanent and unsatisfactory in the long run.

Of course, we prefer certain circumstances or events because we have preferences, but they are not intrinsically better. What we need to do is to awaken to, in English, who and what we are; if you are talking in Dzogchen terminology, to recognize the nature of mind, which is Rigpa, the innate, unconditioned wakefulness, the luminous nature of awareness, not just the shadows, the reflections. They are part of it, but they are secondary.

Whether there are reflections or not, the mirror remains luminous. With or without reflections, the mirror does not improve; more reflections don't mean it is busier—it doesn't get tired; if there are no reflections, it doesn't get bored. That is why it is called "mirror like" wisdom, equanimity wisdom, the "sky-like" nature of mind—the sky can accommodate all forms of weather, they are just transient phenomena. So, in your open heart-mind whatever comes is a joy. You can enjoy all the seasons and all forms of weather. The winter is not really worse than the spring, it is just different.

LML: *Is it coming to experience that sky-like nature directly and to know yourself to be that?*

SURYA: To recognize the mirror-like nature of your being, yourself. Every thing is clearly reflected as it is, and if nothing is reflected, you are not missing anything. It is beyond birth and death because birth and death, change, up and down, health and sickness, are also temporary conditions of the conventional, physical level of our experience. But the Buddha nature, the clear light, nature of the mind, is immanent, always here, the innate nature, the intrinsic awareness.

JLW: *So, this is the understanding one is introduced to in Dzogchen, at the beginning. Then, there is a whole set of practices for stabilizing this understanding. What is the difference between the introduction and enlightenment, or realization?*

SURYA: That is a good question. That's like what is the difference between the sleeping Buddha and the awakened Buddha?

JLW: *Well, the introduction is the awakening, isn't it?*

SURYA: It is.

LML: *So why a path after that?*

SURYA: Well, in one way there is no path, and in another way it is like I always say, "It seems easier these days to get enlightened, than to stay enlightened." A lot of people have an enlightenment, or an awakening experience, but then what happens? The sun of reality might break through the clouds of obscuration, confusion, egoism for a moment, or five minutes, or an hour, or a day but then the clouds, the habits, the mind, the concepts again appear to obscure that sun of reality.

But after having seen the sun once, you know better. You have experienced reality for yourself. You know what the sun means. You know why there is light here even though there are clouds. You know how things work. So you get more and more used to that. By practice you might thin the clouds; you might see through the veils of illusion more easily, naturally, and clearly. In this getting used to the way things are, you mature your view.

The first awakening is like an initiation, not just an outer ritual or empowerment; it is really the meaning of initiation. You are really initiated into things as they are. A satori is an awakening. A breakthrough to reality or emptiness is an awakening. Then the path is stabilizing that view, getting used to that view. In Dzogchen terms, the idea of meditation is understood as "getting used to it." It is not defined as crossing your legs, closing your eyes, and quieting your mind.

JLW: *In other words, the path is to abide as that aware presence through the vicissitudes of life?*

SURYA: Yes. Get used to how that is and how that manifests. But getting used to it means in every day, in every action, in every moment getting used to this innate wakefulness, this primordially pure perfection, this Buddha nature, and how it manifests as the display of phenomena in all of its changes. Because in itself it doesn't change but like the ocean, it has different modifications, waves, whirlpools, icebergs; mists, and clouds rise from it—the ocean doesn't really change; these are just superficial changes on the surface. So, when you glimpse the primordial ocean, the infinite sky-like nature, then you have a bigger perspective on temporary weather conditions in that sky.

JLW: *In the glimpse, isn't a part of what is realized the emptiness, the non-entityness of self and all things?*

SURYA: That is why it is called "sky-like" nature of mind; it is not called "sun-like." It is not even the blue sky; it is space itself; that is why it is called emptiness. It is not a thing, it is more like space, or spacious or open, not empty like empty glass, but open like open window—open eyes, open mind, open hearted, so there is more room for everything to occur.

In Dzogchen it is called cutting through or seeing through, Trekchod. This is cutting through solidity, seeing through the forms and recognizing the essence, the nature, and seeing how form and emptiness arise together, inseparable. Like it says in the Heart Sutra," … form is emptiness, emptiness takes form."

You don't have to get rid of form, you can just see through forms. They become more transparent, workable, non-claustrophobic; you are not so attached to what form things take, what is the form of your emotions or your mind. So, that is the meditation path. From getting used to this view, this wisdom understanding gets more and more mature, more stable so that you don't fall in and out of it so much.

JLW: *Can you talk a little bit about how this occurred for you?*

SURYA: I'll just speak more generally — this view, actualized or matured through meditation, and stabilized through the practice path, becomes the result, the fruit, which is actually the view. Rather than a linear progression, Dzogchen begins with how things are. The path is getting used to it and it arrives back at that same view, but stabilized, so that you never stray out of it. Therefore, the path could be extremely short.

There is really no distance from the fundamental ground, the beginning, the primordial perfection. It is the clear-light nature of things as they are, the Dharmakaya. The path is just that, Rigpa practice, getting used to the view. The fruit as well is Rigpa, but stabilized; it is the same view. But it is no longer the view as like a breakthrough, or introduction — it is not like you introduce me to Lynn Marie, it is like, now I know Lynn Marie, or even, I am Lynn Marie. It is not that you need to break through, have satori, or have an experience; you realize you are there and you have always been there. You are That. You really don't have to become That.

It is all interconnected. That's why the path really has no distance and no development, no stages. But we can still recognize that there is introduction, there is getting used to it, and there is stabilization. Some masters are obviously more wise, more stable, unconfused, and more unselfish than other people.

So, there is a difference between sleeping Buddhas and awakened Buddhas — or a snake that has been tied in knots or that same snake after it has effortlessly untied itself and is slithering around naturally — but, realize, it is still just a snake. Whether the mind is tied up in knots of confusion and identification or free, open and clear, it is still primordially perfect. Essentially it is what it is, and it is not improved by getting straightened out.

LML: *What is day-to-day life like once the view has become stabilized?*
SURYA: It's like this. Everything gets done by itself. Relationships with people are perfect. It's like saying, "How do enlightened people live? Do they have preferences or emotions?" These are good questions; in one way they are speculative questions, but what's underneath them is like, "Does that mean I have to get rid of my preferences and emotions?"

JLW: *Or, "Can I have relationships? Will I be able to make decisions?"*
SURYA: Right. "What will I do? How will I take care of my children? They need money; I need to work," or whatever. So the point is, how does daily life fit in with all this high falluting, philosophical talk? It has to fit in because otherwise it is not the view of Dzogchen. It is just a bicycle lane rather than the great highway; it is too thin, too narrow.

Every aspect of life can be part of this spiritual path and must be if it is going to be a full path. That is again why I think Dzogchen is really the Great Highway of awakening for today. It is very relevant to us today because it does not require you to go on the monastic path of total simplicity and renunciation which is for very few in today's world and very, very few in the West.

We have much more of a lay American Buddhism, and contemporary Western Dharma. It is much more experiential. It is very egalitarian, anybody can do it. You don't have to be smart. You don't have to be a philosopher. Whereas in some schools of Buddhism, you have to become an expert in philosophy, epistemology, or something; Dzogchen can enhance any kind of practice. So, we can use these pith instructions, these Dzogchen teachings, this technology of awakening, this manual for an awakened life, an impeccable life, today in America, in the West, to awaken ourselves and to awaken the best that is in us; that is what we call the Buddha within. Not to become Buddhists; it is better to be Buddhas!

JLW: *We are putting this book together because it seems to us that there is an increasing number of people in the West who are awakening. I am wondering if that is your observation as well?*
SURYA: Yes. Definitely.

LML: *It seems that there has been a maturation.*
SURYA: Right. But I don't know what part of the West we are talking about, or what segment of the culture, or the counter-culture, or the

whole of modern society. Because in one way our modern technological society is becoming more and more alienated and fragmented. I would say, more akin to the Buddhist understanding, a sort of more enlightened vision would say things are more cyclical—it is not just a progression. So, looking at it that way, it's hard to say there is more awakening today; it is also hard to say these times are worse than they used to be.

But if you look at America since the sixties... in America the pollsters say there is more religion today—if that is connected to awakening—it probably is. There are five million Buddhists in America today and there are all kinds of people in other awakening practices.

JLW: *I guess I am wondering if you are encountering more people who have recognized and/or stabilized in the view you have described here?*

SURYA: Well, I am encountering this, but I live in a Buddhist subculture. But yes, definitely, it is an increasing phenomenon in my experience. People are getting more sophisticated, more subtle and deeper, and less fascinated with the side effects and the special effects of spiritual life and more interested in the heart of the matter.

There is a lot more access to the authentic teachers and teachings and good translations, and real ways to train. You know, not just the Buddhist Club on Sunday night at Cambridge University or Harvard University. Now we have real retreats, monasteries, training centers, things for families and children to do. There are Buddhist universities, like the Naropa Institute where young people can study and get degrees combining Buddhism with psychology, or philosophy. Almost everybody in the world knows about the Dalai Lama and his teachings on compassion. This kind of awakening is coming. It is not so obscure, and it doesn't have a bad name. It is seen as a good influence.

JLW: *It is not seen as something that is isolated. It is increasingly seen as something that is available.*

SURYA: It is available and also, it is relevant for today and not something that is totally backward or anachronistic. It can be used in all those fields and others; it is something that we can do ourselves—the Dharma is a do-it-yourself Dharma. Buddha's last words were, "Work out your path with diligence." It is a practice path. It is a do-it-yourself path. You can do it. The teacher and the teachings point out the way only to teach the one who walks it. It is provocative, and so, that also is awakening. It gets your attention; it arrests your attention; it requires your attention, also, so it works both ways. It awakens your imagination.

LML: *At least in the United States, people are all seeking and searching whether it is for material things, the right relationship, a fit body, or whatever they believe will alleviate suffering and disconnectedness. Would you say that the source of suffering is ignorance of the view?*

SURYA: Yes. Absolutely. Not just in the United States, but in general, the source of suffering is ignorance. Ignorance meaning not knowing, ignoring reality, resulting in confusion, illusion. So, you can say suffering results from not knowing the view—ignorance of how things are, ignorance of how things work.

For example, everybody wants happiness. We could say everybody is seeking something; it looks like they are all seeking something different. But really most everybody is seeking the same thing through different means, including us, including people on a spiritual path, including monks and nuns, including people who want to be a millionaire—why do they want to be a millionaire? Because they think that will make them happy. Why do they want to be whatever else they want? To be famous? To have children? Finally, it is to be happy.

It is not so confusing then when you understand the pattern of motivation. Since we are not always really in touch with how things are, we are caught up in ignorance, delusion, illusion. We are wanting things to be different, better, or more. "Yeah, maybe more material things, then we'll be happy." These are the illusions. These are the dysfunctional myths we live by. They backfire on themselves.

JLW: *They are myths we believe, but they are not actually the truth.*

SURYA: Right. Right. More is better, bigger is better. More technology is better. What is better? Will it make us happy? Maybe in the process we are using up the whole world's resources, and we are really ruining future possibilities of well-being and happiness, but we don't want to know about that. In fact, we are just starting to look at that. This is another little awakening too, the ecological awakening, the green awakening, the democratic awakening. We have been moving during the last two hundred years from theocracy and totalitarianism and kings and queens and tyranny toward democracy, egalitarianism. Now it is a little more toward gender equality, racial equality, and ecological equality. This is another little bit of awakening, in the social fields.

So, things are brightening up in one way, and I am an optimist. But in another way the world is very fragmented and speedy, and it has gotten increasingly easy to blow everything up by one madman, or just kill your neighbors. It seems to be a precarious balance. But in the bigger vision it is not just about this world. There are many mysteries and things, perhaps, beyond this world, so we need to keep that in mind when we judge things.

LML: *It seems that everyone is seeking happiness when our intrinsic nature is happiness. The love, peace, fulfillment, happiness are our intrinsic nature.*

SURYA: That's us. "Those R Us!" We all are that. Everybody says this—it's embarrassing; I am talking about clichés. There's a book titled *I Am That*, by Nisargadatta Maharaj. People have been saying for thousands of years in India, "Tat Twam Assi," "Thou Art That." So that is not new news, but it is big news. It is like a secret teaching, not a secret, but it is a big surprise. It is esoteric. It is not in *Reader's Digest*, not on Madison Avenue billboards. It is a "self secret." Trungpa Rinpoche used to say, "When you recognize it, you know it has always been there, and you laugh at yourself." That is why in Dzogchen there is text called *The Primordial Buddha's Twelve Vajra Laughs*. Because it is a big laugh—you are looking for the Buddha, and the Buddha is you. Not just the Buddha is on your head or in your pocket; the Buddha is not even within; the Buddha is you.

Humans are funny you know it? We are always trying to get love. Love comes from being loving. We have to bring it out. It is like getting it by doing it. What do we mean we have to get love? Where are we going to get it from? Everything is available and sufficient within—although there is really no within/without. Everything is here! The problem is that although it's always here, we are not always here; we are usually elsewhere. We are distracted, scattered, or half-asleep.

LML: *Yes, we are what we are looking for. We are missing it because we are distracted by thinking we have to look for what we already are! That is the joke.*

SURYA: So it is—a joke. We are what we seek.

JLW: *So, these teachings, Tat Twam Assi—Thou Art That—have been around for thousands of years, since the Vedas and the Upanishads, and there are individuals who* *awaken, but there are many more individuals who know about it, or who can describe the view of Dzogchen than who embody it. Is there a possibility of it becoming an intellectual construct that is irrelevant?*

SURYA: It is not really irrelevant but an intellectual understanding which might be a part of the unfolding of the Truth within oneself. You can progress, as the Tibetan commentators say. You progress, and that's why some schools emphasize study, understanding, and analysis. It is not irrelevant; it might be connected to deeper experiential realization. You can progress from learning about something, theory and intellectual understanding, to experience and then to realization. But on the other hand, knowing about some of these things could also be an obstacle. Because it can happen that we think we know a lot, but we don't know a lot; we think too much, but we don't know that much.

That is why the most mystical teachings are sometimes called "secret" or for initiates only because, if you give it too soon and people don't appreciate it, it makes an intellectual obscuration. In simple English, it gets in your way. Just like giving adult food to babies or if the children were to see the parents having sex. There is no secret or sin about sex, but you don't want to do it in front of your children because they don't understand, and it can become a confusion or maybe a perversion. They might think that the one on top is beating up the one on the bottom. They don't understand what is going on.

LML: *So there needs to be a certain level of maturity.*

SURYA: Yes, maturity. That is why it is often called, highest, or advanced, or secret, or for initiates only. But it is no big secret—it is around everywhere and you can read about it. There is something that we call in Dzogchen an intellectual obstacle.

An intellectual obstacle occurs when you have too many ideas about emptiness and emptiness becomes just a concept for you. Or you might become a nihilist like Nietzche. You can go crazy that way. He understood emptiness, but he didn't get the other part, the fullness, the compassion. He got the emptiness but not the full wisdom. So he became a nihilist, an existentialist, and everything was meaningless for him, and he went crazy.

That is a mistake that we see quite a bit of today. In general, Westerners get a hold of some Eastern philosophy and drink themselves to death. The Truth should show up in people's lives as some form of higher sanity not insanity, some form of peace or fulfillment, not madness, not nihilism, but impeccable behavior. You don't become a criminal. Just because you go beyond good and bad, why be a criminal? You might say, "Why be a saint?" Well, you wouldn't necessarily be anything, but you wouldn't necessarily be a criminal either.

LML: *Could it be said that the view cannot be understood through the mind?*

SURYA: Yeah, exactly. The view is beyond mind; it has nothing to do with what we think of as the mind. It is more the nature of the mind. We always say it is a pitfall today if people know too much too soon, and it impedes their liberation. You get intellectually jaded rather than experientially transported or realized. You start to hear all these things, "Nothing to do and nowhere to go," and then you think you know it all, and then why meditate? You stay being an addicted, alcoholic, stoned, wife-beating, couch potato. I mean, why do that practice? If there is nothing to do, why are you doing the couch potato practice instead of meditating? That is also a practice; it is a way of life that has its own results.

Again, I think this awakening is coming, and this is good news for the West. We already had our churches and temples, and we got disillusioned with what we felt were empty words, so we want more the mystical, experiential meaning. The Dharma culture of awakening is more experiential. Whether it is meditation or prayer or self-inquiry or devotion or chanting or whatever it is, it is experiential, not about belief or dogma or converting, not about study. It is not happening in the universities; it is really happening in the streets, in the meditation halls. It is happening in action, not just being studied like some dead thing from the past, like the Egyptian mystery schools, something that once, long ago was alive but now, maybe not.

So, I think it is an awakening, and it's juicy. It's happening in many ways and it's a creative awakening also. The heart of the Dharma moves to new countries and takes on different forms. It's the same luminous heart of the Dharma that takes different cultural forms appropriate to time and place. That's happening today in the West. In European Buddhism the Dharma is a little different than American Buddhism. I think that this is also something that is awakening. The Dharma is finding new expression, new ways of being, and that's very exciting, relevant and meaningful to the way we can connect with it. It's hard to connect with it in its oriental forms. For example, in China it's mixed with Chinese culture such as ancestor worship, Confucianism, etc. That's not what's happening here. What's happening here is a little different. It's not like some social conscience that they have maybe in some Eastern countries.

LML: *The Eastern cultures have long held traditions of what the Dharma is and what the spiritual paths are. In the West, particularly in America, that hasn't been established yet. It's just now forming.*

SURYA: That's right. This is the borning time. This is like birth. This is a marvelous moment to be alive. There is an old Chinese saying and blessing, "May you be born in interesting times." I hope everybody felt like this when they were alive throughout the centuries, but I certainly feel like this is the most interesting time to be alive.

Not just because of the new millennium, but this is the time that these things are coming out, and we're a part of that. We're a part of the emerging face of the contemporary Dharma, awakening or new sanity—whatever it's going to be called—maybe some new term we don't even know about. The Dharma has many gates. It's not a mousehole you have to squeeze through. The Dharma has huge gates, an infinite number of gates. It's everywhere. You can't miss it.

LML: *Is it true that at this time there are very few Western Dzogchen lamas or teachers such as yourself?*

SURYA: Yes, there are very few Western lamas. There's some dozen or so. The Dzogchen teachers in the West are also very few. I hesitate to say I'm the only one, but if you look around the books, magazines, and the lists of retreats and see who's out there... I don't know, hopefully more are coming.

It would be a great service to facilitate people accessing these teachings, to create a sangha. Sangha means community, but sangha also means that the teachers and bodisattvas have to come out of the woodwork and out of the ground and create a rooted American tradition of the Western Dharma—the Future Buddhas of America. [Laughter] That's why I always say, "American Buddhas, awaken! Throw off your chains, your neuroses, your hang-ups."

People always ask me, "Where can I study Dzogchen? Where can I learn?" I wish there were more teachers and, I don't want to make this into some kind of put down, but I also wish there were more students. Where are the students who really dedicate? Where are the students who stay, not just the dilettantes and workshoppers in the spiritual supermarket?

LML: *. . . I want to say that a lot has been going on inside of me as I've been listening to you speak. I haven't studied Dzogchen; John has. He's read shelves full of Dzogchen books. But in listening to you, I noticed a profound resonance. By some great grace, recently I have been experiencing a new dawning of the understanding you have been describing. It has been so validating to hear your words. What it has seemed like for me is a long journey just to get right here and now.*

SURYA: Yes, it's coming home.

LML: *And home is being fully present here and now with what is, as it is—absolutely as it is. Everything is just perfect as it is. Totally perfect as is. All of it, the good, the bad, and the ugly. Resting with what is is not something boring or any idea of what the mind might think of it. It is absolutely ecstatic, an infinite ocean of beauty and love right here in present awareness that is completely overlooked. It is the most obvious, self-evident thing.*

This is the view which is now dawning for me. As you have said, Dzogchen begins with this view. I can see now how helpful Dzogchen could be for me. Right here as I listen to you speak a deep appreciation for Dzogchen is being born.

SURYA: First of all, I noticed as you were sitting here that something deep was going on. It seemed as if you were going to start to cry. As you say, it's not passive or static; it's very ecstatic. It carries us away, beyond our self; but in a positive way. It's hard to go beyond our self. So it's good to get some help in whatever way that comes, whether it's from a teacher connection and darshan, or practice, practice, practice, schlepping to enlightenment the Dharma soldiers way, the Dharma boot camp and the Dharma war, then Dharma victory. [Laughter] That's the male way, actually.

LML: *Right, and it was completely developed and created by and for men.*

SURYA: Exactly. That's just one way.

So, tune into what you are, I don't want to say feeling, but what you are opening to, what it really is, where it is, where it's coming from. Like you said, you are experiencing That and recognizing That. The next step is getting used to That. Check it out. Notice if there is anything else. Is there anything better? Is there anything outside That? Is there anything that you need besides That?

LML: *You mean to contemplate That?*
SURYA: To check That, to meditate on it, to contemplate, to inquire, to see if you need help, to see if there's anything better than That. Is there anything else? Check and see if it seems like there's anything else when you're with That, when you are That. What else is there?

It's like being at home. You love your home. You get used to being at home. It's easy to be at home; it's no big deal. That's much deeper. You don't have to brag about how many hours you stay at home. Like I've bragged that I did a three year retreat—that's bullshit. It's like war medals. Who brags about being at home? When you come home to who and what one truly is and how it is, you're at home wherever you are with whomever you are with or when you are alone. It gets deeper and more stable. Just keep awake to That which is not really a state. Then it gets much more stabilized—wisdom, understanding, freedom—it sort of grows.

JLW: . . . *Surya, I am noticing as you are speaking, I'm oscillating in and out of noticing the emptiness of everything. For me it's a kinesthetic sense. It is not like you are not there, but rather it is like you are here and you are empty also. There is a perception of this fundamental emptiness here [gestures toward himself], there [gestures toward Surya] and in between its the same. It is as though I can let my attention drop back and that is what I notice. Is this the kind of thing you are talking about as the meditation?*
SURYA: Yeah. The meditation is something like that. It is the meeting place of that empty, diaphanousness you are describing, where everything is not there, but it is still there, like rainbows, it is vivid, but it is insubstantial.

JLW: *It's like everything is happening, but nothing is happening.*
SURYA: That's why I say it is the meeting place of the Absolute, the great expanse of shunyata, where nothing happens, and the relative where everything happens by itself. At the same time, it is not either/or. It is only the mind that has to say, "either/or," like we are the same, or we are different. It is more like both and sort of neither, also.

Things are not what they seem to be exactly, but nor are they otherwise. So, it is just is-ness in a way; tathagata, shunyata, it is just is-ness. We are not what we seem to be, but we are not something else either. It is not like we are really angels, we're not people—that's just another label.

It is is-ness, like the moment of creation is now, reality; the world is being born every moment. There is a freshness, and the first moment of creation is just is-ness. It hasn't become a world yet, or a depleted world of samsara or nirvana yet. There is a flash or the shimmering; there is luminosity, it hasn't become anything yet. Subject and object have not yet evolved, dualism, "I like," "I don't like," "I," "you"—none of that. That is all devolution into forms. But it hasn't yet happened in the is-ness, in the first moment. That is the meditation, being in the first moment.

It is always, only, ever now. Past, present, future are also always, only, and ever now. Remembering or forecasting is a now activity. That is why the introduction to the nature of this innate great wakefulness is always nowness.

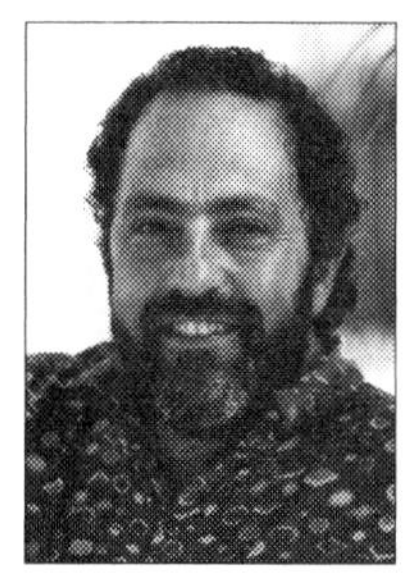

ISAAC SHAPIRO

"BY ITSELF, THERE IS AN INTEREST IN WAKING UP COMING TO MORE AND MORE PEOPLE... BY ITSELF PEOPLE ARE POPPING UP THAT HAVE DIRECT EXPERIENCE OF TRUTH... IT HAS TO HAPPEN NOW... WE ARE NOW AT A POINT WHERE THE STAGE IS SET FOR A MASS AWAKENING."

Isaac Shapiro has been a significant teacher for both of us. His clear, direct pointing to the Truth cuts through the mind's obscurations with incredible precision. No matter what someone asks Isaac, he brings that person back to right here, right now, "Who are you?" With Isaac it's always, "First find out who you are." This inquiry can begin with something as simple as, "Are you your hair?" "Are you your body?" And then lead to, "Are you your thoughts?" "Are you your feelings?" Upon close examination, the answer to these questions is "no." After everything we identify with is eliminated, what is left? What is left, which can be called awareness, space, consciousness, etc., is what we are. And That is directly experienced by many in Isaac's presence. We have witnessed person after person directly experience the Truth of their own being in his satsangs.

It was during one of Isaac's satsangs that Lynn Marie's recognition of awareness grew more and more clear until it was undeniable. She can not point to a particular moment when this recognition took place. She just remembers one day sitting with Isaac and realizing that she no longer felt like she was on the outside of what was being said. As Isaac spoke about awareness, it was clear that this was who she is. So began the fire that he speaks of—the fire of all the mind's tendencies burning and dissolving in the presence of awareness.

Isaac points out that where we put our attention is what we experience. If you put attention on thoughts you experience the thoughts and their corresponding feelings. If you rest attention in awareness itself, there is beauty and peace. Thoughts, feelings, and sensations come and go in the sweet presence that we are. This serves as a constant reminder for us to remain resting as awareness.

Isaac's deep devotion to his late Master, Poonjaji, is apparent. His life has been dedicated in service to Poonjaji and the Truth he revealed. Isaac gives satsangs around the world to large audiences and has published a book of his satsangs titled, *Outbreak of Peace*.

CONVERSATION *with* ISAAC SHAPIRO

JLW: *It has been a real pleasure to be in satsang with you again. It has also been a revelation of how much has shifted for us since we last saw you a year ago.*
ISAAC: Excellent. Excellent, yes, that's clear. I can see this. I see it in your eyes—both of you. I can see it in an instant in people's eyes. I see that you see who you are. For me everything is so visible, really, there is nothing hidden anywhere. People can be awake and still have areas of their lives that are troubling them and you can see it—it is plain. Nobody can lie to you.

LML: *It is funny; what has seemed to have occurred for me since I last saw you is the recognition of the idea that I was seeking for something I didn't yet have. I have been so caught up in being a seeker, fully believing that something is missing, that I missed what has always been here!*
ISAAC: Yeah. That's all.

LML: *As I said in satsang the other night, there is a growing interest in just being here. If I get stuck anywhere, it is in a preference for being present in awareness and a resistance to any distraction away from it. Out of that an "I" gets constructed that is supposed to do something about it and make attention stay here.*
ISAAC: All these subtleties of mind start to reveal themselves. They have to; they don't stand a chance actually. There is the simplicity of here, just being here, and something comes up—relationship-wise, money-wise, something that has some juice—to engage in some way and then again, somehow, by grace it just becomes clear that here, everything is okay. Then by itself, the running after things starts to fall away. What could be added to this? It is really so beautiful. Just here.

LML: *I appreciate your saying that this falls away, just by grace. The running after things has fallen away more so for you and that opens the way for this to occur for me.*
ISAAC: That's really why there is this whole idea of transmission. It's like if you want to learn to play music and you go sit with someone who has played music a lot. Your musical abilities can improve ten times faster because they can show you a few things that might have taken them a long time to develop—style, different chords, different progressions, different ways of understanding what's going on that you can get in one minute what took them a long time to master. It is the same thing with

satsang. We come around a master or someone who is a little—can't even say further along in it—but in a way you can say that because there is a revealing process of the mechanisms. Certain things have been seen, and it might have taken them a long time. It is a deeper relaxation into being, and when it is pointed out to you, it is yours. It is not even in the words; it just happens by itself. It is a strange thing actually. But I know that with Papaji [an affectionate name for Poonjaji] this has been very strong for me.

JLW: *It seems that being around a teacher may be indispensable.*
ISAAC: Yes, and even though you are awake... because you guys both know you are awake—it is clear—but now is the time that all of your hidden vasanas, everything that has been hidden, will be revealed by association with the teacher. When I get around Papaji, every little nuance is revealed—relationship stuff, any idea of good and bad, the way people should be or shouldn't be, preferences, subtleties—they can't be hung onto anymore.

JLW: *Generally, Isaac, these interviews have been structured around a set of questions we felt would be useful for people in terms of hearing different expressions of who we really are. Probably most fundamentally, what is "enlightenment" or "awakening?"*
ISAAC: I'd say it is very simple, all of us actually are That. So, what's been happening is that culturally we have come to value our thinking process, and so we have been giving our attention to this process. This has been so highly valued that everybody is involved with it, so to speak. By this I mean that we have our perceptions and ideas, and basically our attention has gone to these perceptions and ideas and our interpretations. We live in a conceptual world, and it is not a happy world; it is a world of duality. It is a conceptual reality.

So you can see, for example, a husband will have an idea of who his wife is and he'll relate to that idea, not to his wife anymore, or vice versa, or parents about their children. We form an idea of someone, and we relate to that idea. In this way we call someone a friend and it doesn't matter what they do, or even how they are actually impacting our lives because we have labeled them as a friend, and we don't see them fresh. This is what goes on a lot. As long as we are relating like this, there is fear, and there is all the rest of the stuff of suffering.

At some point, an urge comes, usually through some tragedy when something goes vastly wrong and there is enough pain that the person wants to look deeper. Or it happens by luck, or an acid trip, or ending up in satsang without even knowing why the hell you are there—some friend invited you, perhaps. Who knows? Somehow the urge for freedom comes, and eventually there is a direct experience of who one is.

Usually when a person has this experience without a teacher, it is frightening for them. All of a sudden there are no boundaries, and they don't know how to relate to it. It can be terrifying and actually, quite a lot of people end up in mental homes because they talk to someone about their experience. Those people don't recognize what it is, you see.

So, once we bring our attention to its source, to awareness itself (which is a strange way of talking because it is not totally precise in the sense that awareness is not an object), we find that we can't find awareness, and at some point it dawns that this awareness is simply being, just being—not doing anything. I mean, there is no movement anymore, no awareness of any movement of attention, of mind or anything. This experience is very natural. In the East it is actually called, sahaja samadhi, which is the natural state. It is called the highest samadhi there is. There is no sense of personal "I," even though the sense of personal "I" can arise within this and can be appreciated and can function. But there is no identification with this personal "I" anymore. There is a recognition that everything that is happening is appearing in you—the entire universe, time and space, everything. For such a person, there is not even an experience of enlightenment or not enlightenment. It is just the natural state. There is actually no distinction any more of, "I am enlightened and you are not," or anything like this. Clearly we are all consciousness itself, and some people seem to not recognize it and suffer for it. It is like that.

JLW: *This implies that the recognition of who we are eliminates the suffering that comes with living in a conceptual reality.*

ISAAC: Yeah. Well, this is not only an implication; it is a direct experience. Once it is directly experienced, then, you don't need to read any more books; you know for yourself.

JLW: *One of the most amazing things to me is that it is so immediately available.*

ISAAC: That's the beauty of it...

This is another thing—a moment ago, we started speaking about how there seems to be a quickening towards Truth in the world today and...

JLW: *... is that your perception also?*

ISAAC: Well, one of the things that has been interesting for me is exploring when the self-referencing "I-thought" first came about. Language only happened for human beings thirty to sixty thousand years ago according to archeologists, which is not a long time. When you think about it, agriculture, which is what our whole existence now is based on, brought about the big change from hunter-gatherer societies which was a very different form of life. There were no villages. We were living in small bands like monkeys basically, picking from nature whatever we wanted. I would say that this is the era that is referred to in the Bible as the "Garden of Eden." Agriculture was invented ten to twelve thousand years ago, only. Then the next thing that happened was Cain killed off Able. If you look now, there are no more hunter-gatherer societies around.

JLW: *They have virtually been decimated.*

ISAAC: Yes, they have virtually been decimated. We don't have to rely on the gods anymore for finding our food; we grow it ourselves. We have usurped the place of God in our taking care of ourselves. The discovery of agriculture facilitated living in villages and towns. From there things moved reasonably rapidly. A lot has changed from twelve thousand years ago to now. From hunter-gatherer society for millions of years—and then you look in the historical context, Buddha was two-thousand-five-hundred years ago which is like a blip on the screen of history.

Always when there has been an evolutionary change, you get a few forerunners, and two-thousand-five-hundred years ago is just a forerunner. Christ was only two thousand years ago. So Buddha and Christ were the forerunners. Now we are at a place and time where we are ready for a mass awakening on this planet. Ramana said it in a very beautiful way, he said, "When there is a nightmare, everybody wants to wake up. When it is a pleasant dream, nobody wants to wake up."

Awareness can't go anywhere; it never did go anywhere; it's always here. What we call mind is an ability that's developed in human beings to make distinctions and comparisons and relationships. This has been very valuable to us. It's very highly valued in our culture. Now somehow the next wave is happening. People have really explored this ability to make distinctions very fully. Now somehow the interest is coming to wake up, to go beyond it. This is the next wave. By itself, there is an interest in waking up coming to more and more people. By itself, people are popping up that have direct experience of Truth, and then they tell somebody else and this is how it's happening. It has to happen now. As a society and a culture we have now brought ourselves actually to the edge of extinction.

JLW: *Ecologically we are now beginning to face the catastrophic consequences of our ignorance and our arrogance. Also culturally, socially, it is getting chaotic...*
ISAAC: Everything, everything is getting chaotic. Yes, we are now at a point where the stage is set for a mass awakening. We must change for our survival. We are wired up for it—throughout the whole world, instant communication is here. So there is the possibility for a really rapid shift. You know before, if there was a Buddha somewhere, how would people know about it?

JLW: *Yeah. More people know about Ramana now than when he was alive because communications are so much greater.*
ISAAC: Books and videos, e-mail and satsangs—Ramana is on the Internet, you know! I just look at my own life. I go around the world every year. I can hit twenty countries and be on e-mail and audiotapes and videotapes. Look at how many people have been touched by Gangaji in five years. Or how many people have come to satsang with me. It is phenomenal! Six years ago, Papaji had only four or five people with him. Towards the end of his life there were three hundred at each satsang.

JLW: *We have a tape of Papaji speaking about this phenomenon. He says it was never like this before. He doesn't understand it, but he would see two or three people a week waking up in his satsangs.*
ISAAC: Now, in my own experience—and you have been to my day-long satsangs—I have seen fifty to a hundred people waking up in one day.

LML: *Do you have any idea how many of those awakenings "stick?"*
ISAAC: I'd say most.

JLW: *Well, I think "stick" is an misleading term because what happens is that someone wakes up, and then there is the stuff that comes up to be cleared. That is what has been happening for us.*
ISAAC: I call this clearing a fire. I am in a very good circumstance to watch this because I come to a country for two or three weeks, and then I am gone for a year, and I come back. So I can very easily see what happened

in that year. I can see how much has been burned off in the fire of awareness. I am watching a quickening in people. They'll get a taste and come back. And maybe some doubts have crept in and it takes a few instants for them to see what has actually happened; if they haven't already caught it themselves in the interim. Then the second year I see so much more. It is quickening and happening so fast for people.

JLW: *This is very good news!*

ISAAC: What is happening is amazing, actually.

Getting back to what I was saying about the formation of the "I-thought"... when agriculture came then it was, "I grow the food," and "I own this land," and "I am going to fight you for this land." This is my own feeling of it, when you look at how language functions you see that every idea we have in language creates a different reality. For example, if we don't have a word for inside and outside and suddenly it dawns on me, "Okay, look this is inside and that is outside," now I have a concept, inside and outside, which applies to space. Then the next thing that happens is, "Oh, inside of me and outside of me." See, each concept generalizes and creates different possibilities. These concepts create conceptual realities which then build on each other. Somebody will come up with a word to articulate a concept, and then consciousness shifts with the discovery of that word/distinction. In the hunter-gatherer society you don't need a lot of memory; you don't have the complexity of society.

JLW: *But you do need a collective connectedness to operate as a team.*

ISAAC: Very much so. It was a collective intuitive consciousness that was functioning—like with lions hunting together. They are very in sync.

LML: *Now we live as though we are all so separate.*

JLW: *We believe we are separate, and we experience ourselves to be separate. At some point the "I" got concretized.*

ISAAC: So now there is actually a lot of research going on trying to figure out what the "I" is. It is amazing to try and find that because... you take a plant, it is evolved and organized in a certain way to function. Even this whole thing of evolution is such a strange thing because again we have got this concept of time and we are indoctrinated to see time as a linear thing, and so the way we perceive time is in this linear fashion. But our actual experience is a little different than our conception. We live in this world where our direct experience doesn't fit into our conceptual models, and we develop new models to deal with all of this.

JLW: *Could you say something about what you mean by "our actual experience of time is not the same?"*

ISAAC: When we enter this instant, it is eternity. All time is here, you see. Yet in our operational mind, our functioning of yesterday, today and tomorrow, there is a different time sense. For example, here with this interview, we are having fun and time flies, but when we are not having fun, time is very drawn out. It seems like something solid, you know, but this is what is so phenomenal about Einstein's theory about time being relative. When you hit this instant, just right here, all of a sudden there is a direct sense of being everywhere at all times. The doors are opened in a way. You intuit things and you see things.

It was so interesting being around Papaji because he would speak sometimes, and even he was not sure which time he is speaking about. I'll give you an example. I went to say goodbye to him one day. I said to him, "Namaskar, Papa, I am leaving." He says, "Oh, you are leaving tomorrow?" I said, "No, Papaji, I am leaving tonight." "Ah, yes," he said, "you are leaving tomorrow." I thought, "Oh he's a little bit out of it." You know, maybe he's taken his blood pressure medicine, or whatever the thing is, because he was kind of disjointed in his speaking with me; he didn't seem very present with me. So, we go to the train station, and the train was at seven o'clock. And it is delayed for two hours. We come back at nine o'clock; the train is delayed another few hours. Finally the train left at two o'clock the next morning.

LML: *So it was the next day like Papaji said.*

ISAAC: Yes, and this happens enough times around Papaji that you just start to go, "Oh, okay." He speaks to someone about something that hasn't happened yet, and that person is confused. The next thing you know that something happens—and Papaji doesn't tell them, "This is going to happen." He just spoke as if it had already happened. But they don't recognize it until later when it happens. It is a strange thing. We all have intuition or precognition, and we blow it off because it doesn't fit so easily in with our construct of time.

LML: *Yes. It seems difficult to accept the immediacy of the understanding of Truth; people would rather take years and years and years doing practices than accept that it is just right here, right now. It is somehow difficult for the mind to accept that it is just that simple and that available. It gets overlooked. "That can't be, I have to practice more years." [Laughter]*

ISAAC: Well, this is the beauty, too. We can know this intellectually, but as people have it in their own experience; then, they speak with authority. Then when you say to somebody, "Keep quiet," now suddenly it pierces. This is an interesting phenomenon, because, like J. Krishnamurti spoke and spoke and spoke, and nobody woke up around him. There are many teachers around with whom people have not awakened, but they have served because they have brought many people to an interest in true freedom. It is clear that it is all working together, somehow. Again, there was a phenomenon happening around Papaji. And all those who awakened with Papaji are having a profound effect around the world.

LML: *Yes, more people woke up around Papaji or those who awakened with him than anyone else we know of.*

We have also noticed that some of the people who have had a spontaneous awakening without a teacher seem to have a much rougher time of it.

ISAAC: Very much so. I can say that was so valuable for me with Papaji. Even after he asked me to teach, because I had seen what had happened to others.

JLW: *What happened?*

ISAAC: Somewhere their mind tricked them. I can talk about what has come up for me in this whole thing, you know. As people started to wake up around me, and as much as I wanted to be careful and be true to Truth, some identification came with that. Some identification of being someone who was doing something crept in. Through the grace of being around Papaji, this got nailed and nailed and nailed in so many different ways. Not directly, because Papaji was always very indirect, you could say. But it became so clear where there had been some identification. So, I would say that with these others there has been some strong identification with being someone, a teacher, someone who is enlightened.

LML: *But people can see that arrogance. It shows itself.*

ISAAC: But the teachers don't always see it for themselves.

JLW: *This posture that some teachers assume of being someone and others are not someone really gets taken care of in the way you conduct your day-long satsangs. I appreciate the way you spend half the day sitting in the audience and whoever feels moved to can come up and sit in the chair in front of the room and recognize that they are the same one.*
ISAAC: Everyone can see it because at some point you look and you see, well, who is giving satsang here? There is nobody giving satsang—this is so clear to me. It is nobody giving and nobody receiving, and everybody is benefited. That is my direct experience of this.

LML: *It's not just that the teachers can get caught up in thinking they are someone, but the students can support this too—by putting the teacher in an elevated place.*
ISAAC: Yes, and it's such a strange thing too. I've watched this so-called teacher-student game go on a lot, and there are a lot of different teachers and students and ideas about this whole thing. Clearly, even though we are all consciousness itself there's value to be gotten in being around someone like Papaji who is a Master—no question about it in my mind. But, I've seen people go to Papaji who I thought would just blow open around him, and they didn't. And nothing happened. So who can say? It's such a mysterious process. So, there's no formula to this thing; that's clear.

I can speak about this in my own experience. There's the formless, and then there's the form, which is a distinction in the mind. When I met Papaji he pointed me to the formless in which form is appearing. I felt such a deep connection and an honoring of that formlessness. But at the level of form, there was a way in which I didn't trust his form. Often I saw such a circus around him, and sometimes it would be one way; then the next day it would be another way. Sometimes his advice seemed to be great and sometimes it seemed to be off. It played in my mind a lot—how to be in this and use my own discrimination and wisdom. There was no difficulty involved in trusting the formless absolutely. But then to trust the form—it was an interesting play for me for awhile. Then I came to a point where I could see that the form and the formless are not separate. I saw that I could actually trust the form of the teacher as well. I can't even explain how it happened, but it just happened that I now trust the form completely also. Even though I don't always understand the play that is happening around the form, there is a seeing that it is absolutely perfect.

LML: *What has happened for me repeatedly with teachers is that I will have a deepening of experience with the formless when I am with them. But then I get confused by the* *actions of their form, which don't always make sense, or sometimes appear to my mind to be "unenlightened" behavior. Then I would go through disillusionment, disappointment, doubt, fear, etc. This happened so many times that I have come to accept that the form will never, ever appear perfect according to some idea of perfection. We can only realize that the form and formless are one and the same; and therefore, both are perfect in some mysterious way that cannot be understood by the mind. The manifest reality will never make any sense to the mind. The mind tries and tries to hold onto explanations only to have them dissipated again and again. Maybe that's the purpose of manifest form—to always throw you and give you nothing to hold onto except what is most true.*

ISAAC: Yes, and that's absolutely perfect. Even this "throwing" is perfection itself. When you see that throwing the mind is perfection itself, the trust in the form starts to happen. It's just like this play happens, and somehow another level of trust happens with all of existence. It opens up that the play itself is perfect. There is no expression that is not That. The form and the formless are the same.

LML: *Since they are the same perfection, one can accept everything as it is. Then there's no need to be anywhere other than where you are, which brings you nowhere but just right here.*

ISAAC: Yes, yes. Beautiful.

LML: *People come to therapy wanting to change what is; that's what therapy has been about, changing what is. I'm not saying that some things don't need to change; they might. But I find myself listening from a place of knowing that even though there is pain, in some mysterious way, it's all okay as it is.*

ISAAC: Just your sitting in that knowing is the best therapy possible. This is what I see happening in satsang. People come and they talk about something, and there's a direct approach of absolutely dismantling their mental trip which works quite well sometimes. And sometimes I talk nonsense to people and all of a sudden the mental trip just falls apart. I'm not even trying to do anything. I just find myself talking nonsense—it doesn't have anything to do with anything—but then the person will finally open up. They can't keep together what they were holding with their mind.

JLW: *That is how we do it, isn't it? We hold our reality together with our mind. When we step back enough to regard that, that's enough for it to begin to dismantle and dissolve of itself.*

ISAAC: Of course, yes. It is so simple.

LML: *Isaac, you mentioned that you no longer have a sense of a personal "I." Some people get frightened when they hear that and wonder what will happen to them if that falls away.*

ISAAC: That's why I like to ask people, "Right now is your actual experience in this moment, 'I am breathing' or is your actual experience breathing is happening, and there is awareness of this breathing?" You can't find an "I" that is actually breathing. The same thing with thinking—we say, "I think," and "I move." But even with movement, like nodding of the head happens, and there's no decision about making the movement. It happens all the time by itself, and yet we say, "I moved." This is just a way of speaking, actually. My direct experience is that there isn't an "I" that's driving action, that's doing it. It's just happening by itself.

Then when it comes to actual decisions, I use a few examples that people can relate to just so that they will have a contextual background for seeing that "I'm doing it" isn't actually what's happening. With decisions, people still have a sense that they're making them. But when you really look closely you'll see that your decisions come out of your programming. It's a response, basically, to what's going on. Your response comes from your conditioning. Therefore, people from different cultures would respond very differently to the same circumstances. It would seem like they made a decision, but it's just a response coming from their conditioning and their genetics. It's just a program which will continue perfectly. You don't have to do anything about it. But without the identification with it, it starts to function in alignment with the power that's breathing you, that's moving everything. You can say that it becomes a living expression of "Thy will be done."

JLW: *Actually it's a living recognition that Thy will has always been done.*

ISAAC: Has always been done, yes.

LML: *Could it be said that things move more smoothly, more elegantly then?*

ISAAC: Well, the experience is that whatever is happening is smooth. Someone who is free can get beat up, but for them it's no wrinkle; it's not a big deal. It's just another thing that happened. So, who can say if it's more smooth that way. People have this idea that if you're enlightened things always go smoothly. One day Papaji came to visit me in Lucknow, and while he was eating lunch, his car was towed away. In India when your car gets towed away it's not like in America; it's a major hassle.

LML: *So, freedom means not depending upon circumstances or states for happiness.*
ISAAC: That's right. Another misconception about enlightened people is that they don't have accidents; they don't get sick, all this stuff. It's a false idea basically.

LML: *Another one is that enlightened people are always blissful. Can you speak about that?*
ISAAC: The truth is that in every moment that you simply rest as who you are there is bliss because this is your natural state. What happens though is that any unfulfilled desires will get played out. They'll come to the surface. Robert Adams had such a lovely image for this involving a bucket of water. If you leave a bucket of dirty water for awhile all the dirt settles to the bottom. The water can then look clean, but it smells dirty. Then you introduce a steady stream of clear water into it, and it stirs up all the dirt, and you start to see the dirt specifically as it pours over the edge. You could say that this is the process of the water cleansing itself. It's a natural process; with the passage of time it all comes clear.

Ultimately, consciousness is already clear. What's cleaning itself out isn't consciousness. Consciousness is already clear. So even this cleaning process is a natural process that happens spontaneously by itself, but not to identify with that even; because people sometimes say, "Oh, I can't wait for it all to be clear." So, experientially things can be coming across the screen, and as they come across the screen, it can be a very strong experience. As long as there is a willingness to meet this experience fully—like what is expressed in Kenny Johnson's letters to Gangaji—then there's another taste of it. Even when Kenny was sitting in the prison van in his own shit and in pain, there was an underlying bliss to it. It's not that you won't have intense experiences, but they are met in a certain way. This is true for everything: death, divorce, sickness. All of that doesn't just stop; it simply continues.

JLW: *Isaac, one of the things we've been asking people is to share their story of awakening...*

LML: *In satsang the other day you said that there was no "big bang" for you...*
ISAAC: No, it wasn't like that for me. Papaji simply pointed me to something that I've always known, that was always there but had been overlooked. So, for myself it was never any big bang or anything like that.

It was just the recognition that what he spoke about was true. It was very simple, actually, very, very simple. It's just that my mind had been busy with other things. What happened was an invitation was given, and somehow it was received. I don't even know how it happened. The experience of not being anybody became very living. It's like that now.

You know one of the tricks the mind plays is doubt. In this doubt, wanting to look to other people's experience and to make some kind of comparison and have some idea of what the experience is like. What I can say is that if you look in your own experience right now, in this instant—by that I mean your own experience of awareness itself—there's awareness here already. This, you don't have to do anything for. There is awareness here of seeing, thinking, of whatever's happening. Normally you don't pay attention to this awareness. We pay attention to what's coming up in awareness.

You know, I could say that the "big bang" happened when I was nineteen years old and took a hit of acid. I had the experience of unconditional love, of being one with everything, of being able to see the future and the past, being able to see what everyone was thinking around me. My mind became like a supercomputer. I went from no interest in philosophy to understanding every philosopher.

I usually don't tell people how I had this experience, but I don't mind if you tell how it happened. I really don't care about it. Actually, when I took the acid I had no idea even what acid was. I was living in South Africa, which was a very repressive society in those days; they didn't even have television. It was 1968, but I didn't know about hippies or drugs. Even *Playboy* magazine was banned in South Africa at that time, but somehow one got smuggled to me. Here I was nineteen years old, horny as hell, and so I read the *Playboy* and in it there was an article by Timothy Leary about LSD and "thousands of orgasms per second." That's what got my attention. One week later I met an American student who gave me some LSD, and I had no idea what I was taking. I didn't know anything about it, how long it lasted or anything. All I knew about was "thousands of orgasms a second!" [Laughter] But instead I had this experience of unconditional love and oneness with everything.

When it happened I knew that that was Truth. I knew without any doubt that that was Truth and that I had been living in a shadow of Reality. I could see so clearly that my thinking was basically conditioned and distorted. I knew I had to come out of it, but I didn't know how. I didn't even have a concept of a teacher. But this experience is what started a long fire for me. Through grace something revealed itself. I certainly had no idea it was going to happen, but it started me on the search, on being a seeker.

Subsequently, on many acid trips I had an experience of being one with the living presence of God. The trouble was that it all became conceptualized. I knew it was true, and I could never forget it, but it was not realized. So, it would turn into idealism and different conceptual distortions of the Truth. But it kept driving me to go deeper and discover it.

At some point it became very clear to me that attention was the key. Then I was doing awareness work with people showing them how they were focusing attention and where they were putting it. It was strong work. When I met Papaji and he told me to bring attention to awareness itself, that was the missing piece for me. It was like the last piece of a jigsaw puzzle. It was so obvious that I was amazed that I overlooked it all those years. When he said that to me, that was it. And not only did he say this to me, but in being around him, every time my mind would pick up another dream it would explode in front of my eyes. So, trying to hold onto a relationship or trying to hold onto wealth or to being somebody or to different subtleties of personality, would just explode in my face, basically.

This whole thing is grace. It really is grace. After the initial awakening, once you taste it, it never leaves you alone. Then there is a natural progression that happens and at some point it must bring you to a perfect teacher. It must bring you to somebody who points you to the Self.

LML: *There are many people who are longing for awakening, for freedom, if not consciously then unconsciously.*
ISAAC: Every longing is for this.

LML: *Yes, and what would you recommend to people who have this longing?*
ISAAC: That they find out who's longing. Find out the source of this longing. We long for something, and we think that this something will make us happy. After one thing has failed to make us happy, then we try another thing and another and another. But eventually we have to find out what this longing is based on. In other words, who is longing? This is not difficult.

We all have the experience in the morning of waking up and immediately thinking of all the things we have to do and a feeling of urgency about getting them done. Usually we spend our whole life in an agitated mode of trying to deal with life. The best way is to want only freedom, and if you can, to find a teacher who can point you to your Self. Invariably, when this yearning comes it will happen by itself, spontaneously, and you will actually run into a teacher.

To do it by yourself means to stay with this interest in who you are. That means you look very carefully and see that everything that comes and goes is not you because you are always here. When you then have the ability to make this distinction, you know that your feelings and thoughts come and go but something is always here. You can always come back your Self.

You can also use the feeling of "I" and look and see what is this actual feeling of "I," not any ideas of who you are, but the actual feeling of "I." As you look for the feeling of "I," you start to notice, who is looking at the feeling? This takes you right back home. You will eventually come to some place where there will be no doubt. Then it's finished. Actually, this is also a start, the first step. It's never-ending in terms of allowing this fullness of love to permeate everything.

LML: *This is when what you call "the fire" begins, when all the habitual tendencies can come up and be burned up in the presence of awareness.*

ISAAC: I'll tell you; that's where the fire begins. That's the ignition. Some people like to pour gasoline on the fire, and that is to be around a teacher, or just to really stay with this inquiry of who's aware. Whatever comes into your mind inquire, "Who's aware? Who's aware of it?"

Self-inquiry is a very fast way of cutting through the impulse to want to get involved in things. To put it in Western terms, what's known as the highest path in the East is called Atma Vichara. It's called the "kingly path," the "royal path," or the "fastest path." We don't have a word for Atma, but the closest English word would be consciousness, supreme intelligence, God, awareness. Vichara means inquiry into, which in a simple way is interest into. Where your mind is, that's what you experience. If your mind is on the future, you experience the future. If your mind is on your foot, you experience your foot. If your mind is on attraction, you experience attraction. You bring your mind to Atma, to the energy that is breathing you, that is seeing through your eyes, where every movement comes from, and you get interested in this. When your mind comes up with an idea or a perception you ask, "Who's aware of this?" This brings your mind away from the object to awareness itself.

LML: *And even when there has been an awakening, the conditioned habits continue.*
ISAAC: Yes, and our conditioning is to value our perceptions and our interpretation of our perceptions. This is a subtlety that continues for quite some time. We are still so interested in what we see and what we perceive and our whole experience of that. To come to an end of this interest so that the attention is not distracted from awareness at all… because all of these perceptions end up distracting you from your own true nature, from the real juice, you could say, from the real direct experience — these are subtle habits. It can take people some time to get quiet enough so that you don't get pulled into these other interests.

JLW: *It happens in its own time.*
ISAAC: Yes.

LML: *I've been experiencing a wonderful unfolding in that direction. There is a growing interest in awareness and less interest in the thoughts, feelings, etc. that are appearing in awareness.*
ISAAC: I can feel it. We sit here and talk and the living presence of God, if you want to call it that, comes so alive just in our speaking together. The mind is not distracted by anything else. We're just here, and I keep watching you two and seeing it happening in you, and I can feel it happening in me, just being with the Truth of our own being.

I can say for myself as this interest has deepened, the mind is almost constantly now resting in its source. So, when I'm with other people, it seems to automatically pull them in that direction without me doing anything. As they are pulled, it pulls me even deeper. It's so beautiful the way it happens!

JLW: *This is the way in which it's contagious and spreading.*
ISAAC: Yes. This is why everyone is benefited. This is the value of a sangha and also of being around a teacher. Someone at the beginning stages, even though there's no beginner and no… it's so difficult to speak about this sometimes. When you come around someone whose mind is very

inwardly directed—even though inward is not the right word, but there's no way to speak about this really—then your mind becomes inwardly directed also.

LML: *That happened for me immediately upon sitting with you this time in satsang. There was a quickening and an increased longing to rest more fully in awareness. What happened was that it turned into a desire that then constructed an "I" that believed it had to do something about this. There was awareness of this, but it turned into a bit of a struggle and a resistance to anything that appeared and distracted attention away from awareness. As we are speaking, I'm feeling that struggle relax. There's a feeling that it's okay as it is, it will continue to unfold as it does, perfectly. In the contact with you, I am seeing that it is possible for the mind to rest more constantly in its source. Seeing this in you is inspiring me. But, somehow the longing for more constant resting in awareness turned into a desire that created some struggle.*

ISAAC: That is how the desire revealed itself. Now someone else meets you that hasn't walked through this, and just in meeting you it can drop off for him or her. That's the beauty of psychotherapy. You sit and your own being communicates. Through your eyes something happens. It's not even a doing. Just your beingness itself is enough.

LML: *Yes, it's the beingness that heals.*

ISAAC: This is such a service. How lucky, how lucky.

JLW: *I feel as though we are among the most fortunate people on this planet.*

ISAAC: So, so, so blessed. So blessed... and out of this fullness comes a desire to serve Truth. A big secret that nobody knows is that you have to serve Truth. It's a natural expression that comes out of a maturing that happens and in that there's a quickening again. In so-called sharing the Truth, you can't be missionary style—it has to be a living experience and letting it live you.

Another aspect of that is serving the teacher. Whoever your teachers have been, even though they don't want anything from you, in the honoring of the form there is a way of serving the teacher. That's a secret that nobody knows about because we don't have this tradition in the West.

JLW: *Isaac, one of our intentions with this book is to honor those who have been our teachers.*

ISAAC: It's important to honor your teachers, even if they haven't taken you all the way to the goal. Honor them for what they have done.

When I first met Papaji, I was busy trying to evaluate if he was enlightened or not—if he was as enlightened as Ramana. "Was I betting on the right horse? Am I with the right teacher? Well, clearly there might be some benefit here but, I am not interested even in benefit anymore. I want to be finished with any kind of benefit, or any kind of anything. I want someone who absolutely knows, who I know knows, and then I can be finished with this whole thing." But it is impossible. You can't know it through your mind. The teacher will reveal himself to a worthy student. It is like that; it happens.

JLW: *That is an interesting concept. What constitutes a worthy student?*
ISAAC: Again, it is not a personal thing because there is nothing you can do to be worthy. But at the same time, when the desire comes in your heart for freedom and freedom alone, then Truth has to reveal itself. Even when there is a vague interest in Truth, you will meet a teacher, and maybe even a perfect teacher. But the drinking won't be complete because the student isn't quite ready. There will be some benefit; definitely there will be some benefit. If the student isn't surrendered, something will happen, but the ability that they have to drink is not there. They can only drink as much as they can. It is not up to them, and it is not up to the teacher, even.

JLW: *It is just grace.*
ISAAC: It is grace. I heard Papaji saying that for a long time but I just didn't get it. I see it now so clearly in my own experience. It is a strange thing to say because people try to be worthy. But it is not like that. You can't do anything about it.

JLW: *It is like a fruit; it matures at its own rate. And it has to go through its seasons.*
ISAAC: That's it. It's not up to the fruit; it's up to That which is ripening the fruit. It is all unfolding perfectly.

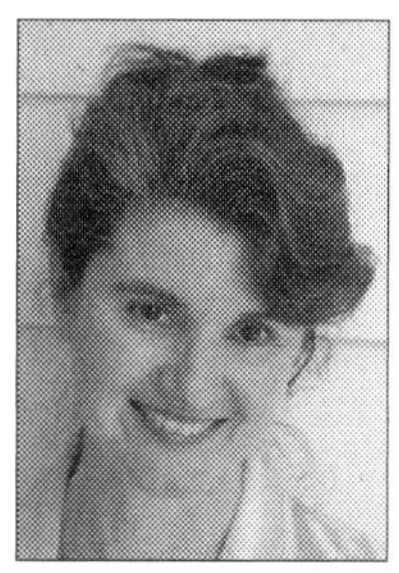

CATHERINE INGRAM

"YOU NEED NOT ACQUIRE ANYTHING TO REALIZE THIS. YOU NEED ONLY SUBTRACT BELIEFS, WHICH OBSCURE YOUR LIVING AS THIS RADIANT PRESENCE, AS LOVE ITSELF... IT IS IMMEDIATELY ACCESSIBLE TO YOU, EVEN AS YOU READ THESE WORDS."

Catherine is one of those who was a dedicated spiritual seeker. Her search began at age seventeen and like many others, was born out of suffering. After a self-described, "miserable" childhood, she was searching for some kind of meaning and purpose to the suffering in herself and in the world. In 1974 she found her first teacher and for nearly twenty years Catherine was committed to Buddhist practices, particularly Vipassana. She did many silent retreats and traveled the world as a journalist for spiritual magazines. During the more than twelve years she spent as a journalist, Catherine interviewed many spiritual teachers herself. But at some point, the Buddhist practices were not enough. There was a longing for something more. This began what she calls the "dark night of the soul" that ended in her meeting the Indian Master Poonjaji in 1991. It was Poonjaji who was able to point her to what she had always known but had somehow overlooked. She discovered that she was already free—and always had been.

Catherine conducts question and answer sessions which she calls Dharma Dialogues in the Western United States, Canada, and Europe. We have been attending these Dharma Dialogues for years. Catherine has long been one of our favorites. She speaks honestly and simply from her own direct experience in an articulate, even eloquent manner. Her presence is sweet and loving and she clearly demonstrates a deep integrity in her commitment to what is most true. Although Catherine is a powerful presence, she is completely unassuming.

Catherine is one of the many women who are now manifesting as spiritual guides and teachers. The feminine has long been denied by all of the world's major religions. This denial has led to an imbalance resulting in a rejection of the feminine, the body, and our connection with the earth. It is an important aspect of the awakening of the West that women are becoming spiritual leaders. The inclusion of feminine principles allows for the trend of relaxing into what is as opposed to striving through effort. As Catherine said in an interview with Marjolein Wolf, "There is a strong feminine voice that needs to be heard—and our time seems to be the time for that."

CONVERSATION *with* CATHERINE INGRAM

LML: *We are going to begin with a very basic question that few people can answer authentically, and that is, who are you?*
CATHERINE: Whenever I have allowed this "Who am I?" question to arise, I am left in silence. It is not a silence of emptiness; it is a silence of fullness. This question dissolves something that is in the way and suddenly, there is just suchness. It is truly just this silence that is the all and the everything.

The power of this is that it just goes to the core; the mind cannot do anything with it. The mind has been telling some limited story, thoughts following thoughts following thoughts. If you are not going to allow the thoughts to define who you are, then there is nowhere for the mind to go. Then what is left is a sense of beingness that is visceral, immanent, and unbounded.

LML: *So, you are this unlimited sense of beingness.*
CATHERINE: Yes. As are you.

LML: *So, what would you say awakening is?*
CATHERINE: I love the word "realization." I include the idea of recognition in this; it is realizing what already is, realizing the truth of what already is. The word "enlightenment," I shy away from; I find it loaded. It presumes this sort of steady state. But realization of the truth, of this suchness that we are, that is very simple and very accessible. What that means is very, very simple. It is to notice, to truly notice in as consistent a way as possible, this shining beingness, this untouched, unbounded beauty that each of us is.

Part of the realization is recognizing that actually, this seeing is the most familiar of all. This seeing is completely familiar to us. The periods of not realizing are simply when we are indulging the story, when we are indulging the nightmare, when we are indulging the belief in our thoughts, the identification with some particular story. But, I would say that many people are actually resting in essence some or much of the time—even people who are seemingly very lost. They just don't recognize or value it as such.

JLW: *You made a distinction when you said you didn't respond so much to the word "enlightenment" because it seemed to denote a steady state. And yet, in the literature about* *awakening there are strong indications that one can have glimpses of the truth of who we are, and then eventually there is the awakening, the realization, the final cut that is permanent.*

CATHERINE: I don't know if that is true. It is not in my experience.

JLW: *Can you say more about your experience, then?*

CATHERINE: Yes. In my own experience, there is a—to borrow from the Dzogchen teachings—"getting used to" this and a stabilizing that is ongoing. If I am very honest about that, lots of identified moments occur; lots of material will arise—for whatever reason, the proclivity, the tendency arises, there is momentary identification with it, and then it goes on its own. I have not a lot of interest in indulging it, of course, because it is so much pain. But nevertheless, the material does occasionally arise. There is also a recognition that even when the material is arising there's no involvement with it at times. There's no identification, but the material arises. Thoughts come, and they can be perverse. The old stuff arises, and it can be ugly, such as jealousy, hatred... the whole gamut of darkness. I find no interest in the engagement with it because I don't believe in the star of the story anymore. Nevertheless, the pictures or the thoughts will come. Though there may be momentary engagement, it doesn't last as long; it doesn't have the "teeth," the power it used to.

JLW: *Yes, and this correlates with my experience also. I have noticed that there seems to be a shift over time in which there are longer moments of disengagement, and they are occurring with more frequency.*

CATHERINE: Yes, there is an ongoing stabilization, an ongoing love affair with one's true Self such that one is not interested in being pulled away from the love affair very much, no matter what presents itself.

We've seen a lot of the dangers manifest whereby someone has an idea that they're in a steady state, that they're not ever identifying, and suddenly they're behaving in ways that might indicate that there is some subtle or gross identification that is now being justified as an expression of enlightenment.

LML: *We've seen this, too.*

CATHERINE: We've all seen it. I would say that it's a dangerous situation. The power of the glimpse of truth is such that it attracts people, and people trust it deeply. People trust being in the presence of someone who has that glimpse. It's the kind of relationship that is very, very delicate. So, it's so important to be true in an ongoing way to that glimpse, to be honest.

LML: *One of my teachers said to me that the most important thing is that I'm honest about what I am actually experiencing. The honesty is more important than any experience, no matter how big or deep.*

JLW: *I find that one of the most common misconceptions about enlightenment is that from then on one is always in bliss. A lot of scripture and literature supports that. I have had that concept myself. This is where the Dzogchen teachings have been helpful for me. As you mentioned, they speak of there being a "getting used to" the recognition of yourself as awareness. This awakening is just the beginning.*

CATHERINE: Yes, it is just the beginning. Then one finds that this manifestation is going on. It's not static; it's "jamming;" it's powering on. So we are continually being called upon to embrace all of it anew every flowing moment if we can borrow some temporal language. This is a stream of now. It's not some stuck, stagnant now.

JLW: *It's not a static eternity. It's an eternally emergent now.*

CATHERINE: Indeed. So we are continually called upon to surrender to this love affair with vastness. We are continually embracing all of its new manifestation, all of its emergent forms.

LML: *We've been influenced a great deal by the Advaita teachings, as I know you have been as well with your teacher Poonjaji. They do not address, as Dzogchen does, the "getting used to it" part.*

CATHERINE: Yes, and I think that we Westerners at this time are blessed to have all of these teachings available and to be able to glean the strengths and weakness from each of them.

JLW: *One of the things we have found valuable is that the experience of Truth is articulated very differently by different individuals.*

CATHERINE: Sure, and certain people are going to be attracted to the way one person expresses it, and that's going to be their wake-up. For others it will be the way it is being expressed by another person.

LML: *We are wondering if you could tell us of your particular expression. What is your story of awakening?*

CATHERINE: Well, first I spent seventeen years in Buddhist practice. I'll have to say that there came a point of tremendous disappointment in my life, exhaustion with striving and the ideas of attainment. After a point I just didn't even believe in any of it anymore. So, I felt this profound dark night of the soul. I felt that I had lost touch with the dharma. Thankfully, gracefully, I met Poonjaji and in his presence I tasted the realization that there was truly nowhere to go, nothing to do, nothing to attain, absolutely here and now, freedom, just this—and it was always this. He would always say that when you see this you will burst out laughing. I did burst out laughing. It was, "Oh, that." "That old beingness that's always been here." The beautiful, ordinary miracle of it was so apparent. You catch that in the presence of someone like Poonjaji. He's sparking what is true in you that you've always known. So, it was truly in his presence that this was seen and seen so clearly. I had heard these words for twenty some years prior to that, but now they were alive. Since that point there has been a deepening in that view... it's a wonderful journey.

I love to quote the Sufis, "There are three parts of the journey: the journey from God, the journey to God, and the journey in God." The journey from God is when we are chasing objects and experiences, trying to find happiness in trinkets and momentary pleasures. The journey to God is when we have grown weary of that chasing; now we want to have a spiritual experience. So, in a way we turn the chasing to the spiritual experiences, which is also more chasing and reaching and grabbing. The journey in God is living in the truth. The journey goes on in the realization. It's not as though there's some lofty detachment that you end up in. There's an intensity to life now. There's availability for the range of joys and sorrows and all of it, which is beautiful. This is the journey in God. It's seeing all of this arise and be celebrated.

LML: *The journey in God is what I'm interested in. It seems to me that this journey just unfolds of itself by itself. It becomes more and more effortless. It slowly just takes over and starts pulling itself to itself.*
CATHERINE: Oh, definitely it takes over. Then too, when you realize the journey is in God, you realize that it was always in God. It could not be otherwise.

JLW: *Do you remember what began your search?*
CATHERINE: Yes, disappointment, suffering, misery—the usual.

JLW: *There are, of course, many, many people who are suffering in this world and a growing number of them are yearning for this awakening. It's been proposed that it take* *many lifetimes or many years of hard practice. People want to know what they can do. When you give your Dharma Dialogues, what do you tell people who are seeking?*

CATHERINE: I see my job as helping with subtraction, not addition. There is nothing to do or add. The only things we ever consider are the obscurations that impede the seeing. So it's a shedding of the beliefs, of the identification. It's not that you need to get rid of thoughts, but you release the investment and the belief in them. We've probably had about a thousand sessions now of Dharma Dialogues in lots of places, and all that goes on is a shedding of beliefs and finding oneself in the silence of being where one is at rest.

JLW: *How do you guide someone to shed his or her beliefs?*

CATHERINE: You see through the belief. A belief arises, for example, "I'm afraid of becoming homeless." "I'm afraid I'm going to lose my job and I will end up on the street." So you take people step by step through all the aspects of the belief—the projection into the future—that's the first problem. They are living in the now which they cannot possibly take one toe-step out of and yet, they are talking about the future and telling themselves a spooky story. Then you get down to the discernment of "Who is this?" "What is this being?" "Who is the entity?"

JLW: *It's the bodymind.*

CATHERINE: Yes, the bodymind and the actual experience that the bodymind can only ever be sensed in the now. You're creating out of your own imagination; you're projecting this picture of bodymind into some other time that doesn't exist and making up a story. The actual experience is always just this. Even if you are on the street, the actual experience is always going to be this open clearing of presence that is occurring all of the time. At that point, there you are again in perfect presence. You can tell yourself whatever you want, "What a drag it is that I'm on the street," or "How fantastic, I don't have any mortgage payments." Whatever it is, it's going to be in the now that you're experiencing presence. So, it's always coming back to just this presence and the actual experience in the moment.

Of course, you may experience physical pain in the now, and I don't make light of that. Some teachers will say you're just experiencing sensations. But some people who come to me live with chronic pain, and that is very exhausting. Unless someone is perfectly stabilized, and I must say

I don't know any people who are, you get thrown because it is so tiring and it requires a vigilance of not buying into the story and the mental exhaustion. It can make it more difficult, but not impossible, to release the identification with the body.

JLW: *Also the release still brings the same relief.*
CATHERINE: Absolutely. The taste of freedom here and now is an instantaneous snap. I title my series of dialogues "Choose Freedom," and I always tell people that if you have to choose it ten thousand times a day, then that's ten thousand tastes of freedom. It doesn't matter; no one is keeping count.

LML: *Emotional pain can also be extremely difficult for people. Loss or trauma can bring about emotional pain that can be as distracting as physical pain.*
CATHERINE: Yes. I say all of that is welcome. In the recognition one allows the expression of the personal from a very vast vantage point. There is a limitless awareness, a great sky of beingness.

LML: *From that vast vantage point it is possible to experience emotional or physical pain without suffering it.*
CATHERINE: Exactly, and without collapsing onto a tiny point of just pain or grief. The grief or pain can be there, and there's a big breath around it.

JLW: *It's there in a spaciousness... I had an experience like that once when I had poison oak so bad my eyes were swollen shut, and I had to go to a hospital emergency room and wait for a long time. The uncomfortable sensation was there, but it was as you say, in a great presence of awareness.*
CATHERINE: Yes, and sometimes pain and grief can just blast you into presence—there's no where else to go. One of my friends once said that freedom is just another word for nothing left to choose. [Laughter]

LML: *We are continually being shown that all choices other than presence here and now only make things worse.*
CATHERINE: All holding, resistance, and drama leads to pain and suffering.

LML: *Back to the concept of enlightenment involving a constant experience... it's tricky because everything is always changing, but it's happening within something that is silent, still, and constant. And one can be aware of this stillness in the midst of it all.*
CATHERINE: The Tibetans call it the one taste. There is a taste that is permeating all, this taste of beingness, of ahhhh... and then there is this wild

display, this outrageous manifestation. That is why I am very vigilant about not creating any tiny separation or duality even with the madness that arises. It is also God shining.

JLW: *Yes, this gets back to something we were discussing earlier. You were speaking about how you perceived that in the West the dharma is taking on another flavor of an embodied consciousness, not a disembodied or separate consciousness believing that the world is an illusion and consciousness is what's real, but that the world is consciousness.*
CATHERINE: I mean, it's real enough. It's just not permanent, but "permanent" and "real" are not necessarily synonymous. I think that there's perhaps some confusion in the translations.

JLW: *What we are speaking of here seems related to what I perceive as a growing ecological consciousness, a mutuality consciousness, and the interconnectedness of all of it.*
CATHERINE: Yes, and a consciousness that embraces the so-called personal. We don't have to believe in the personal as being the totality. We can have a transpersonal vision that includes the personal. To borrow from Ken Wilber for a moment, all transcending orders transcend and include. Otherwise, there is some kind of skipping over, and that's not true transcendence; that's avoidance or disassociation. We are speaking of a fully, radically present, passionately embodied state that sees its totality and is not frightened by it and is not frightened by engagement with it. It's a tantric approach to life.

In the West we have a tradition that has overly honored the personal in our psychotherapeutic endeavors and has tended toward narcissism. Now all of that combined with a non-dual vision, a truly transpersonal vision, is something we haven't seen on this scale and in this context of teachings before.

LML: *Yes, particularly in the United States, there has been a great pursuing of the material and a glorification of the body and of the personal self—we've sort of played that out. We've come out the other end saying, "Something is still missing."*
CATHERINE: Yes, but having played that out is grace. I see that what has happened in the East is that there has been so much denial and repression about this world, the body, sexuality, money—that this repression has turned into obsession. It sneaks around and comes in the back door. This is where a lot of people have gotten into trouble.

LML: *I'd like to get back to the whole issue of the accessibility of awakening or enlightenment. Traditionally, the belief has been that long-term spiritual practice is necessary, and a guru or spiritual teacher is necessary, and that it is very arduous work that takes many lifetimes.*

CATHERINE: Those beliefs are often very obscuring. The incredible joke is that you can't possibly avoid your true nature, not for a second. You can definitely overlook it and miss out on the fun, but all the while it is still shining. As you begin to have a tentative love affair with it, it's constantly beckoning you. The truth is always calling. Truth is constantly demanding a line-up. Anytime there's a chasm there's a pull to it; it's like a universal natural law. See, you can say this superficially, that everyone wants love. Love loves itself. If we really get quiet then we tap into this essence and that's what we discover, an unbounded love. That is what is constantly seducing us. This is everybody's taste. This is what everybody already knows in their heart of hearts.

JLW: *It is what we already are.*

CATHERINE: Exactly. So, to say that it's accessible is not even accurate. It's not that it's accessible; it's that you are drenched in it. You can deny knowing it; you can ignore it. But you are it.

JLW: *I know people who seem to have an intense yearning and hunger for truth. When I talk to them, it seems obvious to me that it's there, but they can't seem to see through to it or recognize it.*

CATHERINE: People can be subtly burdened with thinking that there's something to do even though it may appear that the yearning in them is really intense. As soon as the thought that there's something to do appears, there is a presumption that freedom is not already here. So, just the thought that there's something to do is a massive obscuration, not a little one.

LML: *Some of the people we have interviewed have talked about having a loss of a sense of the individual, personal self. Has this been your experience?*

CATHERINE: No. In fact, I would say that there is a more loose, free, and unique expression of the personal self than there ever was before. In a bizarre way, the so-called personality is flying on its own these days; it doesn't get many flight plan checks on it. [Laughter] But there is a continual sense of a greater context, in which it is displaying itself in terms of its momentariness and sort of see-through rainbow colors. I find the personal level all very amusing and delightful. The personal is happening, and I don't take it personally. [Laughter] There's not the seriousness to it that there used to be. Even though tragedies occur and all that, there is an "ah-so," a suchness that is so compelling and that is always what is most vital. The actual predominant experience of any given moment is the "ah-so," the vastness. Then the personal displays are arising and are mostly amusing and very, very unique. I quoted this in another interview, "There are no two alike, and there are no two at all." It's a bizarre paradox, isn't it?

All of this is very mysterious. We can actually know so little of it. There are just a few things that we can know. It's so important to really be honest to our own direct experience when we speak about this and try as much as we can to jettison our spiritual beliefs. Let's really be honest and say that there is a personal experience and that it is a very unique little expression in eternity.

LML: *It seems that it is a matter of what is more foreground. The experience of beingness and love can come foreground and then the personal self can do what it does, but it is not the primary interest or focus. It's just happening. When the personal self and its story is what is foreground, the presence of beingness gets ignored, and we suffer the story.*
CATHERINE: Yes, that's a beautiful way of saying it. I sometimes say in Dharma Dialogues that I have lost interest in the chatter of mind, even though it goes on. I liken it to riding on a train through some incredibly beautiful country side, just lost in the lushness of the beauty. Some people are talking in the back of the train car and you catch snatches of the conversation, but you're really not that interested, you're more interested in the beauty.

LML: *That's how we can let go of our beliefs; we become more interested in something else. If your attention is someplace else that is more essentially true, vital and present, beliefs fall away on their own. You could say, they "die" from lack of interest.*
CATHERINE: Yes, they do.

JLW: *Catherine, what do you see as the main obstacle to awakening in the West today?*
CATHERINE: Well, it's probably not so different than it's always been... the main obstacle is the simple belief that you're not already awake. I think this is the primary and perennially obscuring factor. There is a story going on that tells people that they need to do something, or that they're this big "somebody" that has to be protected and gotten things for, which is

an on-going wearisome project, or that they need something to aggrandize this somebody-ness. All the world agrees that that's what one does here and that's what people are trained in. It's like a training in suffering, a training in a belief system that will guarantee suffering. The belief is that you need more and you have to protect what you have.

JLW: *And that you're the subject of the story.*
CATHERINE: Exactly, that you're the star and that you have to star in and direct the story, when in fact neither is possible. It is a prescription for frustration and the source of suffering.

Now, I don't want to make light of the suffering in the world. Some people are born into abject misery and suffer real pain. I'm not saying that that does not exist. Again, we're not saying the world is illusion. But, there is a tremendous amount of suffering which is held in place simply by beliefs, and this suffering can be seen through and released.

JLW: *There's another order of suffering that's also held in place by beliefs that has to do with the suffering perpetuated by generations of greed, generations of bias and ignorance which creates the kind of suffering that people are born into and subject to their whole lives. There are things to be addressed in the world that one's heart says, "This is not appropriate."*
CATHERINE: That's right. Truth demands a line-up.

LML: *So, there is pain in life, but there can be pain without suffering. There is a freedom, not from pain, but from psychological suffering that is available to human beings.*
CATHERINE: Absolutely, the taste of freedom is our own essence, the most familiar taste. Poonjaji used to say, "Closer than your breath." I sometimes say, "More familiar than the sound of your own name." What is closer than your own breath? What is more intimate than your own breath? Poonaji means that literally, and I understand it literally now.

LML: *It's your own being.*
CATHERINE: Exactly.

JLW: *For the longest time I searched for the ground of being. Thinking, "What is this ground of being? Where is it?" When actually being is the ground.*
CATHERINE: Yes, yes indeed. [Laughter] You know, this is a thrilling time we live in. I began getting interested in spiritual matters in my late teens and during these twenty-some years I've been watching closely as an

insider in the dharma world, and it just feels explosive these days. This is the most exciting time of the flourishing of the dharma I've ever seen. This truth can speak to anyone, anywhere. This holy ground of being is right where we stand—now and always.

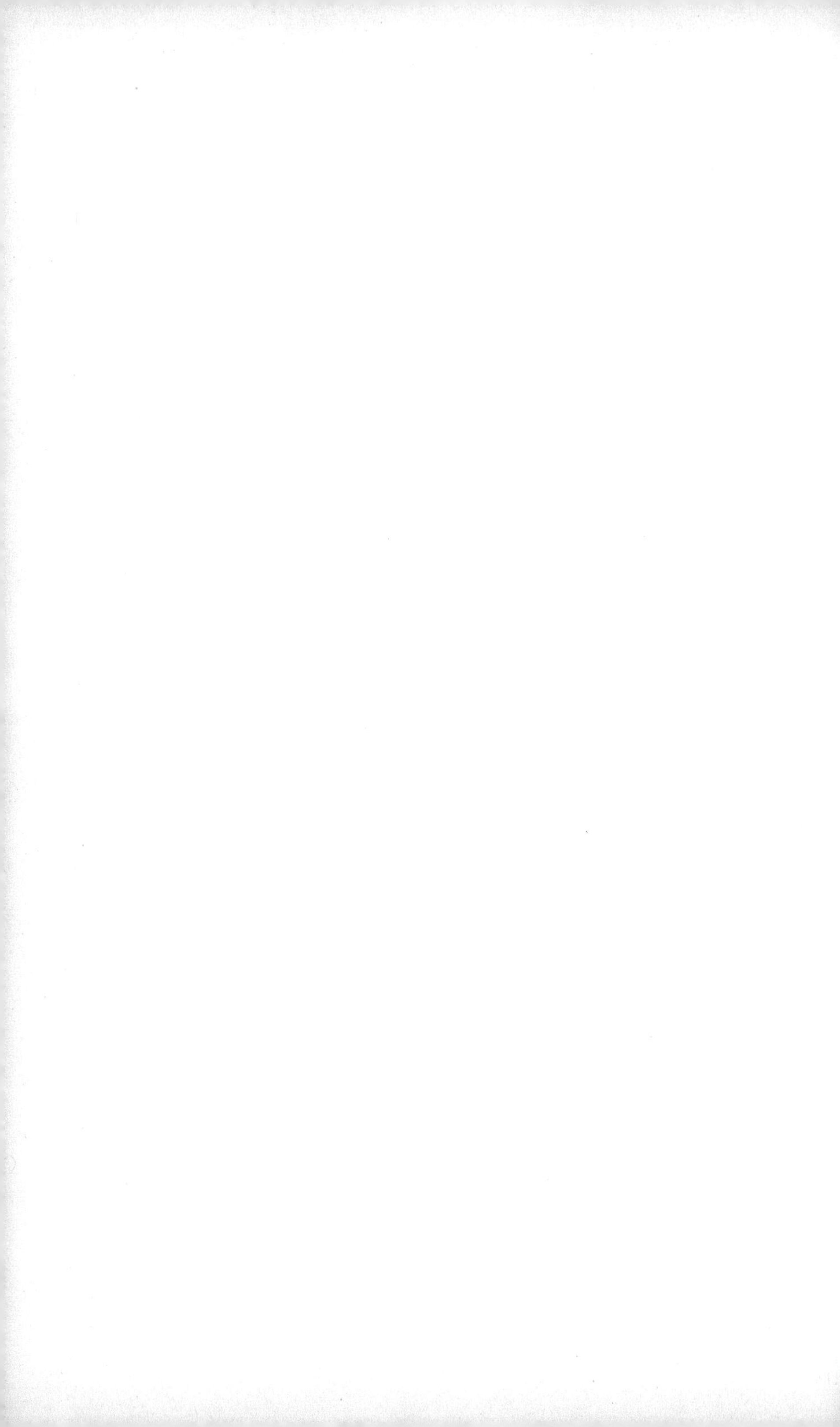

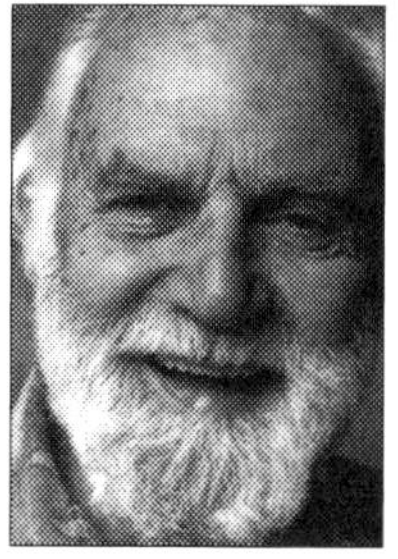

DOUGLAS HARDING

"AWAKENING IS NOT AN ACHIEVEMENT; IT IS SIMPLY REALIZATION OF WHERE ONE HAS BEEN AND WHERE ALL BEINGS ARE — IN THE BOSOM OF GOD, IF YOU WISH... IT IS A WAKING UP TO THE WAY ONE IS ANYWAY, IN ANY CASE."

Douglas is the elder statesman in our collection of spokespersons for *The Awakening West*. He was born in 1909 in England to a family that belonged to the religious sect, Exclusive Plymouth Brethren, for generations. At age twenty one, Douglas left the Brethren and began his own search for the Truth of who he is. In his early years, he practiced architecture in London, India, and his native Suffolk. But, his passion was to develop an accessible and practical way to help others see who they really are. This passion has lead to the publication of many books on this subject, including *On Having No Head* and *Look for Yourself*.

His awakening first occurred at age thirty-three in the foothills of the Himalayas while serving in the British Army in India. Douglas had been absorbed for several months in the question, "What am I?" As he looked out across the mountainous scene, thought stopped, and he looked in at what was looking. Contrary to conventional wisdom, he discovered not a "meatball with two small peepholes" resting atop his shoulders, but a vast, empty openness—as wide as the scene itself.

At ninety-one years of age, Douglas still travels extensively sharing the unique set of exercises he has developed which he calls experiments. When these experiments are sincerely performed and one simply accepts the evidence of one's own direct sense experience as it is, it is possible to immediately recognize our "original face" as it is referred to in Zen. In fact, it was these very exercises that gave John his first direct experiences of the self-evident, undeniable truth that there was actually nothing but aware, empty space, and that the very emptiness of this space allows the whole universe to appear within it.

John met with Douglas during one of his many world tours while he and his wife Katherine were staying with friends in Oakland, California. True to his ever-inventive nature, Douglas shared some of his latest ideas, more ways to share what he had discovered so long ago in India with a wider range of people. A charming, gentle, kind, and brilliant man, Douglas is a treat to be with and a pleasure to know.

CONVERSATION *with* DOUGLAS HARDING

JLW: *I'd like to begin with the question, "Who am I?" Have you found an answer to this question?*

DOUGLAS: Good question. Who am I? Well, the word "I" has two meanings, doesn't it? I use the word provisionally and somewhat improperly for Douglas. But as Meister Eckhardt says, "Only God can say 'I,' really, truly." Who I am in the fundamental sense here at center is not Douglas, but the real "I" which is the one "I," the one first person, the one who is conscious, the inside story of all beings—namely God if you wish, or Atman-Brahman, Allah, and so on. False "I" is attributed to Douglas. So, I use the word "I" in two senses.

JLW: *So what is awakening, enlightenment, realization? What do these words mean for you?*

DOUGLAS: They mean becoming conscious of the fact that you are already there; you are already home and dry in the Father's house, everyone is. Awakening is not an achievement; it is simply realization of where one has been and where all beings are—in the bosom of God, if you wish. It is very important to realize that it is not some kind of achievement on the part of the allegedly awakened one; it is a waking up to the way one is anyway, in any case.

JLW: *I'd just like to say that the particular way you have articulated the awakening and your specific, repeatable exercises that make it self-evident have been extremely useful to me. I greatly appreciate their ingenious, insightful character.*

DOUGLAS: Yes, the exercises are useful. I really believe they are a breakthrough in the spiritual life because they make this experience of awakening to the fact that you are already awakened, shareable. Not only shareable, but on tap. When you want them, there they are! Just pointing here [points toward himself] and noticing that there is nothing here. Or seeing that I am looking out of one huge eye and not two little peep holes in a meatball [gestures, forming the thumb and index fingers of each hand into a circle, bringing the circles up to his eyes like glasses and then, slowly opening his hands and extending his arms so that his hands frame the periphery of his 150 degree-wide view]... being in a car seeing that in truth the countryside is in fact moving while I am sitting still. All these things are available once one has done the experiments I offer and takes the message they offer. These experiments are mentioned in my books and demonstrated in my talks.

JLW: *For myself, it was your experiments that provided me with my first direct experience and insight into the spacious emptiness that has always been here at the "near-end of my neurons." So, I am very grateful to you for this... could you describe how the awakening occurred for you?*

DOUGLAS: I don't know. Sometimes, I say to myself that it was because I was so desperately fed up with Douglas and had to get out of the trap; because I was such a mess. Sometimes I say that, but I don't think this is actually the main reason. I think perhaps I had a gift. If I had a gift at all, it was just a curiosity. It was during the war, and I was over thirty. Things were looking bad in the Far East where I was stationed, and I thought, "Well, while I am still around, I am going to have a look at what is here and not take anybody else's word for it." I wanted to have a look at what it's like being me, being first person; what it's like in my own experience of being myself. I just wanted to have a look. I'll be damned if I was going to live and die without having a look at who is doing so.

JLW: *Rather than just follow the prescriptions and stories you had been handed.*

DOUGLAS: Yes. You see, John, everybody was telling me from birth onwards what is here. But nobody has been here but me. Nobody is literally in a position to tell me what I am here because they are too far away. They are literally too far away, by feet and inches! Nobody has been here but me. What they tell me is a regional impression of Douglas. Whereas, I have the central origins of the impressions I am giving over there. So I said to myself, "Let me look at that."

JLW: *What did you find?*

DOUGLAS: Space, which for the moment includes you, John, as well as the ceiling, walls, piano, etc. When I look at what is here, I find nothing, no thing. It is nothing except empty, open, spacious awareness in which you, John, are appearing.

JLW: *At zero inches from center, what there is is just space.*

DOUGLAS: Exactly; that's it, space—unbounded, aware, transparent, brilliantly clear, empty and, of course, full—brim full of whatever is appearing as the world at the moment because in itself it is empty.

JLW: *Full because it's empty—couldn't be otherwise.*

DOUGLAS: Yes, indeed.

JLW: *So, this next question is almost a loaded question for you because it asks if you have suggestions or recommendations for others who are experiencing a desire for awakening. Obviously you do; you have developed a whole set of experiential exercises to facilitate that direct experience.*

DOUGLAS: Well, I'd have to say this, John, I think it would be mere chauvinism and partiality to say that this is the only way. There are as many ways back to home as there are ways out, perhaps. But, I do think that while "the seeing way"—which is what I call the way my experiments make clear—is extremely valuable, by itself, it is not enough. On the other hand, it does have great virtue in that it is always available independent of one's mood. It is always available and shareable. It is not a mystical experience at all. It is not even what you might call spiritual, but even that is a bit pretentious. As the Dzogchen scripture says, it is our ordinary awareness.

JLW: *Are you saying that perhaps your way, the seeing way, is insufficient by itself?*

DOUGLAS: This is important... I have been on to this seeing way for half a century now, and at times during that half-century my behavior had fallen so far below standard as to be worse than ordinary decency. While I was very clear about who I was, and coming back to it quite often, my behavior all too often was bad in terms of unkindness or indifference to people and all sorts of naughtiness. I also have friends who share awakening experiences, and who are very good at showing people these exercises, whose behavior from time to time has been very shocking. So, it's important to look at the way this chap behaves, look at the way Douglas behaves. The question begged here is, can this be such a wonderful way if the people who travel it behave in these ways; unlovingly and so on? In other words, it is possible, and not only possible but all too easy, perhaps, to see who you are and still behave badly?

JLW: *"Badly" meaning, unethically and hurtfully?*

DOUGLAS: Yes. I have been working recently on this idea. See, if I pursue one path sufficiently, whatever path I am given to pursue—it will lead me to the others. It might be the path of devotion; it might the path of loving service like St. Vincent De Paul or Mother Theresa; it might be the path of the follower of beauty—but whatever path I pursue really, sincerely, with sufficient energy, consistency and time, it will lead me into the others. It is not because the way of seeing has any defect or any limitation; it is because it is an in-and-out thing. It is primed as a coming home to who I am and then out again and not noticing that. It has to become steady. How can it become a steady state?

JLW: *That's a good question. In my experience and also in what I have witnessed, many people have recognized who they are, but they haven't stabilized as That. The patterns of personality take over and they once again believe they are a separate, isolated individual.*
DOUGLAS: That is the big problem, John. The answer to it is not to decide, "Oh, this way is not a good way; I must go another way." Does one say for instance that a particular way is not good enough because there is bad behavior in people who know that way through and do travel it occasionally? Should one therefore abandon that way and try another? I think not. I say, stick to your way. Stick to the way that is your way, or that you perceive to be your way, and see it through to the end. If you do that with sufficient earnestness and regularity, you will be eased into the other ways.

Let me give you an example of what I am saying. In this path of seeing, when I see who I am, which I do now, I am open to you, John. I find that I have got nothing here; there is simply spaciousness with no particular emotional valence. Now, when love is lacking, as it has been from time to time in the case of myself and the other people I am referring to, can I genuinely say, "I love John?" No, it would be an absurd, artificial thing. Love has to be spontaneous and real, or it is not really love.

Well, what do I do? If I look more closely at what I find here, I see that I am space for you; there is no real separation except in an abstract, conceptualized way. You and the rest of the world are the appearances of awareness for me. You appear as the substantial contents of my empty awareness. Thus, upon examination, the self-evident truth of the matter is that we are built as a marvelous pattern, a fantastic, beautiful pattern of disappearing in favor of the other. In this sense, all of us are built to give our lives for one another. Now, as I recognize that, come to rest in that, and enjoy that, I can say that this is a grander love. That is where unbounded, selfless love can spring from.

JLW: *Douglas, that was very beautiful... can you say a little more about the convergence of the distinct paths?*

DOUGLAS: In fact, I have been working on it. [holds up a large sheet of paper upon which he had made diagrams] Let me show you the drawing of the four crossroads. The idea, John, is that this way [indicates one of the "roads" on the drawing], the seeing way into who we really, really are has its defects, as all the ways have their limitations. Goodness, truth, beauty, and devotion—these are the classic values and ways. All these ways also have their disadvantages. In the way of beauty, you can see the beauty and remain cold hearted; you can revel in the beauty of the world and remain selfish. With the way of devotion, you can get hooked on the guru, you know. For example, you can be hooked on the man Jesus instead of what Jesus was on about, which is the Universal Christ. Then there's the way of goodness—to be a determined do-gooder is not necessarily to give people what they need. I mean, God protect me from some of these dedicated do-gooders! Then there are artists—this is a real way through—I mean, Mozart tells me something about God. But off duty, artists, musicians, poets, and dramatists are sometimes very naughty people.

So, each way has its limitations; but, I say, stick to your way. You see, it's like a traffic system. Here is God in the center and we are travelling in by the routes of goodness, truth, beauty, devotion, seeing, etc. But here, in this nearer region, as on the highway, traffic conditions may be bad. There could be roadwork, terrible weather, etc., and one is diverted around to this way or that way. If you go on long enough, you will find it happens that you will be diverted along. We have many instances of that.

JLW: *Along the lines of what you are saying… the direct teachings of Dzogchen, for example, were traditionally not imparted to students until the teacher realized that they were living as exemplary ethical beings, that they had established a pattern of ethical conduct.*

DOUGLAS: Well, that is so.

JLW: *Now, it is a little different. Now Dzogchen is being taught freely. But formerly, these teachings were reserved for very few, selectively chosen students when the teacher felt they were ethical enough to recognize the significance.*

DOUGLAS: Well, I think we are using those scriptures differently now. In a way Padmasambhava predicted that, didn't he? When you are addressing a hundred people, maybe three people will get the point so clearly that they will start living it. And that is worth it, isn't it?

JLW: *Oh, certainly.*
DOUGLAS: But there is something very special about this way, the seeing way.

JLW: *Well, it's so immediate.*
DOUGLAS: Yes, and it is a real journey, John, from there [points out, away from his body] to here [points at his face as he's looking at the tip of his finger]. It's a journey from my appearance, which you have got, to my reality, which I have. It is a real journey from a real place to an even more real place. All of our tools are vehicles for traveling this journey from my regional appearance to my central reality. The other vehicles of goodness, beauty, truth, devotion, etc. are only journeys in a metaphorical sense; these are not journeys in the sense of a road from one real place to another. But the way of seeing is shareable, you can share it as soon as you have experienced it.

JLW: *Yes. It is more objective in the sense of being replicable by anyone willing to give it a fair trial, and so it can be shared and imparted as a direct, recognizable experience very clearly.*
DOUGLAS: It really can be shared. It takes you through to what Meister Eckhardt would call Godhead, not God, but Godhead.

JLW: *The source out of which everything emerges, in which everything exists, and to which everything returns.*
DOUGLAS: Yes. You see, once you have love in the world, it creates a shadow, which is indifference and hate. Once you have music in the world you have noise; once you have service, you have selfishness. In fact, every one of these functions, except the seeing, has an opposite.

This is one of the reasons the path of seeing is special. The Dzogchen scripture speaks of naked seeing, naked awareness—seeing into your essential nature, being naked awareness. Seeing has an absence, which is blindness or ignorance, but it has no opposite. Whereas truth has an opposite, lies; love has hate; beauty, ugliness; goodness, evil but seeing has no opposite. One either looks within and sees the open, empty nature of awareness or one does not.

In our modern world, this way of seeing is agreeable to modern science. It's an up-to-date way that is eminently shareable. Now with beauty... I mean you may find Chopin incredibly beautiful, and I may not, so how do we share this?

JLW: *Getting back to the consideration that in and of itself, the path of seeing is not sufficient, were you referring to its lacking love, devotion, and service?*

DOUGLAS: Yes, indeed. One way of putting it is in a rather personal way: If I had to go on a walking tour, or a holiday, with a person who is a clear seer of who he or she is who had no love, or alternatively, with a really loving person who was rather foggy in their seeing, I would give precedence to love in that sense. All the same, the priority of seeing is very important to notice

JLW: *So, as a practice, what you seem to be recommending in your books is to just notice, again and again what is actually here.*

DOUGLAS: That's right. Attention, attention, attention. Attention in two directions you see, this and that [pointing toward himself and away from himself], in and out. Just telling it like it is without any of our conditioned, preconceived notions about how it is. Attention, or mindfulness, is the name of the game, absolutely. If we do that with sufficient sincerity and regularity, we shall be led to all the other ways such as devotion, truth and service. Also, by living our approach, John, a linear approach of our chosen way, it becomes a lateral approach, and includes the other approaches. Indeed it becomes an all-inclusive convergence on the center if we allow it to.

A quick example from Ramakrishna. Ramakrishna at six years old was walking through fields during the monsoon in Bengal. There were clouds and white birds flying across and he was so overcome by the beauty of the world that he passed out. At twenty, he came in by the route of devotion, and he was appointed the priest in charge of the Kali temple at Dakiniswar, near Calcutta. Ramakrishna was absolutely devoted to the Goddess, who creates with one hand and destroys with the other, absolutely devoted and with the greatest simplicity. Then along came a naked sadhu, and converted Ramakrishna to the Formless God, and that became his chief way. Not that he abandoned his devotion, but that his understanding of and approach to the divine was expanded. Then he founded the order of Ramakrishna monks who were devoted to the service of humanity. This is a model of what I was saying. If we are sincere enough, things will develop that way. If you want to do anything properly, do it. Stick to your way but allow it to mature into convergence.

JLW: *Yes... do you feel that a teacher or a guru is necessary to point out the truth?*
DOUGLAS: Yes and no. I never had a particular guru, but I would say I have had many gurus. I have read many books, and I have gained from hundreds of people. But, the actual vision of the aware openness, no, nothing and no other are required for us to recognize that.

JLW: *As you awakened to the essence of who you are, was there less of a sense of an individual, personal self? If so, how did this effect your relationships and day-to-day life?*
DOUGLAS: There was certainly a huge shift from feeling under inspection as this special person, Douglas, into being space for the world. I can't tell you the relief, John, at being out of this terrible, terrible trap that I was in of morbid self-consciousness up until quite an advanced age. I hated people looking at me because they might embarrass me. I hated them not looking at me because they were ignoring me. When one is free of that curse, one comes into his own because one isn't trapped in that fellow. It is not so much that one is freed of the personality, but one perceives the tricks and the whitewashing of motives and all the funny stuff which adheres to that little guy. You perceive it more clearly, but from a distance.

JLW: *Then, it is seen as just another phenomenon in the field of awareness.*
DOUGLAS: That's right. Well put.

JLW: *Do you perceive that there is an increased interest in awakening in the West at this time?*
DOUGLAS: I don't know. It seems to go up and down. In England, at one time, I was going all over the place, most universities had their Buddhist societies, and I was very busy. Nowadays, very few.

When I return to England, I am going to Manchester University Buddhist Society, but this has become quite uncommon. In France, there is a very big development there. We have workshops there, quite nice size ones, a hundred or two in most of the big cities in France. Also, publishers seem to be very keen to have my work, but that is recent. Everything is up and down. I just don't know what the answer is to that one. I'd like to think that there is an increased interest in awakening, but I am not too sure.

In medieval times, people were crude and uneducated and so on, but there was a general acknowledgement that there was another realm, another world; there was God in heaven. In this modern world, in some ways, John, these are the dark ages. In medieval times, John Scottus

Arrigeina was in the court of Charlemaigne who couldn't read and write, but he was the king of the Western world. John Scottus said, "Everything is an appearance of God." So, which are the dark ages, those days or these?

JLW: *Given your experience, what do you see as the source of suffering in the world today?*
DOUGLAS: Well, I see two sources of suffering. One is the ordinary price of being in the world, the suffering that comes to everybody—from tummy aches to birth pangs, to the inconveniences and pains of old age and death—the inevitable. And there is the other kind of suffering, which is unnecessary and imposed, the suffering that comes with believing that I am what I look like. And I am not. I am the exact opposite of what I look like! If I take on the appearance of that little guy, Douglas, I get parasitized by allowing this specimen to delude me. That is the suffering which is unnecessary and for getting rid of.

But, you see, there is another sense in which we don't get rid of it. When we see who we truly are, we take on the suffering of the world. We really must. I mean, who you are truly is taking on the joy and the suffering of the whole of it, inevitably. Compassion means that your suffering is my suffering. So, one is in a way not offering a nice comfortable way out of a nasty pain by discovering who you truly are. One could say that the cure is through experiencing the suffering more directly and fully without getting distracted thoughts about it.

JLW: *Yes; more of it and none of it at the same time.*
DOUGLAS: More of it and none of it! Suffering is a great mystery. I think that it is only through suffering that the highest joy, the real joy, is found.

JLW: *What you just said makes me think of what you were saying earlier, about how both yourself and others have behaved badly in some moments. In those moments, we are disconnected from actually seeing who and what we truly are. If we are cruel or hurtful, we are not in that moment seeing the Truth clearly.*
DOUGLAS: That's right. The seeing—until we are really doing it with great sincerity, sufficiently and often enough—it is inherently a flying visit.

JLW: *Yes. We notice it, touch it, and then we are gone. We are back in our personal story.*
DOUGLAS: Exactly.

JLW: *Why is commitment to the truth of who we are so difficult for most people? What do you see as the main obstacle to people fully awakening?*

DOUGLAS: The fear of annihilation, fear of disappearing. We all have it, John. I mean, I look in the mirror, and I see this guy over ninety years old whose shelf life is extremely limited. I see crummy, old Douglas, but at least he is; there is something to him. However briefly, there he is. But when I look here [points back to his head] there is nothing. That is scary. That is the real obstacle. We think up all sorts of reasons why we don't want to see who we really are, but I think this is the basic one, fear of annihilation. Of course, what is actually true is that there is nothing and everything! This nothing has a very practical component in that it is an awake nothing, an awake nothing that is full and quite something!

JLW: ... *Well, Douglas, I don't have any more questions. Is there anything that you would like to add?*

DOUGLAS: I think your questions were absolutely super. I would like, John, to include here some of the exercises from my books and suggest to the readers that they actually perform the experiments and experience for themselves the results.

JLW: *I had planned on that because I don't think this will make much sense without the direct experience.*

DOUGLAS: Yes, exactly. The most direct experience and the most obvious one is: "You are now looking at some black marks on the white paper and you see the book, here, in the hand. Now, on present evidence, what is on your side of that writing?" "On present evidence, is there nothing here registering that?" You must say, "On present evidence..."

JLW: *Yes, direct experience is the key to your work.*

DOUGLAS: The key. "What's taking it in here, now?" Another one is, "What are you looking out of now? Are you looking out of two little peepholes in a meatball or is it one huge, huge window? Isn't it all encompassing, as wide as the world?" Another, "Have you ever been face-to-face with any body? Hasn't it always been face-to-space?"

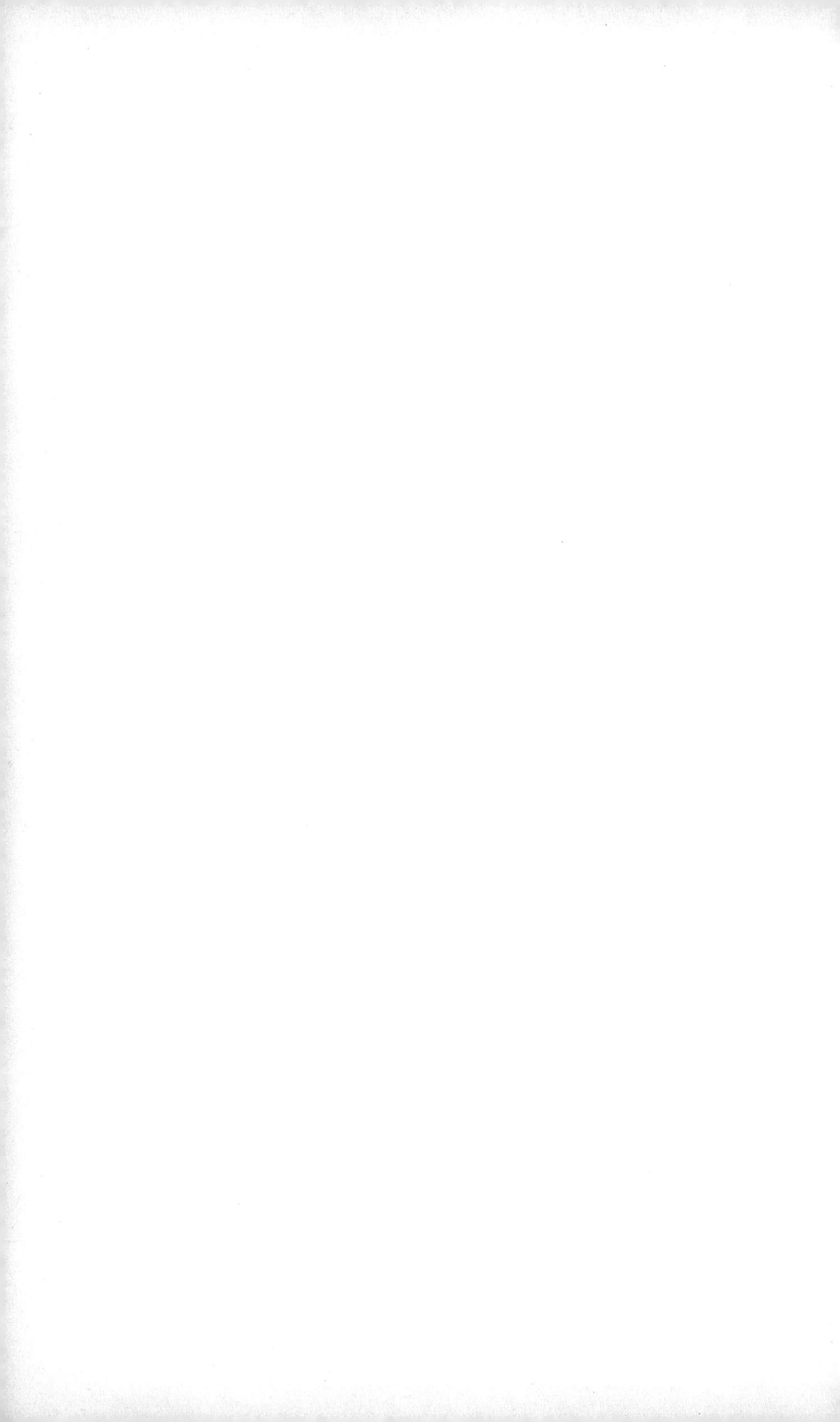

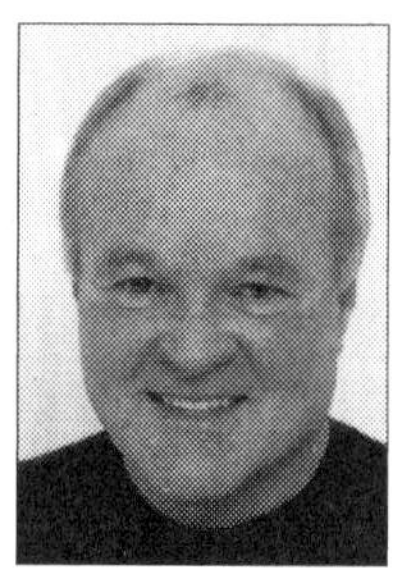

SATYAM NADEEN

"NOW ALL OF THE RIPE SEEKERS ARE FALLING OFF THEIR 'SPIRITUAL TRIPS' OF TRYING TO GET FROM HERE TO THERE AND ARE JUST RELAXING INTO THE KNOWINGNESS THAT ALL IS WELL IN THIS LIFE, EXACTLY 'AS IS!' WHY NOW? BECAUSE IT IS TIME. BECAUSE A SHIFT IS HAPPENING AT LAST. RIGHT NOW! WITHOUT EFFORT!"

Satyam Nadeen was known as Michael Clegg when he awakened in a violent county jail where he was imprisoned for selling the drug Ecstasy. He lived there in crowded conditions with constant noise and experienced his life being threatened daily. It was in this extreme environment that he gave up the search that had propelled him all his life and awakened to what was always here. This search began early in life. He entered the seminary to become a Catholic priest at twelve years of age and did not leave until he was twenty-six. After that he spent thirty years searching intensely through Eastern and New Age practices and—you name it—he did it all, including thoroughly exploring the world of money, sex, and drugs. Now he teaches that the best thing to "do" is nothing; just embrace life fully as it is.

Nadeen, as he is now called, met with us at his beautiful home overlooking the San Francisco Bay. He had recently returned from Costa Rica where he has a retreat center. At the time of our conversation he did not stay in one location for long. He has traveled extensively giving satsangs and is clearly enthusiastic about sharing with others the truth that he has discovered. For years he held weekend intensives three out of four weekends a month, all over the globe. Now living in Georgia, his schedule is curtailed while he is recuperating from illness.

Nadeen is one of the more unique Western expressions of this truth that we encountered. He has developed his own languaging to describe the process of awakening with such terms as "the high five," and "shift happens." Nadeen says he wants to do away with the old concepts about enlightenment that have been passed down for centuries. He offers a fresh, new perspective on awakening in a contemporary vernacular that is fitting for what he terms the "Millennium Shift." Nadeem whole-heartedly agrees with us that a major shift in human consciousness has begun. He says that all you need to be a part of this is a desire for freedom—the rest will happen effortlessly.

CONVERSATION *with* SATYAM NADEEN

LML: *What, if any, answer have you found to the question, "Who am I?"*

NADEEN: Is this a trick question? I don't even know who I am or where I am any more. But there is a shift of consciousness and it involves the simple remembering of who we are. Until that happens, nothing else is possible. I call awakening "the shift" because these words "awakening" and "enlightenment" are so loaded today. Nobody knows what you are talking about when you say those words anymore.

The core event of this shift is the day, when by grace, we wake up and remember that Consciousness is all that there is. Consciousness is all there is and I am That, and so is everyone else! It sounds so simple. It seems that it couldn't possibly be this simple; after all, we've had five thousand years of spiritual discipline. But it is that simple! There is a force field present in the world right now that is allowing this ancient memory to come forward. Infinite intelligence and design have always purposefully, kept it in the background.

So the moment you remember who you are, that you are not a third dimensional, separated being, even though that has been your life experience, the shift takes over. The part that may be sudden is the remembrance. One day you don't remember and the next day you do, but that is only a baby step in this whole process. It is the very beginning. Each month and year after that, you look back at that first day you started to remember, and it really feels like a baby step. After that remembering, what I call the "deliverance" takes over.

LML: *In your first book,* From Onions To Pearls, *you speak of a shift from the third dimension into a fourth dimension. Could you explain what you mean by that?*

NADEEN: First I have to explain what I mean by a third dimension. The third dimension is set up by infinite intelligence to make it seem as if your identity is just the mind and whatever the mind presents. The way it judges, the way it separates into polarities, the way it gives you the illusion of free will, control, choice, and the way it constantly doubts everything from your intuition—that's the third dimension. There is no way to get out of the third dimension by yourself. There is not a discipline invented that can get you out. There is not an enlightened master that can take you with him. The shift into the fourth dimension is the change of identity from the dominance of the mind to the presence of the witness, where you become this observer of life just as it is. You are simultaneously watching in choiceless awareness the third dimension happen with the mind making its same judgments but no longer identifying with them. There is an incredible presence of a witness that produces a deep knowingness—beyond the mind, beyond experience, beyond explaining, like I am trying to do now—which can see through the mind and is not pulled into it.

This doesn't mean we can't feel contraction. Contractions are equally present after the shift as they are before the shift. The difference is that you no longer identify with them. The difference is that there is a simple witnessing of, "Ah, anger is present, joy is present, and that is the mind doing its thing like all good little minds are supposed to do." You don't identify with it. This is the greatest miracle of the fourth dimension.

LML: *Are you saying that it takes a miracle to have this shift take place?*

NADEEN: Yes. There is no way to disidentify from the mind with human intelligence through intentional effort. That is the mind trying to get rid of itself, and it can't do that. Its function is to stay on top, to stay in control. It takes some sort of supernatural power that is greater than walking on water, walking through walls, or any other miracle you can think of, to simply watch life happening and instead of judging it and trying to make it better, to simply allow life, to embrace life just as it is, without trying to fix it. The nature of the mind is to fix and make better.

The fourth dimension is simply watching life unfold without the slightest need to fix it or make it better. That is the only secret of happiness there is. It is not possible to be happy in the third dimension, no matter what the conditions. If you are not in the space of embracing life as it happens, you cannot be truly happy because all of life is an equal balance of freedom and limitation. Every person, no matter how enlightened or dense they are, has the same balance of freedom and limitation—that part never changes. The miracle is this ability to dance "yes" to the "no" in the middle of disaster. That is the shift that is the fourth dimension, and it has never happened before.

Even in the tales of saints and masters, I am not sure how far they got in this because there was still an agenda of shoulds and shouldn'ts, dos and don'ts, still trying to control life. If you look at what history has presented us with the saints and the masters, they didn't always seem like a very happy lot, did they? The saints still considered themselves sinners not worthy of the great grace of mystical union.

Hey, when I woke up, I knew I was totally worthy because I knew I was the Source of it all. There was no possibility of being a sinner or not worthy or of needing to control life any more. So, to the degree that my deliverance has brought me more and more into harmony with embracing every detail of life, that has been my degree of resulting happiness, joy, peace, freedom or whatever else you want to call it.

LML: *You said that the shift to the fourth dimension where there is an ability to say "yes" to the "no" in the middle of a contraction has never happened before. From what I have read and studied, this is not new; it's just becoming more widely known, especially in the West. Teachings that discuss letting everything be as it is and allowing it to be liberated in that acceptance have been available for a long time. The Buddhist Dzogchen teachings, for example, discuss this.*

NADEEN: If that's in there, then how could the Buddhists have ten thousand rules of do's and don'ts about life? You come to such a place of total freedom in this shift that there isn't one single do or don't possible because it's all Source in appearance. That means that everything is exactly the way it's supposed to be, everything is just happening just as it is. To put do's and don'ts in there means you might have a rather limited experience of enlightenment.

JLW: *I think the distinction here is that in Buddhism there are teachings for every stage of development. The Buddha taught for forty-some years, and he taught many people in different stages of development. One thing he taught was right conduct or character development so that people could stabilize in that to enable them to get in touch with their yearning and move towards the next stage. In that, there is a lot of do's and don'ts, a lot of ethical dimensions to that aspect of Buddhism. Then with Dzogchen and Zen, especially Dzogchen, it's not that way. It's a much more direct introduction to the presence of awareness and living from that, letting things be as they are. These teaching are new to the West, however. They have been around for a long time, but have spread to the West only since China's invasion of Tibet.*

NADEEN: There is probably nothing that anybody can say that is new under the sun. Let's just put it this way: in the main stream spirituality that is available to the New Agers, I haven't heard it. For that reason, I quoted verses from *LaoTsu* in the *Tao Te Ching* in my first book. These are three thousand-year-old verses saying exactly what I'm saying. In the second book I have put in verses from the *Ashtavakra Gita*, which are just as old and also saying the exact same thing. The problem is that you have to be shifted to even understand it. If you are not shifted, it doesn't even make sense. So, these truths have been around, but they haven't emphasized the non-doing and accepting of life just as it is. What has been emphasized, however, is the doing, the disciplines, or even less noteworthy, the states of nirvana, bliss, and samadhi, which are really only a minuscule part of it. The sooner they are gone the better; they are peak experiences. What you live with in this shift is the presence, which is not a peak experience, and it never goes away. Anything that distracts you out of that presence, including bliss-outs, is just a blip. It's not part of the shift.

JLW: *In reading your book,* From Onions to Pearls, *we were struck by the paradox of how you found freedom in a situation where your worldly freedom was extremely curtailed. Would you please describe how that came about for you?*

NADEEN: What is even more paradoxical, John, is the fact that when I was living at my mountain top in Costa Rica, with basically unlimited money and power, that I didn't find freedom there. It didn't happen until I found myself confined within an overcrowded, hellhole of a prison. Certainly it is a paradox, and Source's favorite dance in this third dimension is through paradox. The way paradox works is that you figure out how things would work the best through human logic and then do just the opposite. This just seems to be the way Source plays—through paradox.

In prison every freedom was not always taken away, but my life felt like it was always in jeopardy because I was in a violent prison by no accident, by design of the correction authorities. Waking up in those conditions was the greatest validation of freedom I could have imagined. Had I gotten out of prison, gone back to my mountaintop and then all of a sudden had the experience of awakening, I might have thought, "Well, maybe it is connected with being free from jail." I was at the beginning of my prison term when this happened. I hadn't even started my federal penitentiary time yet but had just done two years in a county lockup waiting for sentencing. So, I sat there in this psycho ward and watched guys assault, kill, and rape each other, or commit suicide, and feel such intense hatred and hostility toward each other, but yet, I was feeling the happiest I had ever been in my whole life! I was just crying from joy and freedom. I knew something was happening that went beyond anything that I had ever heard of, and I could only call it a shift to the fourth dimension.

I can remember instances before this in my life when I had done some really good acid, maybe mixed with a little Ecstasy, and created a cocktail that took me out of this feeling of separation for a few hours where I felt some minor sense of freedom. It doesn't compare. The true freedom of the shift is the full nectar that doesn't go away.

The first thing that I noticed in this whole experience of the shift was that all fear vanished. Now, what I have since found out is that fear doesn't necessarily leave everyone. Other people still have fears where I still may have frustrations, at delays, for example. But my memorable experience of this shift in prison was that the fear I had at every moment of being killed just went away one day and never came back.

LML: *Were you seeking freedom at that time of this shift?*
NADEEN: The last thing I could care about in prison was a shift, or God, or anything else spiritual. I just wanted to stay alive and get out of that prison.

JLW: *But previously, you had been a spiritual seeker...*
NADEEN: Only all my life! I was intensely interested in the spiritual. I searched through the Catholic priesthood for fourteen years. Didn't find what I was looking for, so I jumped from Western to Eastern mysticism. There I lived in ashrams, kissed guru's feet and did zazen thirteen hours a day. Doesn't that sound like a typical New Age seeker? Then I went to the other polarity also. I went as deep as you can go into the third dimension in the world of money, power, drugs, and sex. But the longing to go "home" and to know the thoughts of God had never left me until the day I woke up. Until that day, everything I did was part of that search.

You see, the passport to this shift, besides being human, is this intense yearning to go home. The people who are involved in this shift all have this in common, and they don't even know where this home is. It is like that movie, *Close Encounters of the Third Kind*, where the music kept drawing the chosen ones, attracting them, pulling them closer and closer to this one center. Then, when they get there, they finally know what it is, but not before.

Source is obviously having a very different experience in the last ten years or so than has ever appeared in recorded history. Right now instead of only a handful of people remembering who they are, we have millions of people that are attracted to this home of oneness, to remembrance of who they really are. Millions instead of a few!

JLW: *What makes you say millions?*

NADEEN: There are two reasons. One was my first intuitive hit, which I put in the first book, that it was one percent of the population. Then after I got out and checked around, I saw that the seekers in the world actually do make up one percent of the population. When I started to do all these satsang intensives and got to share with people everywhere in satsang, the only people showing up were the intense seekers. These people are not dilettantes or light weights. These are people living on the edge, where the longing is so intense that it is more important than their career, their relationships, or even their health. Such intense longing that only their tears provided the sure-tell clue of the shift in progress.

JLW: *Sounds like us. [Laughter]*

NADEEN: Yes, that's one of the signs we have all shared in common. The other interesting part of this that we all share is the precursor to the shift, lying in the dark night of the soul. I have found that to be virtually universal. The dark night of the soul is this feeling that you go through at some point when you feel totally flat in your business, in your relationships, in your hobbies—it is worse than flat, you feel despair. It feels like God has abandoned you; your common sense has abandoned you; and your value systems are zip.

This is the crumbling of the ego-personality that identifies itself with the mind. The experience of the disidentification that happens seems to use a dark night of the soul as its process. I haven't met a person who doesn't go through some sort of incredible crushing of everything they thought they were. You won't do this on your own! You won't go off to a Zen monastery and say, "Ok, I want to crush my personality now." The mind doesn't give up that easily; it is not supposed to. All the old conditioning has to be crushed and overcome by something other than the mind. I call this the dark night of the soul. This is the part that people don't want to hear about.

JLW: *I want to clarify something. You have traveled rather extensively—you mentioned seventy-eight cities in the last two and a half years and seeing about ten thousand people in satsang—and you are saying that this same awakening process is happening in everyone?*

NADEEN: It is happening to seekers with "the longing," and it doesn't matter what language you are translating from. It is the exact same thing, all over Europe, Canada, the United States, South America. We are talking about the shift, the intensity of the longing, the dark night of the soul, the remembering in the beginning of who you are, and then the gradual embracing of life as it is. Everyone at satsang is shaking their heads, "Yes, this is my experience, too." This is a universal happening.

LML: *You are validating our vision and intention with this book—to show that awakening is a happening phenomenon at this time and that it is possible to experience this. There may be people reading this who have that yearning, and they may be wondering what can I do? It often seems, "Am I going crazy? What do I do about this?" Do you have any suggestions for them?*

NADEEN: Just one; do nothing! [Laughter] It can't occur where there is a doer trying to make it happen. Yet, if the mind is involved, there is a doer, and that is the way it is supposed to be. If you are feeling this longing and you wonder, "Is this my shift or is this my mid-life crisis?" Please know this: if you are a seeker, it is the shift because it is happening simultaneously to every seeker on the planet right now. It is amazing to walk into a room of three or four hundred people where I don't know them, and they don't know me. But when I start talking about this, people are crying and sobbing and getting up and passing the mic and saying, "This is exactly what I am feeling and going through right now." Usually, it is still mixed in with a lot of concepts about how it is supposed to be, but we get past these in the intensives. It is easy to get rid of the concepts. What you can't get rid of is the longing until you are finally home.

Another amazing thing that I'm finding out is that there are people who have been intense seekers their whole life—done everything, been to India, followed masters, doing the whole trip, you name it, until the longing became just unbearable. But then one day, suddenly that longing went away and never came back. This is the only sudden thing in this whole process. The longing just disappears the day you remember who you are. Now, your deliverance has begun. The miracle is this: that something so strong, that has driven you for thirty, forty, fifty years, can disappear in a night, or disappears on a weekend during an intensive. That's when you don't care anymore if you ever shift or wake up. You feel like you are coming home, and there is nothing else to do. I have seen that so many times, I can't tell you. It is such a beautiful thing to see and watch people sob tears and tears of relief that the search is over; there is nothing left to do. It is not because I told them this. You can't recognize anything someone tells you unless you already know it. But when you validate what they already know at some deep level, the shift occurs in the sense that the longing stops. This cessation of the longing seems totally illogical in the face of a whole lifetime of seeking.

LML: *At that point what you call the deliverance begins. Would you say more about what you mean by deliverance?*

NADEEN: What is keeping you from the shift your whole life in the first place are concepts of "how life should be." You have been programmed in a number of ways, the strongest being your predispositions. Everyone has unique strands of DNA that make them totally different from any other person in the universe. (The biggest thing I got out of the Clinton-Lewinski scandal was when they tested the famous blue dress to see if it was Clinton. Sure enough, there was a seven and a half trillion to one accuracy with the DNA sample—trillion! That meant in a million planet Earth's with as many people as we have now, there still wouldn't be a mistake—there is only one Willie Clinton.) That is how unique each one of us is. These predispositions come with us into a world where they are programmed by society in concepts about how life should be. This is the barrier between the third and fourth dimensions, and the breakthrough is the remembering that you are this Consciousness, this Source. Then begins the gradual breaking down of every concept that you have had from the beginning of time. This won't end until the day you die. However, with each new contraction you have, there is an embrace of the contraction and the witness saying "yes" to the "no." In that process a concept dissolves; every time you have a contraction and you meet it with awareness something dissolves and never comes back.

LML: *And by contraction you mean a resistance to what is?*

NADEEN: It's a strongly felt "no" to what is. Your tape recorder isn't working right, and you say, "no" inside. That's a contraction, a little bitsy one on the big scale, but it's a still a "no." And in the middle of this contraction there is a witness saying, "All is well." That's the miracle of the shift. The big secret of the shift is that your deliverance happens, not through blissing out and going into nirvana, but with awareness in the middle of a contraction. In the middle of a contraction there is the "no" of the contraction and the "yes" of the witness happening at the same time. The reason it is so miraculous is that the witness sees through the contraction and doesn't buy it. It just says, "Ah look, anger is present." Only the witness can say "yes" to "no," or even "hell no." That's not possible without the grace of what we call the shift, or the awareness of the fourth dimension. How many contractions do we get in a day? Twenty, thirty, forty contractions a day. You'll never run out of contractions. Your deliverance will always go on. And guess what? It always gets better; it only gets better. It's never as good as it gets.

LML: *What's so amazing to me is that there's no need to get rid of anything we experience or any part of who we are in order to be free. I have spent so much of my life working so hard on changing who I am. It's a surprise and a relief to be discovering that it's all perfect, just as it is. Just leave it alone; just be. It is so simple!*

NADEEN: All of the people who are in the shift are sharing this same experience. The curiosity of the people in the shift is all the same. We all have the same questions.

JLW: *Two or three years ago, the focus of the questions we heard in satsang was, "How can I see what you're talking about?" Now, what we hear is, "How can I stabilize in this recognition?" "How can I keep this no matter what? I seem to lose it in different situations." Now, more people have had the awakening recognition and want to know how to stay with the experience of awakeness in the stress of everyday modern life. Can you address this?*

NADEEN: They're confused! They are expecting a trouble-free existence. What they don't know is that the fourth dimension lies in the middle of the contractions. They're trying to stay in a space where they feel bliss, freedom, joy, and oneness, but it's never going to be that away all the time. The law of balance prevails. This means that your life is going to be as much freedom as it is limitation. This doesn't mean that you identify with the limitation side of it, or even the freedom side of it. These people have had what I would call peak experiences. The nature of a peak experience is that it comes and goes, but then you try to get it back after it's gone. That's not what we're talking about here. That's not the shift; it's a peak experience. It's part of the shift; it's a glimpse. But the real heart of the shift is a deep pervading presence that never leaves you and is always available in the middle of every contraction—a deep safety net of knowing who you are, and that all is well. This never goes; peak experiences come and go. Limitations and contractions come and go. The presence never goes. Whenever you want, the witness is always there. This is the part that you wouldn't trade for anything outside of you in the whole world, this presence that never, ever leaves you.

The deepest experience in this whole shift is just being ordinary and being in neutral. Now neutral sounds like a very boring place. But it's the most incredible, delicious experience available because you are not looking for the highs, and you are not bummed out by the lows. You're in this deep valley that is unaffected by bliss or disappointment. Bliss can be as much a distraction as disappointment. People are looking for the bliss in this shift, and they're looking down the wrong alley. They are still confused but will understand eventually in time.

JLW: *I believe that this confusion happens because very often when awakening first occurs there is incredible bliss at the release. The revelation is then associated with bliss rather than the recognition of the spacious presence, which is just here, no matter what the experience. It's so simple, effortless, and ordinary. But the release into the recognition can be dramatic.*

NADEEN: It's a relief from the pressure of not having to perform, to achieve, or maintain anything. But that goes quickly. I had about a three week bliss out when I just cried from relief and joy at knowing I was home. Then life got back to real again, but it was totally different. Now I wasn't identifying with the judgments. I was shocked when I had my first judgment. I thought, "How could I have experienced this bliss so strongly and still be judging a guard for beating up on that inmate?" I wanted to go kill him I was so mad. My biggest recognition was an acceptance of life as it is. Here is a guard beating up on an inmate brutally; and on the one hand, I was angry and judgmental. But the real identity saw that this is just as it is, and it's okay. The mind was going crazy trying to figure this out. With deliverance I learned, "Forget the mind. It's not going to figure it out." It's not supposed to figure it out. Not now, not ever!

LML: *There are many misconceptions about enlightenment. One is what we were just discussing—that enlightenment is constant bliss.*

NADEEN: Up until recently, no one has ever told the whole story about what enlightenment really is. Everything you've ever read in your whole life about enlightenment that was written before ten years ago is more of a fairy tale than factual reality. Historically, authors have been telling stories about the glory side of enlightenment that aren't true. When you get down to the nitty gritty of what it means to live in the fourth dimension, you're talking about things like embracing, accepting, and dancing "yes" in the middle of "no," contractions... instead of words like siddhis, or supernatural powers, mystical insights, psychic abilities. These are all phenomenon. They come and go and mean nothing to your personal happiness, nothing. The key to your deep, lasting, permanent happiness is accepting life just as it is. And you cannot do that as a human being unless you're shifted.

LML: *It sounds a little extreme to say that everything ever written about enlightenment before ten years ago was a fairy tale. The old masters knew something.*

NADEEN: The problem here is that it wasn't the masters who were necessarily writing about their own experience of enlightenment. It was their devotees or investigative kind of biographers putting down on paper what they imagined the master was experiencing, as interpreted through their own filters of the mind and their own third dimensional experience of life. For whatever reasons of destiny somehow even the masters managed to slip into their message of enlightenment enough do's and don'ts to lose the total freedom side of this message. Until now it hasn't been time or appropriate for Source to completely reveal how consciousness can simultaneously dwell with a foot in the third and one in the fourth dimension. Source has finally come clean with this shift!

JLW: *Saying "yes" to everything that happens in life brings up the issue of suffering. There is an incredible amount of suffering in the world today; really horrific things are occurring everyday to many people. How do we say "yes" to this too?*

NADEEN: All suffering in the world, without exception, is the mind judging that life should be otherwise. Even something like physical pain is not suffering; it's a grace. If there are people suffering out there because their mind is doing the job it was designed to do, then they don't need fixing. That's destiny; that's what's happening just as it is. That's Source operating at a level where the mind can't understand, but it's going crazy trying to understand it. When you shift, nothing changes as far as the number of contractions you are going to have every day. The difference is that because you don't identify with them and you don't try to fix them, you don't suffer. When I cannot relate to my own suffering, then I can't relate to other people's suffering. I don't see people suffering. I see all the craziness going on in the world right now and I know Source is whipping it up into something juicy. I don't know why. I'm not supposed to know why.

"Don't know, don't care," are the favorite words of the witness to my mind. Every time someone asks me a question in satsang about the suffering in the world I say, "Don't know, don't care." It has nothing to do with me. It doesn't mean I don't empathize or feel compassion, but there is nothing I can do to fix it.

Every question you are asking me is so relevant that I applaud your clarity. I have gone into it very deeply in my new book, *From Seekers To Finders*, exactly the same line of reasoning because these were questions that challenged me.

What is interesting in my second book is that I discuss the myths of enlightenment. There are five different kinds of people I meet in my intensives. There are those that say, "It could happen to others, but it can't happen to me," or "This could happen some day, but it couldn't happen now." And I meet people that say, "Everything I know about spiritual enlightenment says that you have to do something to get it. You're not saying anything about doing or meditation. So, this is too simple to be true because there's no doing involved." Then there are the people who are tradition-oriented and say, "This isn't traditional." And in traditional spirituality you have a master or a guru and a teaching and you do disciplines and when you are a good boy long enough. Finally you have those who question this shift because either I or the others describing their experience don't look like the image of what they had expected an awakened person to look like. I just go through all of these objections which are basically all stemming from the one central point that this is too simple to be true.

LML: *There is something I would like to address about the many concepts about enlightenment. Your second book is all about this. Yet, it seems that in establishing set ideas about how it occurs, such as shifting to the fourth dimension, dark night of the soul, deliverance, etc., and saying that this is the only way it happens in all cases, is itself a creation of new concepts. You may be getting rid of some old concepts, but aren't you creating new ones?*

NADEEN: First of all, every single word out of my mouth is a concept, meaning that whatever I can say, the opposite is also just as true. That is the universal law of polarity that defines the third dimension. I would never, ever say that the norms we talk about in this shift are "the only way" it can happen. Source loves diversity and contrast. Anything is possible. What the book describes are general norms that happen to most people caught up in this shift.

JLW: *Is there anything else that you would like to add?*

NADEEN: In my life within my own shift, which is over six years now of deliverance, I am more and more grateful every day for whatever it is that keeps cranking up the awe and passion in my life. This is the understanding and knowing everyday that there is a process going on within me of embracing life as it happens. This is not something that I can do. It is just happening more and more. Embracing life just as it is and watching this mind that was going crazy in the beginning with objections, fade into almost nothing. Life is so funny and so simple. The real mystery of life lies in its simplicity, not in its complexity.

This is so simple that people can't believe it. You would never have looked here in the middle of contractions for perfect happiness. You would have looked in fixing the suffering of others or in fixing your own suffering as the logical place to go. Then when you embrace the events of life just as they are, life has a way of turning right around and provides you with your own happiness from within. This is the most surprise ending you could ever put in a comic book about the soap opera of life.

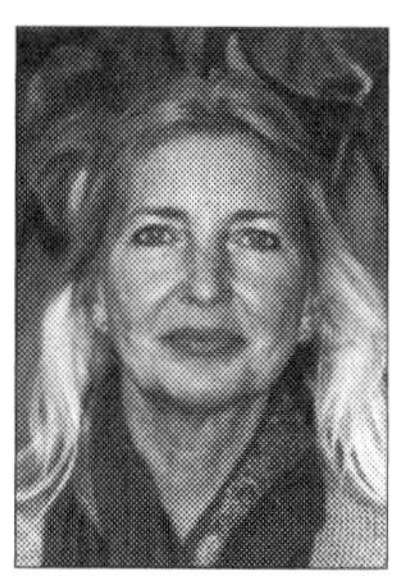

MIRA PAGAL

"NO ONE HAS TO BE READY FOR FREEDOM BECAUSE THEY ARE IT. THEY DON'T HAVE TO THINK, 'THIS IS NOT FOR ME.' NO, THEY CAN REALLY HAVE A GLIMPSE, JUST NOW, WHILE HEARING ABOUT IT. TIME IS URGENT NOW...IT IS NOW POSSIBLE."

Mira is a beautiful expression of the Truth that we all are essentially. She is an embodiment of this Truth in an ordinary and humble form. Mira is almost continuously joyous and expresses unconditional love for everyone she meets. We felt truly loved and accepted as we sat with her. Something inside naturally relaxes and lets go in the presence of such a being. Mira sees others clearly, as they are, awake and free. She once said, "When I look out at people in satsang, all I see is free beings." Because of this, contact with Mira is very empowering.

With the bright, clear eyes of a child, Mira's warm inclusive embrace, earthy laughter, and her unmoving truthfulness made this conversation thoroughly delightful. In her satsangs, she responds to questions very simply from her heart. But it is her loving presence and the silence of the heart which emanates from her that touches people. Her Master, Poonjaji, was right in saying he foresaw her inspiring the world.

Mira's life truly is an inspiration. Her unrelenting dedication to the truth led her to leave everything at age twenty to follow her longing and search for a teacher. Since meeting and recognizing Poonjaji as her Master, her life has been dedicated to him and the Truth he revealed. She had a long-standing close relationship with this great Master as a disciple and a wife.

Mira appears to be one of the rare few who has taken her spiritual journey to its end. She wanted only complete freedom, nothing less. In his biography, Poonjaji comments on meeting Mira: "I recognized the fire in her, the fire for freedom. That fire is very rare. I don't see it on many faces, but after one look at this girl I could see that she had fully dedicated her life to finding freedom."

CONVERSATION *with* MIRA PAGAL

LML: *John and I have been going to satsangs for many years and we started to notice that there is now a phenomenon of awakening occurring among Westerners.*
MIRA: Yes, this is happening now.

LML: *Something has shifted in the past five or ten years. So we wanted to write about that and speak with people who are experiencing awakening. The ones that are most accessible are those that are making themselves visible as teachers. As you know, prior to* *maybe ten years ago enlightenment was something that none of us really thought about. Even those of us who were meditating all the time—we didn't think it was possible! Or it was just for Easterners or Himalayan sadhus. But now it is coming to the West and this seems to be where it is happening.*

MIRA: Yes. Now we Westerners go to India and give satsang. When I went back there two months ago I felt, "This is incredible!" I went there searching thirty years ago, and now I go there to give satsang. I really feel it is an incredible time.

LML: *A number of the people we have spoken with are students of your Master, Poonjaji. He was such a big force in all this.*

MIRA: Yes. And he knew that too. He told me that he hadn't seen anything like the number of people waking up in his satsangs before. He told me that it was happening with Westerners.

JLW: *He knew that there was going to be a big awakening in the West?*

MIRA: Oh, yes. He knew it. I tell you, in 1976 or so he started to speak about that. He knew. Only Westerners were interested in his teaching. It would not be alive today if it weren't for the Westerners coming to him for this.

LML: *Why do you think the interest in awakening has shifted from the East to the West?*

MIRA: Well, we are kings from the material point of view. It is only to the king that this thought can come in the sense that we tried all that the senses and the outside world can give us.

JLW: *We have experienced it and found it didn't bring fulfillment.*

MIRA: Exactly. And in the East this is true only for an elite which is wealthy, and so in general, their minds are really craving to fulfill their material desires.

LML: *Even though their culture is so steeped in spiritual traditions?*

MIRA: Yes, but they make it a religion now.

JLW: *Can you explain what you mean when you distinguish a religion from a spiritual search?*

MIRA: Religion is something based on a belief; it is stiff. It doesn't ask you to have your own experience of what is indicated, of where the religion comes from. It is not alive; it is just a belief.

JLW: *You are saying there may be dogma, ritual, and lifestyle but no vitality, no living spirit that is directly experienced.*
MIRA: Exactly.

LML: *So, maybe another reason these teachings of awakening have become more alive in the West is that our culture isn't as steeped in religion and tradition as they are in the East.*
MIRA: Well, the sacredness is really inherent to humankind. So if you don't have a religion or your religion is not responsive to you, you have that need to find what is sacred in life, what is reality. And we are part of this generation that moved away from the empty rituals of our parents' religion as well as all the traditional structures and institutions of our culture.

JLW: *Yes. The sixties were a crack in human consciousness; we would not accept the habits of mind our parents' assumed and tried to hand off to us. And who knows why us? Why then?*
MIRA: It was a collective.

JLW: *It was a collective movement, and it is still a collective movement. This phenomenon that we are documenting is that same movement refined and revisited. It carries the same themes of universal love, equality, peace, and justice.*
MIRA: And it is funny; it does have a link because today it is the same revolution but more inner. Now we experience it at a deeper level. But in its first expressions we had to be rebellious. This same revolution has matured now.

LML: *It has matured to include a discovery or a waking up to who one truly is, to a freedom found within.*
MIRA: Perfect! This is the end of all. Discover this; only then can you live. Only then is the offering of whatever life presents to you seen simply as what it is. It is an enjoyment, too. It is not based on suffering as the religions told us. It can be based on what it is, and at times there is real divine enjoyment.

JLW: *What can you say about what it is you have discovered?*
MIRA: Not being separated from everything. In other words, in finding oneself, that sense of separation with all the rest is no longer real. Of course there is the play that you see differences, you are reacting and acting with differences, but the sense of separation is not there. It totally

changed the vision; the world is no more a world of danger. It makes all the difference, you see; everything comes from here, and all is included. For me, that was the biggest insight which changed all. All is included in this.

There are no more questions arising about what is life, what is the world, and who are you. Because it has been recognized that you are this beingness—it is hard to describe—it is the substratum. You are it. It is not that you became it, but you are it and you see that there is nothing apart from that.

LML: *There aren't any words to describe what that is.*
MIRA: It is absolutely indescribable. Not because it is an experience like indescribability, but it is indescribable because you are it. Whatever you describe, you separate. It is totally inherent to being.

LML: *Maybe you could tell us about your journey, how this awakening occurred for you.*
MIRA: Well, it is a long story because it is thirty years. But I will just tell the main points. I was searching desperately for freedom, enlightenment. In 1968, I decided to leave everything because that was my priority. I knew that I would recognize a master or that he would come to me. That determination, that faith was there. And in fact, it happened like this. He came to me.

A few days before I left, I was studying for my philosophy exams and I read Socrates' words, "Know yourself." It jumped in my heart like a tiger and spoke directly to me. I realized that I really didn't know myself and it was that knowing that I must search for. I left for Greece immediately, three days later. I went to find a living Socrates, a master who could show me who I am. I didn't even finish my exams. I could not wait. I dropped out of the university the same day I read Socrates' words. Three days later I was on the road hitchhiking to Greece. With onions, a bottle of wine and brown bread in a bag and sixty dollars, that was all. [Laughter]

JLW: *Amazing!*
MIRA: Times were like this in the sixties. I went and I was already quite impatient, because I had already asked my teachers of philosophy, and nobody could satisfy me. There, in Greece, I didn't meet anybody who could help. It was just philosophy always, or some religious mysticism, but somehow I knew it was not that. I felt, "So there is no living Socrates,

there is only a living Buddha then, and it is in India." So I continued on the road to India and went immediately to the Ganges.

I was given many addresses of gurus, but I didn't accept any of them because I knew it had to come from a recognition between us two. So I went to the Ganga in the Himalayas knowing that yogis live there. And after living with different yogis or saints for three months and learning their techniques, I was really puzzled about which method is true. I was wondering if the bhakti path was the true one or the jnana path, and so on. So, I decided to live in a cave just to digest and see for myself. My visa was finished after three months and my money was finished. I had only one rupee was left and a book of Kabir in my hand—nothing solved. I was blissful in meditation, but the search was not done.

With my last rupee I went to a chai shop and a man asked me if I needed any help understanding the Kabir poems and I said, "No thank you." I had had enough of people trying to help me. He said to me, "If you need me you can find me every morning at 5:00 AM by the banks of the Ganga." The next day I did my regular life which was washing clothes in the Ganga, meditating, and taking food in the ashram. But at night this man's face came in a dream and he said, "Perhaps I am the man you are searching for."

So, I went to the Ganga at 5:00 AM to meet him and he laughed and asked, "What do you want?" I said, "Cosmic consciousness or if you know more than that, I want that as well!" He said, "What do you do for that?" I said, "I meditate." "Show me." And I just closed my eyes; I don't know how long, and when I opened them I looked to the Ganga, the sky, a few birds, and to him... so simple. I had the insight that things are just as they are. Something that was so simple and obvious made itself known to me. Everything stopped, you know. Everything stopped. It was not a dramatic explosion. It was more like suddenly becoming aware of something that had always been there.

I recognized this man as my Master. I had the strong feeling that I had known him for a very long time and that I had just temporarily forgotten who he was. I knew that I had found the Master I had been looking for. Then he shocked me and said, "You can go now. You have got what you came for. You can go now." But I completely recognized him! I knew this man for so long! I mean I really recognized my Master. But he said, "No, you go. When you need help I will be there." I had to go. I did not know his name, and he didn't know my name—nothing. And I went. I had to go.

I was in a state of ecstasy. I was not in my senses. I was totally desperate that I was not with him and at the same time the insight was the fulfillment of my life. In ecstasy I went to the cave in the forest. But I became obsessed about being with this man and the only common knowledge we had was that spot by the Ganga. So, I decided to wait for him and live there until my death if it was needed. I lived there for eight months meditating and waiting for him. I had only one dress and one blanket. I was meditating only—very nearly not moving at all. I was in such an ecstatic state...

LML: *What determination!*

MIRA: Absolutely, yes. I was determined. Then one evening while looking at the Ganga and meditating, I turned my head and saw him coming. From that day on, he came to see me every day at about noon to give me food and answer my questions or just to sit together. Then one morning he woke me up very early and he said, "Today you can walk with me." We walked to the Phool Chatti ashram, and I was alone with him. I had to laugh because all these people were crossing the Master on the road and were not recognizing that Buddha was there! I started to understand that unless your eyes are open, you can't see this. So then life started to be lived with him all of the time.

LML: *You spent how many years with Poonjaji?*

MIRA: Poonjaji and I were together almost all the time up until 1976. I accompanied him on his first trip to the West in 1971 and several other trips. So, we were together in India and in the West. In 1976 our daughter had to be educated, so we decided to educate her in the West. But that was a dilemma because it meant a real physical separation. Then circumstances put me in Venezuela for five years, living quite a paradise life. I lived with one of Poonjaji's disciples who I fell in love with. I was always welcome to come and see the Master and received letters from him often. Then there was a letter that had one sentence that struck me. He said, "I wish you a very, happy, ordinary life." I felt that I had already had ordinary, happy lives and to be with the Master breaks that. So, I just left. After five years I left my ordinary, happy life. I went back to India to visit the Master and then went to Belgium to be alone and to educate my daughter and work.

JLW: *What kind of work did you do?*

MIRA: I did several kinds of work. There was a big problem because I didn't have a diploma. And I didn't know Flemish and to get a job in Belgium you have to know French and Flemish. And I was thirty-five years old, which was at that time too old to get a job. There was an economical crisis. So, I worked with a friend of mine who was a doctor as a secretary, then I worked for old people, and again as a secretary at a school. Five years later in 1981 I visited the Master. I always wanted to come, but he said, "No, I will come to the West." And somehow I always believed him, but five years past so I decided, "I go!" It was perfect. When I met him in 1986 there was already a big change because he started to become well-known. And we were no more the holy family that we were before. I was no more coming to him as an intimate relationship. I was a disciple, and our child was accompanying me to see her father, but in totally different conditions than it had been before.

LML: *You had a unique experience. You were not only his disciple, but you had a personal, intimate relationship with him as well.*

MIRA: Yes, I had a child with him. But this changed. I can say that I had golden days up until 1981. Then it was quite a strong challenge to go to work in the West in 1981. I was absolutely not prepared for this. To be away physically from him! But we had a very tight correspondence. We wrote a lot, and he replied to me always.

Then in 1986 he became a Zen master with me. It was really the dark night of the soul. I was no more recognized as a close intimate; I was one of the many. I started to have a deep, new understanding of his teaching. I remember that at that time what struck me was that if you see light it's because you keep darkness in you. That was an extraordinary understanding. Whatever I could experience, it was based on its opposite. It was a big thing to see that. I began to see the falseness or relativeness of all experience—of even the experience of freedom.

Then at the end of 1991, something started to happen on a bus. I had an insight and all revelation started to pour out like a volcano. Revelations came which describe what the past, present, and future is about. So, I had to get off the bus and I had a big fear that I would not be able to do that. There I saw, "Oh, the mind is tricky." I saw that the thing to do was to surrender that fear. I just got off the bus. So, that was quite a good experience to see that mind wants to spoil even the perfect moments.

Then I started to write many times a day to the Master describing those revelations to him. It started in December 1991 and lasted until February 1992. And for the first time, the Master never replied to my letters. I wanted some confirmation, but he never replied. I had to go to him. In February 1992 I went there, and I was in a kind of samadhi. The month I spent with him then was the most sweet, beautiful time I had ever had with him. I was in a natural samadhi — nobody could notice, but I was in that.

When I came back to Belgium I realized, "It's not yet That." I saw that I still was not completely free. I wrote to the Master and said that finally I want to finish this journey completely. Then he phoned me, which he never did, and he requested something very hard for me. He requested that I leave my daughter to come be with him. Because in February during that beautiful time with him I told him, "Only one thing remains which is my attachment to my daughter in this world." At the moment I said that my hair stood up on my skin because I knew that he would touch that. He didn't touch it at that moment, but a few months later he made this request. That was the challenge of my life! You have to understand; I am a two on the Enneagram. I am very motherly. I had to choose. But you know, even a child is illusion, is maya. So, I decided to obey him and to leave everything to go be with him.

LML: *How old was your daughter at that time?*

MIRA: She was old enough to be by herself. She was nineteen. But she was not having an easy time, and she needed me badly. It was not appropriate as a mother for me to leave. But I decided to obey. At one point I had my ticket in my hand, and I asked that if there is any reality it has to show up now because this was too hard for me to do. It just didn't seem possible to leave and I also felt it was not a good example to the world to abandon my daughter, even for the sake of Truth. And you know what happened? I lay down, and I went through all the layers of whatever is in oneself, and at some point I really died. The moment I got up to sit, only this small movement, I really realized that attachment is just the mind's twisted translation for love; it doesn't exist. So, I phoned the Master and told him my insight and said, "I do not need to come." But I was full of gratitude for this understanding, and I asked if I could come and see him for only fifteen days. And he said, "yes," so I came for only fifteen days.

It was from October 1992 to March 1993 that I was in Belgium taking care of our daughter, Mukti. She needed it at that time. Then for twenty-three days in 1993 again this volcano of revelations came out. I could not sleep. I wrote down what came up; then it left me. I had thought that this is enlightenment. But then I again said, "It's not yet That!" It was still not the final completion. Then I became very quiet. No more experience came to me. Nothing, totally nothing. I became very happy, totally free, no problem. The search was totally gone.

Then in 1995, I wanted to pay my respects to the Master and to serve him. I was totally detached from my own story then. So, I went to India for two months to serve him, and he allowed me; he really fulfilled this wish. When I came back to Belgium, everything was perfect. My personal story was finished, and there was no trace. So, when he left his body, I did not expect that something else could happen. But somehow, when he left his body it was a reunion, total reunion. The first impact was when I met him for the first time and then also when he left his body. In between those times was just a burning. It was a burning up of all that I thought I was.

LML: *It may not be possible to describe that reunion, but if you would try, at the time of the Master's death what occurred? And was this the final completion?*

MIRA: Yes, it was final. After his death I couldn't speak for three months. When finally I spoke again, I didn't come back to the previous life I knew. And I have never come back since then. Life totally changed. Life took care of me, and I didn't have a personal life anymore at all. The seeker went away completely and also at the moment of his departure, I felt a tremendous urgency to listen to what he always indicated to me. One sentence came, "Dedicate a quarter of a second to yourself," which was done and the entire structure of myself changed. I also felt that my karma was burned with his ashes, and I really, really realized what was meant by "Now." That is all I can say…

JLW: *I have a question. What in your opinion happened to some of Papaji's first Western disciples who became teachers? It seems that a few of them have gone astray into the ego.*

MIRA: You see, when you get a glimpse of the Truth, even if this glimpse doesn't look like a glimpse because you abide in it, it's a very, very critical period. If you immediately go and teach and don't stay quietly with your master, or give some time, maybe months, maybe years — it depends on each individual — to just keeping quiet, it can create problems. Don't teach! Don't teach! You need to ground.

I know of one case of a person, who the Master really loved and said, "You are my son." But he went away and didn't come back because it seemed that all was fulfilled. It's so tricky. It was my luck to spend so much time with the Master. I even indirectly heard the Master say, "Mira cannot be washed away because she spent those years with me." It means something. In India there is a tradition about this. I have seen that in most the cases, one has to be very vigilant. I've seen too many washed away because for me, they left too early. When you have that glimpse, mind may be totally burned or some very tiny layer of a latent tendency may be there. So, after some time if you don't keep quiet, these tendencies become stronger.

LML: *What's beautiful about your story is that you refused to settle for anything less than the total freedom.*
MIRA: I could not settle. It was impossible. I could not. And I tell you, when Papaji left the body, I was totally left by myself. Then someone asked me to give satsang, and I said yes. The yes was out of my mouth before I realized it. I didn't want to fall into that trap of teaching.

LML: *So, Papaji did not ask you to teach?*
MIRA: No, never. Well, I can say that he said a few sentences. He said, "I will never make you a teacher, but I want you to inspire the world." And when he asked me to leave my daughter and I told him my experience, he said, "It was a bit too early to ask you this, but I will come to your own house with the bowl and the robe." [In the Zen tradition when the search is completed the master sends the monk out of the monastery bestowing the bowl and the robe.] And when he left his body, I was not with him. I was at home in Brussels. He said this to me in September 1995, and he left his body in September 1997.

JLW: *You've given satsang in the U.S., Europe, and India...*
MIRA: Yes. And I will go to a few other countries next year.

JLW: *Have you discovered in your travels that more people are awakening?*

MIRA: Yes. There are people coming to satsang now who are free beings. And I never saw that years ago with Papaji. In those days nobody who went to see him was already free. But people have been to see masters now, and if it didn't happen when they saw a master, it happened later. I see that more and more. And I see that people are having glimpses. No doubt. No doubt. What they do with that, I don't know. But, it's wonderful. When I was with Papaji I saw this also. People were getting glimpses like popcorn.

LML: *But is it still rare that people take that glimpse and deepen it until they fully embody it?*
MIRA: Yes, this is still rare. But it is less rare.

LML: *There are also many people longing, yearning for freedom.*
MIRA: Yes, and I believe that nature balances because more insanity is also here.

JLW: *The shadow is being revealed more and more. We see that everyday. But the light is coming to the foreground as well.*

LML: *What do you have to say to those people who are longing for freedom?*
MIRA: They just need to hear this Truth. They don't have to be ready. Maybe it's because of these special times we live in, I don't know, but no one has to be ready for freedom because they are it. They don't have to think, "This is not for me." No, they can really have a glimpse, just now, while hearing about it. Time is urgent now. We are in Kali Yuga. It is now possible.

LML: *They might wonder how. How can they have that glimpse?*
MIRA: Let them come to satsang to be in the presence of one who is free. Just by that presence or by a word, it will sink in their heart. And it will be enough.

LML: *Are you are saying that awakening is occurring more easily these days?*
MIRA: Yes, yes. It's needed. It's needed now.

JLW: *Many of the people we are encountering, including ourselves, have had glimpses, sometimes very profound experiences, and there is a deep desire to give everything to That, to abide as That and to be free of the latent tendencies that arise. What do you have to say to those of us who are intent on stabilizing in Truth?*

MIRA: Not to worry if any tendency arises. You cannot control that; and, in fact, it doesn't stain your Self. You still abide. You still abide. Remove the belief that vasanas should not be arising. Don't be thinking that they should not be there. You cannot control this. Just don't be swept away by them.

LML: *You are speaking of an acceptance of everything as it is, including the vasanas...*
MIRA: Yes, surrender to what is.

JLW: *Yet, part of "what is" is a tremendous amount of suffering in our world... what can be done about this?*
MIRA: Yes, my God. [said with great compassion] But, you see, when a saint is passing by there is a fresh breeze even when he walks in hell. So, let's awaken. And I would like to say that it is important that the children in the world hear of this Truth. They should hear once. They should hear this Truth once. Not as a teaching, telling them everyday, "You are That." No. Once is enough so that the seed is there. Then they can remember one day. This is very important. So, it has to be introduced in families and in education.

LML: *What do you see as the main obstacle to awakening for Westerners today?*
MIRA: Thinking! Wanting to understand. Wanting to grasp it with the mind. The discrimination should be there, you have to have very clear intention and have a good mind, but at some point to realize your own being, the understanding has to leave you. At some point, this has to let go into silence. That's all.

JLW: *It is recognized in silence and yet, it can be experienced even if thoughts are moving.*
MIRA: Yes, of course. People have these ideas about how you can't function in the world if you don't think. It's not like that.

LML: *This is a common misunderstanding of Papaji's teaching, "Be quiet."*
MIRA: Yes, I know. I have to clear this often in satsang.

LML: *In closing, is there anything that you would like to say to seekers?*
MIRA: As Papaji said, it is really the birthright of everyone — everyone, let it be a rascal, let it be a saint — to be free from ignorance, from suffering. Let each one rest in his or her own natural beauty.

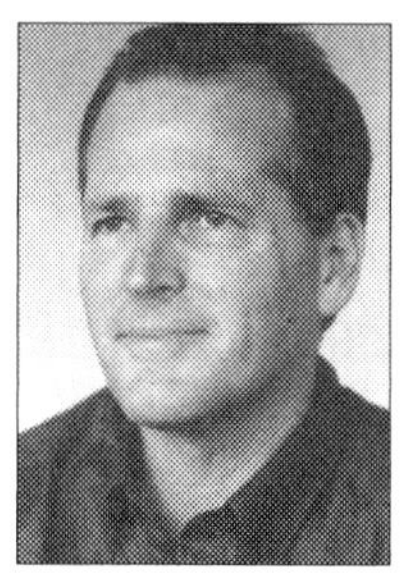

PETER FENNER

"IF WE TUNE IN RIGHT NOW TO THIS MOMENT, THERE IS NOTHING, ABSOLUTELY NOTHING MISSING...IT SIMPLY CAN'T BE ENHANCED ANY FURTHER BECAUSE THERE IS NOTHING TO ENHANCE. IF WE ARE GOING TO USE THE TERM 'AWAKENING,' THIS IS WHAT I AM REFERRING TO."

When a friend of ours first invited us to an evening dialogue with Peter Fenner in 1996, she couldn't really say what he did. She did, however, assure us that it would be interesting. We did indeed find Peter interesting as well as a little disconcerting. Within minutes the ideas and beliefs we had woven together concerning our spiritual and psychological insights and development were shown to be flimsy concepts that we had taken to be real and solid. We repeatedly found ourselves with no place to stand and nothing to hold onto. Yet, there was something very refreshing about entering into dialogue with this man. Although it can be frightening, it is quite freeing to see the long held beliefs that have formed your reality just pop like bubbles.

We continued to attend Peter's courses and evening dialogues whenever he came to the Bay Area, and he also became our friend. We found that Peter's presence, perceptive distinctions, and willingness to confront anyone's most preciously held conceptions was a little startling and somehow quite attractive. Although we would be hard pressed to succinctly describe what his approach of "deconstructive contemplation" is, suffice it to say that an encounter with him reveals mental constructions to be both true and false and neither true nor false, leaving only the emptiness of being and then deconstructing any ideas that we may have formed about that.

We have had the pleasure and benefit of watching Peter's work deepen and expand during the time we have known him. We have observed him "doing" less and less as a teacher and just "being" more. Simply being in the unbiased and open space he creates opens up the same possibility for those sitting with him.

Peter was a Tibetan Buddhist monk for nine years. He is the author of several books and has taught Buddhism at institutes and universities for over twenty years. He is the founder of Timeless Wisdom, which offers workshops and retreats. He has designed a practical programs that translate the essential wisdom of Asian spiritual traditions into contemporary Western frameworks. Peter lives in Australia and teaches in Europe and the United States.

CONVERSATION *with* PETER FENNER

LML: *We'd like to ask about your unfolding, the story of your journey. We know that for some people there seems to have been a dramatic shift that they can pinpoint in time when something occurred for them. They'll say, "This is when this recognition occurred, and it has never been the same since." And for other people, there was a gradual wearing away of old constructions and at some point there was a recognition that things were different from how they used to be, but they don't know exactly when that happened. How has it been for you?*

PETER: My journey?

LML: *Yes, the exploration of who you truly are.*

PETER: The truth is that I really don't know what has brought me to this point on my "path." My interest is more focused on what is happening now. I'm wondering what "this" is.

LML: *What do you mean by that?*

PETER: Well, we're sitting here talking, but is this all that's happening? There are sounds, colors, feelings—the movement—but something else is happening that can't be identified, that can't be located. There's an immediacy and a freshness to this that we can't point to. It isn't sensory. Yet, without all of this happening, it doesn't exist. This is alive and vital and vibrant, but at the same time it is continuous and uniform, like space. And whatever this is, it can't come into existence—nor can it disappear—because it doesn't exist in the same way that other things do.

This is why the non-dualistic spiritual traditions say that the experience of presence or awakening can't be gained or lost. This experience has no structure, so there's nowhere for it to go. It can't be enhanced or degraded. Nonetheless, for me this experience does come and go. This is the wonderful paradox. At some point this experience seems to stop. At some point I suddenly think, "I'm not there; I'm not in the nothingness that is everything. I don't feel as spacious and clear as I was a few minutes ago." I look back on this "nothing" and think that this was "something." I think that I have lost something quite incredible.

But also, as the years go by it becomes easier and easier to re-enter this space where "nothing is missing." I have some methods of inquiry that help to re-activate the experience. Sharing this space with others also strengthens the experience. Overall, I think it's a question of becoming more and more familiar with a pressureless and problem-free way of being. At a more practical level, access to the state is also a function of learning how to live in the world so we don't make problems for others or ourselves. So that is my "spiritual story."

LML: *You say you don't know how this ease of being came to be in your life, yet you have a history of extensive spiritual study and practice.*

PETER: Yes, I do, but I don't know how much of that has actually contributed to the process of "transcending the conditioned mind." When I began my search, I sought out a path that was predicable and well mapped out. I needed to know that I was on an absolutely foolproof path to the total eradication of suffering. I studied and practiced the "stages on the path" as these are described in Mahayana Buddhism. The Buddhist path gave me confidence and trust, but I'm sure it also supported my basic insecurities. It must have because I was constructing a path designed to fulfill my "needs." I was attached to the path and this stopped me entering the space where everything drops away and there is nothing to strive for.

My study and practice of Tibetan Buddhism has definitely contributed to my journey, but a lot of the real learning has also come through the challenges of parenting, teaching, and especially my relationships with my spiritual teachers. I still recognize a preference for a safe and sanitized spiritual path and continue to be challenged by situations that reveal my desires and expectations. More and more I see what is meant by the Vajrayana expression that "the world is our guru." And more and more I see that the only effective practice is to be authentic in the moment with whatever resources are available to us.

LML: *This requires learning to trust the unknown.*

PETER: Ultimately it involves going beyond trust and reaching the space where nothing can go right or wrong. In some ways our need to trust in the unknown is just another dimension of the search for security. In the unknown there is no need for trust because there is no one to be helped or harmed and nothing to help or harm us.

JLW: ... *You were saying that being present and authentic seems to be more useful than searching for another tool or device in the face of life presenting you with situations that went beyond your study and training. How does this experience of authenticity relate to that sense of well being in which nothing is missing?*

PETER: By "authentic" I mean that we are simply who we are, without any complication or contrivance. We learn to be with ourselves without any trace of pretense or embarrassment. In the Complete Fulfillment or Dzogchen tradition this is spoken about as discovering our "natural condition." We aren't preoccupied at all with who we are, so our identity, in fact, our very existence ceases to be a concern for us. We are so free of problems that we are simply not in the picture. We become completely integrated with our environment so there is no division between our self and others. We are nothing and everything at the same time.

JLW: *Some people say that the experience of being an individual is an illusion.*

PETER: But this is an illusion too. If we ignore our conditioning, if we deny the fact that we have a particular psychophysical structure and live in a particular culture, we reject our own unique path to awakening. Everyone's natural condition is different. The fact that we have different bodies and different histories guarantees this. It is natural for some people to have a high profile. It is also completely natural for others to live in relative obscurity. By accepting who we are without any pretense or embarrassment, we release ourselves from all preoccupations about who we are. Then we can connect with our natural condition as boundless, unstructured consciousness.

LML: *Our karmic conditioning continues to unfold as it should—and much more freely—when we stop struggling with it.*

PETER: Just as it is unfolding now. From one point of view this is conditioned. We are speaking in English and through human bodies, but this conditioning in no way interferes with the experience of unconditioned consciousness. We are aware that in the midst of this conversation, nothing is also happening.

JLW: *Yes, what a paradox that so much is going on, this whole display is occurring, and simultaneously, nothing is happening.*

Peter, as you know, self-inquiry is a key element in most, if not all, of the essential paths. The acceptance of who we are, it seems, must follow on some kind of inquiry into who we are, really. Does inquiry play a part in your work?

PETER: When I first began teaching I used a very penetrating form of inquiry that was inspired by the powerful deconstructive methods of Madhyamika Buddhism. These days in my work, the deconstruction of people's problems and fixations seems to happen much more easily and often without any intervention on my part. When I sit with people it seems to stimulate a type of natural koan inquiry into the nature of the present experience. I don't impose questions on the group; the questions seem to arise naturally as people move into less structured states of consciousness. Sometimes the inquiry happens in the open—in the public space—but increasingly it happens as a silent mind-to-mind communication with people.

LML: *From what you have said so far, it seems that for you awakening means to be fully present with who you are in the moment, to be authentic and present with whatever is occurring, just as it is.*
PETER: If we tune in right now to this moment, there is nothing, absolutely nothing missing. It is beyond deficiency or plenitude, and beyond perfection or imperfection. It simply can't be enhanced any further because there is nothing to enhance. If we are going to use the term "awakening," this is what I'm referring to. Awakening is just "this" and I don't know what this is.

JLW: *When you say awakening is "this," and you don't know what "this" is... what I see in you is an alert presence in the face of the incomprehensibility of the present moment.*
PETER: You are trying to make sense of this. You are trying to understand or "know" it. You are also locating this experience outside of yourself.

All I can do at this point is share my stream of consciousness with you. When you ask the question, "What is this?" the question echoes in my mind: "What is this?" but there is no answer. No response is formulating in my mind.

Right now at the level of sensation we are fully present to each other, but something is also happening that is completely beyond thought and totally indescribable.

JLW: *I know that many people are longing for this indescribable space beyond thought and may not know how to find that. What can you say to them?*
PETER: The first thing to be aware of is that the experience people are finally seeking turns out to be totally different from what they think it is. Whatever we might think about awakening, those ideas dissolve along with all our concepts and needs. We are going to be left with nothing other than "what is."

Whatever we might think awakening is, that's only an idea, a projection. That thought has nothing to do with the experience that satisfies all seeking. At some point the lesson in this begins to dawn. We see that we aren't getting anywhere by trying to understand this so-called "state" of awakening. The grip of our intellect begins to loosen; we let go of the need to know what it is and how to get it. We relax and begin to let things be, just as they are. "Perhaps there is nowhere to go!"

As our emotions settle and our thoughts thin out, we begin to wonder where we are. It's clear that we are fully functional, but we also seem to be entering a space that cannot be known. We might think, "This is it." But we don't know what "this" is. We cannot know, because "it" isn't anything. In this way, people can easily enter into the state that is known by names such as "pure awareness," "witness consciousness," and "contentless wisdom." Once people have a taste of this, the next task is to deepen, expand, and prolong the experience. This deepening and expansion can involve a complete readjustment of our lifestyle and relationships. As they say in Zen, satori is just the beginning.

In cultivating this state, it can also be very helpful to share in the energy field that is offered by different teachers, such as those you are interviewing for this book. In different ways all of these people can help lift us out of the structures of consciousness that produce our problems and introduce us to a level of consciousness that transcends all pain and suffering.

LML: *It has been my experience with the work you do that you create a space that allows people's ideas and concepts to deconstruct.*

PETER: Yes that's what seems to happen. Basically I share a space of "unknowing" with people. People present their problems and beliefs about who they are, what shouldn't be happening to them, the spiritual path, enlightenment, and so on. I listen and respond from a space where I cannot discover what they are talking about.

At one level I'm very familiar with what people are saying because I have experienced similar problems and I've also studied psychology and Eastern philosophies quite extensively. But at the same time, I can't find anything solid or real in what people share with me. I can't find anything in my own experience that corresponds to what they're talking about—nothing. I'm available to be with people as they share their constructions and interpretations, but I don't hear any limitation or problem in what they are saying. I'd say it's neither a passive nor an active listening. I'm certainly not disinterested in what people share, but nor do I encourage or energize their constructions.

I provide a listening that stimulates a deep and gentle exploration of the reality of people's constructions. This exploration leads people into less structured states of consciousness. Their problems dissolve, and they enter a space that goes beyond the cycle of pleasure and pain. This is the state that is spoken about in non-dualistic traditions of Buddhism as "transcending the duality of bondage and liberation." We then work at deepening this experience and expanding it into our lives.

LML: *I have experienced this myself in working with you. In the space that you create, I saw that I had so many spiritual ideas and concepts about what awakening is, who I am, what I am supposed to be experiencing, and so on. It became apparent that they were empty ideas. I particularly remember believing that something was missing and then seeing "something is missing" as just another belief. This has allowed me to see more clearly what has never been missing.*

PETER: And what is happening now?

LML: *[Silence] I'm thrown back into the present moment. Nothing is happening now.*

PETER: I don't try to stop people's constructions or alleviate their problems. If you interfere in this way, people can easily become defensive, and this just prolongs their suffering. I never know how long someone will hang onto a limiting construction, and I'm not concerned. I create space around it and let it have its natural life span. When we don't interfere by imposing our own need about how things should be, the dissolution of problems comes about very quickly.

LML: *Your work is very unique. We haven't seen anything like it, and we have been with many teachers, both Western and Eastern. In some subtle and sometimes less subtle ways, by talking about the Truth, other teachers can't help but present concepts. This is not to say that what they are doing is not useful—it is—it's just different. The complete neutrality that you are expressing is not there in the same way. What you are doing in your teaching, if you can call it a teaching, is being a living expression of the teaching rather than talking about it. Much of the time spent with you is in silence. I also experience this silence and neutrality to be challenging. There is nothing in it for the ego. It is uncomfortable for the ego to neither be validated nor invalidated. It feels lost in the face of that.*

JLW: *One of the aspects of your work that I really enjoy is the way in which a natural silence just happens. Everything naturally falls off into silence and then just as naturally, without any force or tension, dialogue begins again, and then silence again. It's organic and effortless. There is a very beautiful quality about that.*

PETER: Yes, it is very smooth and natural. In part, I think this happens because I have no preference for whether we are in silence together or in public dialogue. Also, as you've experienced, the silence is very rich. I can feel people conversing with me, conversing with the space that is arising, without needing to talk. I am in deep communication with people in that silence.

LML: *To me, what you are describing about your work is the same as what I am learning about living life. To be at ease with life is to be in a place of neutrality with whatever experience arises, not to struggle with it, not try to get rid of it, not engage in it, just let it all be as it is.*

PETER: We do not have a model for what we should or shouldn't be doing… [Pause of silence]

JLW: *What happened just then? It's as if the energy for thinking just dissipated.*

PETER: Most of our thinking doesn't contribute to the quality of our lives. You could say it is an epiphenomenon or by-product of the attempt to establish a solid identity and give ourselves a point of reference and certainty.

LML: *Thinking maintains a sense of an individual, separate self.*

PETER: But, as we said earlier, being separate or one, it doesn't make any difference. I can be myself and not have any problems. How can I not be myself? If I try not to be myself, or to be no one, then I have a problem.

JLW: *Compared to the norm, it's radical to suggest that life is unproblematic, that we can simply be with whatever occurs.*

PETER: It's completely radical, and often surprising at first, because it's effortless, natural, and totally ordinary. Everything changes—it becomes impossible to construct, or even resurrect a problem—yet everything is exactly as it has always been.

The task you have set yourself with this series of interviews is interesting. I appreciate the dilemma you find yourselves in. It is beautiful. You feel some need to elicit information, descriptions, about this so-called state of awakening, but at the same time you sense, you know, that it is nothing. The question is how to share that dilemma, how to be present and honest to the paradox.

LML: *Right. That's what we're doing; talking about something we can't talk about.*
PETER: It is quite strange, isn't it? You sense that you're talking about nothing at all. At times it's quite an elaborate presentation of nothing, and you know that too! [Laughter] You're even making decisions about who has this nothing, and who hasn't!

LML: *I don't know how we can know whether or not someone knows that "nothing." It's an experience that happens in someone's presence, a knowing, but it's not describable how it occurs.*
PETER: I don't know why people come to sit and talk with me. They must think I have something to offer. They must know more than I do! [Laughter]

LML: *We have known you for several years now, and it seems to me, Peter, that you are more in a space of not knowing than ever before.*
PETER: I am experiencing a deeper, more profound unknown. I prefer to say unknown rather than not knowing. When we say not knowing it gives the idea that there's something to know that we're not getting. By unknown, I mean that there is nothing to know—it's the experience of knowing nothing. There is no interpretive thought, no meaning, and no understanding.

JLW: *It's not that you're not comprehending what a person is saying, but there is no interpretive response. Is that what you are saying?*
PETER: I understand, and I don't understand. At one level I identify with people's problems and achievements. I hear what they're saying. I understand what they would like me to understand, but I don't see what they are describing as a problem or an achievement. If they engage with me, they can also experience that they have no problems.

LML: *I think many people are afraid of awakening because they are afraid of the unknown. Have you experienced that fear?*
PETER: Yes. We fear being who we are. We fear the destruction of our ideas and fantasies about spiritual awakening. We fear the possibility of

having nothing more to "work on." We prefer the experience of loss and gain, rather than going beyond the cycle of conditioning.

LML: *Again, it's a paradox. Awakening is both ordinary and extraordinary.*
PETER: Yes. Awakening is natural. It is also completely uneventful. There is nothing to write home about, nothing to prove, nothing to take credit for. And it is totally extraordinary because in this state we see that we have never suffered and will never suffer again.

LML: *Even though it's still rare, would you say that there are more people interested in awakening these days?*
PETER: In the West, certainly. But the experience we are talking about is still extremely rare. Even tasting it is rare. Most people on the planet can't relate to what we are talking about right now. But in the West, more and more people are experiencing the bliss of unstructured consciousness. When I sit with people here in California, and in Europe, and Australia, I'm profoundly aware of the tremendous amount of work that people have done, in working with their emotions and purifying their minds, to the point that they can enter the space that removes the very possibility of suffering.

I feel a tremendous sense of respect and gratitude to people for this preparatory work because it lets me work with people at a quite refined and subtle level in dismantling the beliefs that block a clean experience of pure consciousness. I'm deeply touched when I join people in the mutual recognition that we are sharing exactly the same state of pure, unstructured awareness. In this experience, the details of our respective journeys become irrelevant. Our paths may have taken us to Indian ashrams and Himalayan monasteries, or we may have journeyed the path through our work and relationships. Our journeys may have been rough and arduous, or smooth and gentle, but here, history dissolves in the mutual awareness that there is nowhere we have come from and nowhere else to go.

And of course I include you both in this experience. I really appreciate how easily we can join in this space together and enjoy the freedom of "going beyond the need to know." Thank you both very much.

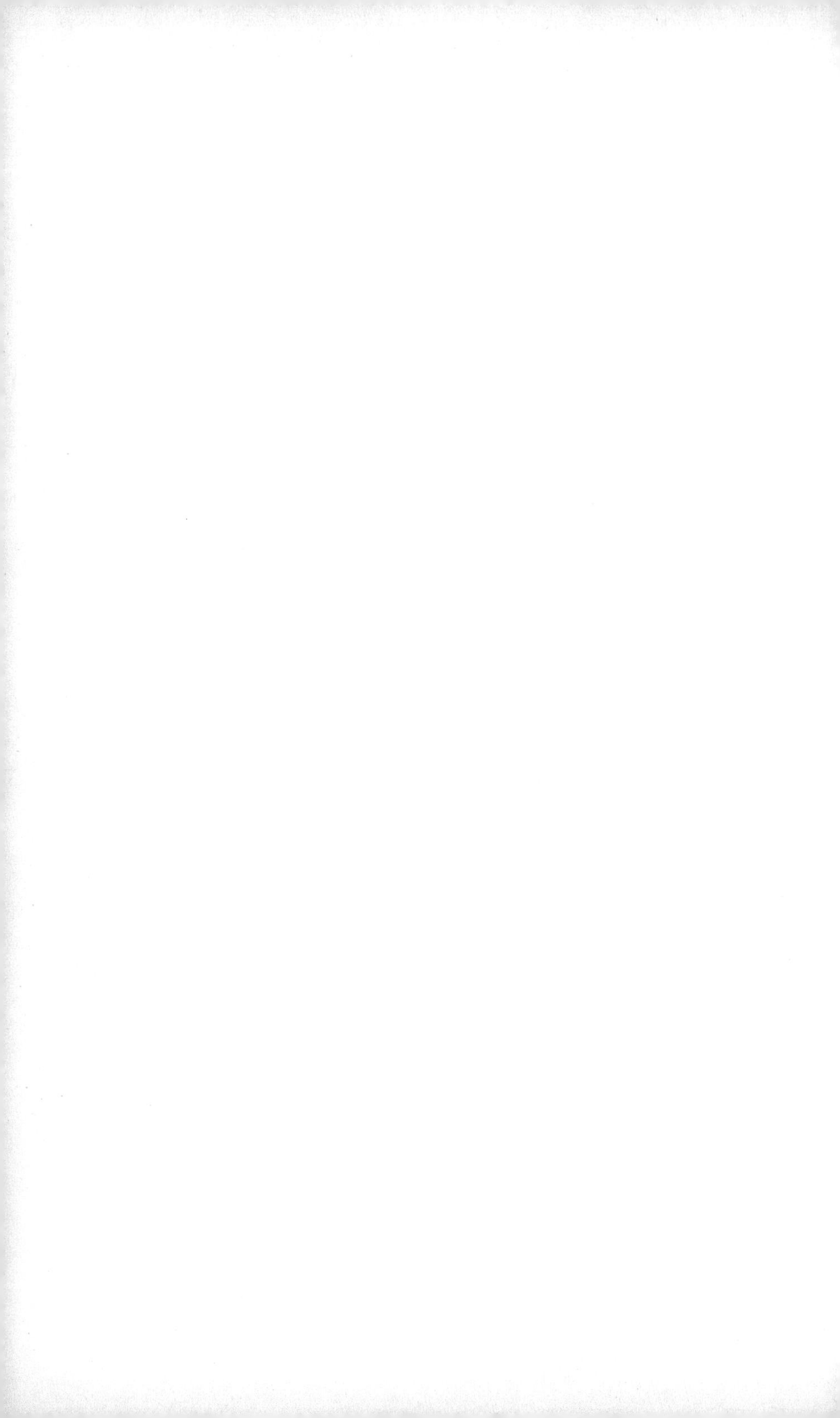

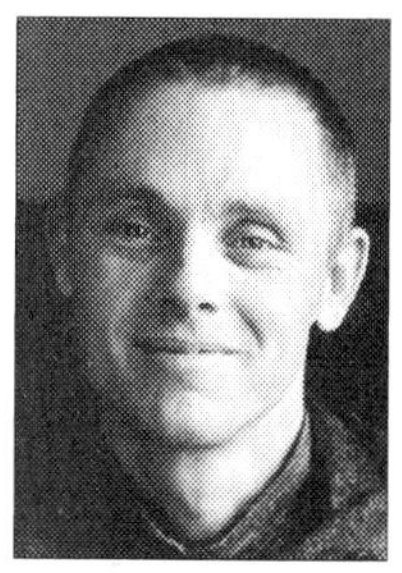

ADYASHANTI

"STOP ALL DELAYS, ALL SEEKING AND ALL STRIVING. PUT DOWN YOUR CONCEPTS, IDEAS, AND BELIEFS. FOR ONE INSTANT BE STILL AND DIRECTLY ENCOUNTER THE SILENT UNKNOWN CORE OF YOUR BEING. IN THAT INSTANT, FREEDOM WILL EMBRACE YOU AND REVEAL THE AWAKENING YOU ARE."

Adyashanti truly exemplifies the primordial peace that his name denotes. He was born Steven Gray and raised in a loving family in the northern California suburbs. For many, the yearning for Truth is born out of a life of suffering, but Adyashanti had a happy childhood and a very "normal" life. Yet, for some reason, there was a burning, passionate desire for Truth. He frequently had experiences of awakening beginning in childhood but kept these experiences to himself. In fact his journey was very much a solo one. Although he studied with two Zen teachers, he relied on and trusted only his own direct experience. As a young man, he became quite dedicated to his Zen practice, which he was involved in for fifteen years. His first major awakening occurred at the early age of twenty-five. This awakening deepened for eight years before his teacher asked him to teach.

Many of those we have interviewed have been our teachers, and we are grateful to them all. However, this interview is special to us because Adyashanti has become out primary teacher. In our admittedly biased opinion, he is extraordinary and exceptional. Although an unassuming man, his embodiment of freedom is evident. Out of this embodiment comes an impeccable integrity and tremendous love.

Adyashanti is also an exceptional teacher. When his teacher asked him to teach, she told him that "teaching is in his blood." We experience this to be true. He has a way of meeting each person where they are at with great compassion, clarity, and precision. This invites the student to relax into a profound acceptance and insight into themselves. Adyashanti speaks only from his own direct experience and his most powerful teaching is his presence and example.

Adyashanti worked as a machinist at the time of this interview. He now teaches full-time and lives in Los Gatos, California with his wife Annie.

CONVERSATION *with* ADYASHANTI

LML: *At the core of all spiritual seeking is the question "Who am I?" As far as we know, that inquiry was extremely rare in the beginning of this century. Now, as we are at the turn of the century, this inquiry is becoming more popular, particularly in the Western world. So, we'd like to begin with what, if any, answer you have found to that question.*

ADYASHANTI: Aware space. [Silent pause] I am aware space—that same aware space that gives rise to everything that is.

LML: *Could you say more about this aware space?*

ADYASHANTI: Aware space just is. It's just consciousness, without that consciousness taking a form. Before it takes a form, it is just awake. Everybody shares the same fact of being awake. We all know, "I'm awake." Everybody knows they are awake, except when they are asleep. But most people go on to define themselves. They define themselves as what that awakeness sees, thinks, and feels. I think that finding out who you are is simply not taking that step to define yourself. It is finding the awakeness before any definition, or before what the awakeness sees.

I think the "Who am I?" question is a step backwards into that awakeness away from what we see and perceive and into the mere fact of awakeness itself. To call it awakeness, of course, diminishes it greatly because this limits it to something almost static. But it is that awakeness that is the source of everything that is manifest—worlds and human beings, thoughts, emotions, cars, and plants, and animals—everything. When that formless awakeness takes form, that is the world, the universe and all its contents. So, in that sense, it's very pregnant with an infinite number of possibilities, but, in and of itself, it is empty of all qualities.

LML: *As I have heard you say many times, people get confused about the question "Who am I?" in that they think there is supposed to be an answer to that question.*

ADYASHANTI: The answer to "Who am I" is when you burn the question out so that there's literally not a question anymore. You couldn't possibly answer the question with any words or thoughts or feelings, or even any experiences. When the question has worn itself out to that degree, then there's the absence of even the question. And when there's an absence of the question, then there's an absence of the questioner, the separate somebody or me. Then, what is left is what you are, and that's undefinable.

JLW: *But it can be called aware space.*

ADYASHANTI: Yes, it can be called aware space. Or it could be called consciousness, or spirit. In the West it might be called pure spirit.

JLW: *The terms awakening, enlightenment, and self-realization have been applied to the recognition you are speaking of. What do these terms mean to you?*

ADYASHANTI: To me they mean different things. To me, awakening is awakening "out of" what we are not. When you finally find out everything that you're not, what you're left with is what I am calling aware space. So, when you awaken out of the identification as a separate individual, that is awakening. I personally don't call that awakening, in and of itself, enlightenment. To me, enlightenment or the term I often use, liberation, is when that awakening has become a permanent state of being. Usually, when people have that awakening they do not stay awake, they keep contracting back into the identification with the personal. To be liberated, or truly enlightened, one is no longer contracting back into the personal. It is when, to the core of their being they know that they are that awakeness, or aware space. They have left the personal behind.

JLW: *This is when you see that everything is who one is, everything is the Self.*

ADYASHANTI: Yes, because that aware space is where everything returns back to the One. Everything turns back to its source. That source is always the same. It's much the same as saying that the substance of every wave is water. Every wave is exactly the same as every other wave, in its most fundamental nature. It's all the same source. In the appearances, it appears to be different. Each wave has a different appearance. The appearances themselves are beautiful and as soon as you realize that you are not the appearances, then you are free to enjoy the appearances without getting lost.

LML: *So, you are making a distinction between awakening and liberation.*

ADYASHANTI: Yes, but it doesn't necessarily need to be a distinction, because one can awaken and not contract back into a sense of a personal self. But, usually this does happen to some extent. When you are actually liberated, the awakeness is exactly the same as when you awaken. In that sense, it's no different except that the liberated person has ceased to contract. That awakeness has ceased to contract back down into a misidentification of an individual "I." Then what you are liberated from is that contraction. That's what you are liberated from.

LML: *There is a common belief that awakening is something that occurs all at once, then it's finished.*

ADYASHANTI: Yes, but in most cases that doesn't happen to be true. That belief is the source of endless confusion and misunderstanding. A gradual letting go of whatever is left of the tendency to contract into a personal "I" often follows the sudden awakening. Often times, that process is something that's more gradual and happens over time. It doesn't need to happen over time; it just usually does. Even if it does happen over time, it can come to a final completion. That completion is what I mean by liberation.

LML: *Is that completion of coming to liberation still relatively rare?*
ADYASHANTI: Yes, as far as I know, it is relatively rare. The reason I say that is because one can even have no more tendency to contract into a personal "I" and actually have that become a permanent condition, and in that sense be liberated, but to me, even that's not really enough. That's not the full expression because one can do that and still have the personality that's in the relative world of time and space not express that. The personality could still express that liberation in a very distorted way, and often does. That is how we can end up with people, oftentimes teachers, that can actually have a very powerful and pure teaching and be able to help people, but yet their daily life, in ways they move in time and space, do not reflect that realization. I continue to find that it is extremely rare for that realization to be reflected in daily life. This is rare because it demands everything. It demands one's entire life. It even demands one's personality. It demands the end of all excuses. It demands that you not make any excuses anymore for acting other than from that liberation. It seems like very few people are willing to do this.

LML: *This is what you call the full embodiment of liberation.*
ADYASHANTI: Yes that is the full embodiment. To me, what we are speaking about is actually the evolution of consciousness itself. This human drama is not a mistake. It is so often implied in Eastern teachings that this human life is somehow a mistake or some second class act. I don't see it that way at all. Consciousness, or aware space, has come into form for a reason. It has come into form so that it can be conscious through a form. That's the beauty of the human birth. Consciousness can become self-aware through this human form. It can not only become self-aware, but can finally manifest that liberation through the form, through the humanness, in the way that we act in the field of space and time.

So, to me, just to be liberated from being a human being is not enough. The consciousness or spirit or aware space itself literally has an impulse, or you might say an urge, to manifest itself in the world of time and space. Why? I don't know. But it certainly seems to be the case. This is where so many fall short. They think that just to have the realization is where it's all at. To me, it's being able to have that realization function in the world of time and space that's truly important and the true call of the evolution of consciousness.

JLW: *When you ask why consciousness manifests in the world of time and space, what comes to me is that it's for the experience of the expression of love.*

ADYASHANTI: Absolutely. That's beautiful. Ultimately, the manifestation is a creation. It's a birthing. It's an act of love, as you say. It's not some horrendous mistake that we need to escape from into some transcendental state as quickly as possible. That is the ultimate dualism. And yet, so many of the non-dual teachers teach this incredible dualism. And of course they make all sorts of excuses for why they do it, and seemingly really good excuses. But, nonetheless, if it's truly all one, then it's all one. There is no reason why that Oneness can't express itself in the world of time and space just as much as it can express itself in the transcendent world of eternity.

LML: *What about violence and evil and destruction? Is that also an expression of the Oneness?*

ADYASHANTI: Yes, it does that too. That's called confusion, ignorance. There seems to be an inherent, great danger when consciousness comes into form and then tries to become conscious, self-aware. When you look through nature, the more self-aware the animal or the organism, the more propensity it has for a sort of schizophrenic violence. It seems to be a risk that consciousness takes on its maturing, or evolving into becoming truly self-aware through a form. It's taking this incredible risk. It's probably simply a natural maturation, and that is to get confused about its ultimate identity. It comes into form; and then, it thinks that it is the form. That is the first confusion, and from that confusion all hate, ignorance, evil, greed, violence comes out of that innocent misunderstanding. It just seems to be the price to be paid.

LML: *The purpose of it all seems to be to make the discovery of its true nature.*

ADYASHANTI: It seems to be. The purpose seems to be to discover it, and then to manifest it in this world.

JLW: *How did awakening and liberation occur for you?*

ADYASHANTI: I had my first what traditionally would be called awakening experience when I was twenty-five years old. This was very powerful and full of emotion, release, joy, bliss, and all that it is suppose to be full of. But, because there was so much emotion involved, it obscured the simplicity of awakeness itself. Like so many others, I continued to chase certain emotional experiences and certain ideas and concepts of what that awakeness was supposed to be. That caused years of misery. Gradually over time I had the same experience reoccur, but each time with less and less emotion. I could see more and more clearly over time what was the actual essential element. Then finally an awakening occurred where at the moment of awakening, there was no emotion in it. It was just the pure seeing of what is. When there was the pure seeing of simply what is, unclouded by emotional content, it was obvious. It was very obvious that consciousness recognized itself for what it really is—aware space before any emotion or thought or manifestation.

JLW: *Would you say that this is the point at which the distinction between awakening and liberation occurred?*

ADYASHANTI: No. Even though there was a freedom and an incredible sense of fearlessness and release from not being confined to the dream of a separate "I," I started to feel somewhat discontented with that. I didn't know why I felt discontented, and it didn't bother me in any way. The discontent didn't touch that freedom, so it didn't bother me, but I was interested in it.

Then one day I was sitting and reading a book, and I folded the book to put it away and realized that somewhere in some magic time, something had dropped away, and I didn't know what it was. There was just a big absence of something. I went through the rest of the day as usual but noticing some big absence. Then when I sat down on the bed that night, it suddenly hit me that what had fallen away was all identity. All identity had collapsed, as both the self in the ego sense of a separate me, and as the slightest twinge of identity with the absolute Self, with the Oneness of consciousness. There had still been some unconscious, identity or "meness" which was the cause of the discontent. And it all collapsed. Identity itself collapsed, and from that point on there was no grasping whatsoever for little me or for the unified consciousness me. Identity just fell away and blew away with the wind.

JLW: *When you noticed that the identity had collapsed and was gone, what remained?*
ADYASHANTI: Everything just as it always had been. There was just the lack of any "I," personal or universal, or of the fundamental unconscious belief in any identity or of fixating self in any place. The mind can continue to fixate a subtle identity of self even in universal consciousness. It can be so incredibly easy to miss. To say "I am That" can be a very subtle fixation of consciousness.

JLW: *It's still a landing, a form of identity.*
ADYASHANTI: It's a slight landing, a slight grasping. It's very subtle. But when it collapses, you are even beyond "I am That." You are in a place that's indescribable. You can't describe it.

LML: *And that is what you call liberation?*
ADYASHANTI: That is what I call liberation. Right. Really, in the end what you end up with is that you don't know who you are. You end up in the same place you started out. You truly don't know who you are because it's impossible to fixate self anywhere.

JLW: *But this not knowing is not the same as ignorance.*
ADYASHANTI: It's not the same not knowing of ignorance. It's the not knowing that comes from recognizing that the whole issue of a self, personal or absolute, is fantasy. Both the self and the Self are interpretations upon perception, and nothing more. And when that interpretation ends, thought ends. There is nothing to say. What could you say? There's nothing to say.

LML: *At that point you are in the complete unknown.*
ADYASHANTI: The complete unknown.

LML: *Have you have found comfort in that complete unknown?*
ADYASHANTI: Absolutely. Right. When all identity collapses, you abide in the unknown. There is no tendency left to fixate identity anywhere—even in a universal somewhere. So, you are literally resting in the mystery as the mystery. It is only then that you can be truly and absolutely free of all concern.

LML: *That is completely incomprehensible to the mind!*
ADYASHANTI: Yes, to my mind too. I can speak it, and I can know it, but my

mind doesn't comprehend it. It couldn't. However, because it's been there and it comes from there, the mind can reflect it in some pale way.

LML: *Adya, you've been a spiritual teacher now for over three years. Could you describe your teaching?*

ADYASHANTI: I think my teaching has several elements. I won't describe the teaching itself because that would be much too involved, but the basic message of the teaching is that this awakening to the true nature of your self is available to everybody. Nobody is excluded from that. In order for that to happen, it requires the letting go of all ideas, beliefs, concepts, hopes, and dreams. Everything has to become unknown, if even only for a split second. That possibility is a big part of the teaching. I continue to have it proved over and over again that this is actually the way it works. It is possible for everybody. It's not just for yogis up in the caves in the Himalayas. In fact, most of those yogis are probably hiding more than they're being enlightened. Put that in your book!

LML: *We will! [Laughter]*

ADYASHANTI: The other part of the teaching is the more challenging part. This is the evolution that consciousness is having, which is the expression of that transcendent realization through the individual, through the personality, in the realm of time and space. That expression will, of course, never be absolutely perfect. Manifestation, which means things, bodies and everything of the world, is relative reality. That relative reality will never come up to our conception of perfection. It simply is not part of that reality. But, it is incredible the extent to which that transcendent realization can manifest itself through the human form. It is possible. That is the aspect of my teaching that people have the most difficulty with. I say, don't only realize, but actually manifest it; be it; embody it. I say embody it in your body, in your personality, in your entire being, not just in transcendental states three feet above your head while making excuses for your behavior. Manifest it through and through the whole being, as well as it can be done in human form.

LML: *What is so beautiful and powerful for me is being able to have you as an example of the embodiment you are speaking of. You do embody that in your personality and day-to-day life as far as I can tell. I am grateful for this lived example, which for me is the most profound teaching.*

JLW: *And we've talked to your wife! [Laughter] [Referring to a Zen saying that if you want to know how enlightened the Zen Master is, ask his wife.] And we've also talked to your mom and dad!*

ADYASHANTI: Well, I am in a very interesting position as a spiritual teacher in that I have my aunt, my wife, my mother and my father as students. These are all people who knew me well before I got into spiritual life and know me well now. They know all the personality traits, some of which are quite quirky and funny, but these are people who truly know me. I have never had the luxury of being able to fake it because the people who are closest to me know otherwise.

LML: *So, having your family as your students has been a gift for you.*

ADYASHANTI: It has been a real gift. I'd feel very uncomfortable saying one thing in satsang and then coming home and being a complete S.O.B. If someone comes to know you as a spiritual teacher, it's easy to sort of consciously or unconsciously justify whatever your behavior is. But, you can't pull the wool over someone's eyes if you came out of that person's body and they changed your diapers. They know better. So, it's been a real gift.

LML: *Adya, I'd like to go back to what you said about awakening being available to anyone. There is such a wide spectrum of people in this world. Some are actively seeking Truth, some are actively seeking money and material objects, some are actively being destructive. Are you saying that freedom is available to all of these?*

ADYASHANTI: Let me say this… freedom is available to anyone who has the yearning for it. It's possible but rare to awaken without the yearning. But, usually it happens as the result of some yearning. The mere fact that the yearning is present is proof that it is possible. This is what consciousness gives to the human being when they are ready. In most cases, the individual has to come to the end of a line where they start to see the ultimate futility of seeking happiness in any material object or external activity. By that I mean not only things like houses and money and cars, but also the perfect job, the perfect mate, and so on. There has to be some recognition that ultimately none of these will satisfy the deepest yearning in the human heart. When that happens, that person in one sense has reached a state of spiritual maturity.

JLW: *During the time that you have been teaching, have you noticed a growing interest in awakening? Have you noticed an increase in the number of people who are having glimpses or some degree of recognition?*

ADYASHANTI: Oh, tremendous. Many, many, many more people are actually experiencing awakening than they were ten years ago, fifteen years ago, twenty years ago. A lot of the reason for this is the current movement in some spiritual circles, which says that this awakening is possible. Simply the power of that message that this is possible breaks down the conceptual barriers to it actually happening. The barriers to awakening are all conceptual. The biggest barrier to awakening is believing, "Not me, it couldn't possibly happen to me." When that barrier is dropped, then the awakening is almost a forgone conclusion because you suddenly run out of excuses. When an individual runs out of excuses, they tend to get very serious and stop wasting time. As long as we say, "It's only for the few," we have an unconscious excuse not to take on the possibility ourselves and live up to what that possibility may ask of us.

JLW: *Yes, awakening hasn't been seen as a real possibility in Western cultures, until very recently.*

ADYASHANTI: Yes, and I don't think that any culture that we know of in the modern day has ever believed that it is available. You go over to the East where these teachings originated, whether it's Japan, China, or India, and actually the belief that it's for the few is even deeper there than it is in our own country. So, this phenomenon of actually seeing it as possible has really taken hold in the West more than it has in the East. The Western mind doesn't have as many centuries of being enculturated into believing that it is for the few. It's not that we thought it was only for the few in the West; it's that we strictly haven't even thought about it period, up until relatively recently. So, in that sense, we are at a very advantageous point because we don't have as much cultural conditioning as the cultures that have given us these spiritual teachings.

LML: *One of the primary purposes of this book is to put out that awakening is possible. We want to show that it is in fact, increasingly happening to ordinary people. And, it is most certainly possible for anyone who is interested enough in awakening to read this book.*

ADYASHANTI: Yes, that yearning would have to be there for anyone interested in picking up this book. And yes, it is happening to very ordinary people. I think that quite a few of the spiritual teachers in the West these days look like ordinary people. They don't have beards or long flowing hair down to their waist, and they're not all dressed in robes. They look like ordinary, everyday people.

JLW: *Also, most of them are not playing out the whole guru role.*
ADYASHANTI: Right, they're not buying into that so much. And I think that the mere fact that ordinary-looking people, literally just the look of them, really helps a tremendous amount. People look at you, and they see they look like you do.

LML: *Then the spiritual teachers are not so separate from the people they are talking to.*
ADYASHANTI: That's right.

JLW: *I love the fact that you work as a machinist.*
ADYASHANTI: Well, it has become advantageous in my teaching. If someone starts to complain about the fact that they don't have time because of work and other excuses, I can say, "Well, I'm a machinist, and I support myself and help my wife, and I teach anywhere from four to seven satsangs a week." That I have a lot of these elements that everybody has in their life takes the excuse away. If I have a favorite thing to do, it's to pull the rug of excuses out from underneath people's feet.

JLW: *Then they plummet right into the now!*
ADYASHANTI: Plummet right into the now, that's right.

LML: *People who have a yearning, or at least curiosity, about awakening may wonder how they can find this freedom we are speaking of. "What do I do?" "How do I get it?" These are common questions.*
ADYASHANTI: There are two important elements as far as I am concerned, maybe three. Number one is, before you get too involved in teachings and teachers and conforming to the way you think things should be spiritually, connect with the raw yearning at the core of your own being. Basically, this means, "What do I yearn for more than anything else?" For most human beings there will be conflicting yearnings, but see what the core yearning is in you. That very deepest core yearning is your red carpet to freedom. It's the place that you follow. You follow backwards into that yearning. This is something that many spiritual students don't take the time to do. They just jump into the teachings and start imitating and doing practices that they don't understand. They miss that the divine call is in their own heart right from the very beginning. That's the really important part.

Once you hear that call, the other important question to ask is, "Who am I really?" "Who am I really, truly, after all is said and done, who am I really?" To go into the unknown of that. The fact is that when someone asks, "Who am I?" the first thing they notice is that they don't know, and they usually run from the fact that they don't know. It's this running away from the fact that they don't know who they are that is the cause of so much suffering. So, simply to ask who I am and not to know, then to rest ever deeper in the fact of not knowing. It's by resting in the fact that you don't know who you are that you come upon the direct experience of who and what you actually are.

These first two are the most important by far. The last one, which is not a necessity—and it's very important to understand that it's not a necessity, but it can be very useful—is to find an enlightened teacher. I stated these in the order of importance. Because, unless you've taken care of the first two, the teacher is not going to be able to do a whole lot for you. If you know what you want and you know that you don't know who you are, then when you come into contact with a true spiritual teacher the relationship between you and that teacher can have a very dynamic quality.

JLW: *What is the role of the teacher?*

ADYASHANTI: The role of the teacher is to simply be him or her self. That's really ultimately the role of the teacher. The role of the teacher is to respond to the questions of the student in such a way that the question is used to point back to the student's true nature, which is exactly the same as the teacher's true nature. So, ultimately the true desire of all authentic teachers is to put themselves out of business as quickly as possible. This means to have the student rise to the same level of consciousness that they are so that they are no longer needed. As long as a true teacher understands that, then their motivation will be very pure.

JLW: *And what is the role of spiritual practice in awakening?*

ADYASHANTI: It depends on the nature of the individual. By practice I assume you mean some sort of meditation, prayer, or devotional practices. These practices either will or will not happen. You will find yourself drawn or not drawn to them.

JLW: *They're not necessary?*

ADYASHANTI: They're not necessary in and of themselves. But, if you happen to do them, then maybe they're necessary for you. They can become a barrier too. "I don't do enough meditation; how can I possibly awaken?" That's not to say that spiritual practices can't be very useful. They can be very, very useful as long as they're not used as unconscious defense mechanisms.

JLW: *You mean a defense against awakening?*
ADYASHANTI: Yes, because most often that is what they are used for. What I'm saying is that most meditators are avoiding their own experience rather than trying to truly understand it.

JLW: *I think there is also a way in which spiritual practice actually does play a role in awakening. You have spoken about the balance between abiding in awareness and inquiry, that the inquiry or curiosity needs a calm state in order to go deep.*
ADYASHANTI: Yes. In one way, the two biggest prongs of what I teach are number one, to abide and number two, to inquire deeply. To abide simply means to let everything be as it already is. For most individuals it is extremely challenging in the beginning to simply let everything be as it is. In order to do that, we cannot hold onto any preference for our experience to be any particular way. Most spiritual people are doing anything but that. They are trying to make their experience be a very specific way. So they end up with a sort of spiritual slavery. Abiding is simply letting everything be as it is. Paradoxically, when we let everything be as it is, even if our experience is very uncomfortable, the first thing that starts to come into our experience is a great peace and calm. When this peace and calm comes into our experience, there is a sense of not being so hemmed in by our experience. There is an experience of more vastness.

It's from that place of true abidance that we can begin to inquire. Abidance without inquiry usually doesn't produce much, except a good feeling. But when abidance is coupled by true and authentic inquiry... what I mean by inquiry is curiosity, a real curiosity about the true nature of one's self, or who am I, or what is life? When those two are coupled, the inquiry adds a very dynamic quality that simple abidance doesn't necessarily have in and of itself. It's the dynamism of simple abidance coupled with a passionate inquiry into the true nature of one's self or reality that provides the ground for awakening to be most likely to occur.

LML: *So, it seems that meditation could either help or hinder that process.*
ADYASHANTI: Right. Exactly. In my own teaching, in my retreats, there is

quite a lot of meditation just for the reason of being able to abide. If someone cannot sit still, then they find it very difficult to inquire in any concentrated, single-pointed way. They inquire in a very messy, conflicted way.

LML: *It helps to know how to quiet the mind.*
ADYASHANTI: Yes. Spiritual practices are not bad. It's more the attitude that we're doing them with than what those practices actually are.

LML: *You yourself did fifteen years of intense Zen meditation practice.*
ADYASHANTI: Right, and for a lot of that time I did exactly what I am telling people not to do. I did a tremendous amount of meditation and a lot of that meditation was an unconscious hiding from myself, or it became a grasping at an ideal that I had of what enlightenment was. In both cases it was a horrendous waste of energy. It was useful in the sense that I finally got tired of it, but in and of itself, it was a real waste of energy. It wasn't until after many years of this that I actually got in touch with my true yearning. We can literally go through this for years before we really get in touch with our true yearning. The true yearning was really two things: "Who am I really, finally?" and "What is the Truth?" "What is the ultimate nature of myself and the world." "What is that?" These are deep inquiries. And when those inquiries came, everything became very one-pointed and had a direction that it didn't have before. It didn't take long for a lot to start happening once that inquiry came in a focused way.

LML: *There seems to be a lot of fear in many people about awakening to who one truly is because to do so requires giving up everything we think we are. It requires giving up an individual, separate self. As you said earlier, this is part of the experience. There is a lot of fear around this; fear of the unknown, fear of not being able to function in the world. "How will I do my job and take care of my family without an individual, separate self?" "How can I have relationships without an individual separate self?" Would you talk about how the experience of awakening has affected your day-to-day life?*
ADYASHANTI: Well, actually it has been a removal of all fear. It has been a removal of all fear of what happened in the past, of what's happening in the present, and fear of what might happen in the future, including death. All that fear evaporated. It does evaporate when you awaken to who and what you truly are. When you awaken to the fact that you are not this individual, separate "I," then you are released from all fear of whatever might happen to that "I." As far as how life is lived, all I can say is that

this realization for me has had a call from the very beginning for integrity, for that transcendent realization to be manifested through the body, mind and personality in the way that life is lived. In that sense, it has really transformed my life.

Being in the rare position that I am as a spiritual teacher, it's paradoxical that the discovery of freedom itself stole my life away from me. I don't really have a life that belongs to me any more. I used to have many hobbies and be very athletic and like everyone else, needed a lot of my own space, whether it was quiet time or just space for me to be me. But all that has been given up. If you are not identified with a personal I, you don't need that space. You need to take care of the body, but that's very little maintenance. What is paradoxically found is that when you become a slave to the way the Truth wants to manifest through you, the revelation is that you don't need all that "me time."

You don't need to do what you like to do. You just do what that truth of Self manifests through you and you're actually not only happy, but you are as happy as you could possibly be. That's why it's freedom because it is free of all need in a personal sense. You get back to more of a functional need of the body itself and the functional need of relationships, which are time, energy, and commitment. But those functional needs are miniscule compared to the needs of the personality that most people are burdened with.

JLW: *Yes, people really are burdened. There is an incredible amount of suffering in the world today. What do you see as the source and solution to this suffering?*

ADYASHANTI: The source of suffering is ignorance. Ignorance means misunderstanding about the true nature of one's self. It's actually pretty simple when you get down to it. At the inception, before it snowballs into some of the horrors of modern life, it is something very innocent. It is just an innocent misunderstanding of the true nature of one's self. The only hope for the end of suffering is for that ignorance to be rectified, which means for people to wake up to the true nature of their self.

LML: *You could say that there is only one problem and one solution.*

ADYASHANTI: There is only one problem and only one solution, right. It's actually very simple, and there's not more than that. Ultimately, when you go back to the real true nature of suffering, it's very simple. If that awakening is authentic (and that's a big if) and expresses itself in the world of space and time as selflessness, as true love, as tremendous intimacy, as peace and joy, then these very expressions are the answers to the world's problems. These answers can only come in a very natural way once the awakening has occurred. It doesn't mean that we can't be loving and kind and compassionate when we haven't awakened, because we can, but we can do it in a way that is truly selfless when awakening has occurred.

JLW: *It is the nature of who we are to express itself as love, kindness, wisdom, and compassion. It's just how it is.*

ADYASHANTI: That's the unfathomable glory of it. It has all of these beautiful attributes. It's just who and what you are. This is a whole other subject, but many people in the West who have terrible self-images find this so hard to accept. When they even begin to come into contact with the true nature of their own self, they have such a hard time accepting that they could naturally be something so positive and beautiful. In the West, many people struggle with negative self-image.

LML: *This is an important point. In my work, I see that most of the suffering and problems people have can be boiled down to that one thing, negative self-image. And, that negative self-image was learned. It is only conditioning, but it's believed to be true in such a deep way for most people. It is taken on as an identity, and as miserable as it is, it's held onto because many people believe that a negative identity is better than no identity. They don't know who they would be without it.*

ADYASHANTI: Yes, I have seen that negative identity held onto even in the midst of profound revelation. It so easily contracts back into, "It couldn't be me." "It couldn't be who I am; it's just too good." If I had a dollar for every time someone told me that, I'd be a rich man!

LML: *Aside from the tendency for Westerners to believe they are not good enough, what do you see as the main obstacle we have to awakening?*

ADYASHANTI: Pride. Pride in the form of an unwillingness to admit that all the avenues that we try to pursue to make us happy don't ultimately end in happiness. Yet, we continue to insist that they do in the face of overwhelming evidence to the contrary.

JLW: *We continue to bang our bloody head against the wall!*

ADYASHANTI: [Laughter] Yes, and that's a lot of pride. The other kind of pride is being unwilling to admit that you simply don't know who you really are and that you don't know what life is about. Pride will keep somebody from being able to say something that is so obviously true. When someone's willing to call into question these most fundamental beliefs and ideas that is the birth of a true humility.

LML: *Pride keeps people from telling the truth, from being truly honest with themselves.*
ADYASHANTI: Yes, we have to protect our pride rather than tell the truth. It's difficult for people in the West not to be prideful because we have an unconscious belief that to be humble is to feel bad about one's self. It may be unconscious, but when we think of humility, we usually think of something that's rather depressing.

JLW: *More like shame.*
ADYASHANTI: Yes, shame. Absolutely. And it's unfortunate because shame is not humility at all.

LML: *Actually, shame and pride are two sides of the same coin. On one side is arrogance and inflation and on the other side is shame and worthlessness.*
ADYASHANTI: Yes, and we can have a lot of pride wrapped up in being worthless. "Don't tell me I'm not worthless. My whole existence depends on it!"

LML: *You said it right there, "My whole existence depends on it." This is why that negative self-image is held onto so tightly.*

JLW: *It can feel like the whole structure of your world is wrapped around it.*
ADYASHANTI: Right. This whole dilemma of the human condition is really an avoidance of emptiness, an avoidance of the unknown. There is an emptiness in the midst of the human condition, but it's not the threatening, empty emptiness that the mind thinks it is. When one finally gets the courage to go into it, it's found to be empty and at the same time pregnant with every possibility there is.

LML: *It definitely takes courage because the mind will be frightened of it no matter what. Even if the mind has the intellectual understanding that it's okay and a good place to be...*
ADYASHANTI: Even if the mind is convinced that the emptiness is all okay, it's not nearly enough.

LML: *It's only by knowing through direct experience, beyond the mind, that we come to see what a safe and beautiful place this emptiness is that we try so hard to avoid.*

ADYASHANTI: It's not only some place good and safe, but this is actually the true nature of myself and everything else. The paradox is that in order to know this, you have to go through the gate of not knowing. In order to find true security, you have to be willing to dive right through the gate of tremendous insecurity. You can't avoid insecurity and find that which is ultimately secure. You can't avoid the unknown and expect to find the known. You have to dive right into those areas that are the most frightening. Otherwise, it's not going to happen.

LML: *Once we take the risk and go through the gate, we find that we go right through it, and that there was nothing to be afraid of after all. Once that is known through direct experience, we can begin to relax and begin to let go of the negative, conditioned identity.*
ADYASHANTI: Yes, but not until then.

LML: *It can't happen until then because we need to know there is something there to let go to. When it's not known that there is something else, we will hang onto anything, even something that's causing tremendous suffering.*
ADYASHANTI: Yes, but to find that out you have to be willing to take a risk. Your desire to know what's true has to be more powerful than your desire to avoid what's frightening.

LML: *And more powerful than your desire to be comfortable.*
ADYASHANTI: And prideful, and all the rest. You have to find what is deeper than the impulse for survival. We think that the core impulse of any species is survival, but actually for the human being there is a deeper impulse, and that is the impulse to be. This impulse to be is more powerful than the impulse to survive.

JLW: *Is there anything you would like to add before we finish?*
ADYASHANTI: The only thing that comes up that I would really like to add is not something to say, but a plea. It is a plea that in many ways I am always pleading with my own students, which is to please take this awakening all the way. Take it all the way. Don't stop with anything short of really being liberated and being able to manifest that liberation in your day-to-day life. There will be a great tendency all along the way to stop short of the true possibility. Don't settle for anything less than the Truth itself.

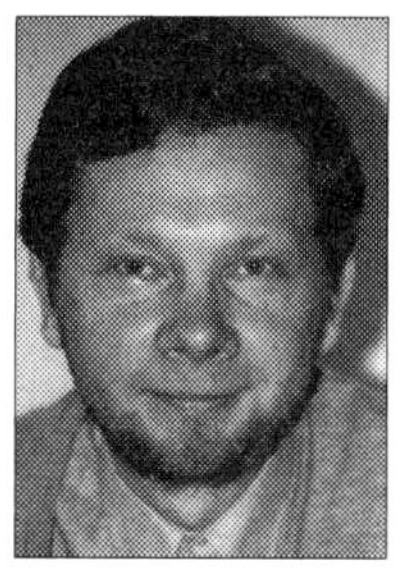

ECKHART TOLLE

"A PROFOUND TRANSFORMATION IS TAKING PLACE IN THE THE COLLECTIVE HUMAN CONSCIOUSNESS OF THE PLANET: THE AWAKENING OF CONSCIOUSNESS FROM THE DREAM OF MATTER, FORM, AND SEPARATION... WE ARE BREAKING MIND PATTERNS THAT HAVE DOMINATED HUMAN LIFE FOR EONS."

from The Power of Now

The manuscript for this book was completed when we learned about Eckhart Tolle through his book, *The Power of Now, A Guide to Spiritual Enlightenment*. We both agreed that his book would have a profound impact on many people. John is a prolific reader who has averaged about a book a week his whole adult life, and yet he found *The Power of Now* to be the most important book he had ever read. Eckhart's simple, clear expression of the problem of the human condition and its solution is so accessible and free of jargon and dogma that it can be related to by anyone with or without a spiritual or religious background.

After reading his book, we wished he had been included in ours. Then we heard Eckhart speak at a conference, and we knew for sure that he had to be included in this book. The power of his presence is such that it draws everyone into the Now. When listening to Eckhart, you are not just hearing words, you are experiencing what he is speaking about.

We found Eckhart to be sweet and timid in personality. He is soft-spoken and gentle. Written words do not convey the playfulness of his presence and the delightful humor that is expressed through his gestures and in his descriptions of the "little me." He is a rare, precious, and pure being whom we are grateful to share with you here.

Eckhart Tolle was born in Germany. He later lived in England where he was a research scholar at Cambridge University. His spiritual awakening occurred at the age of twenty-nine and changed the course of his life. For the past ten years he has been a spiritual teacher in Europe and North America. He now lives in Vancouver, Canada.

CONVERSATION *with* ECKHART TOLLE

LML: *In one of the talks you gave this weekend you distinguish between the "little me" and the stillness of the Now in which the "little me"and its world arises and disappears. You said that the Now is what we truly are. Could you say more about this—that we are the Now?*

ECKHART: [Long pause of silence] Unfortunately this stillness doesn't look good on paper! [Laughter]

I am the Now... that is a strange statement that came to me not long ago in a talk I gave; I never wrote it in the book that I am the Now. If you look at your life as constantly fluctuating and changing conditions, every moment seems different. Forms come and go; they appear and disappear. Yet, there is something that underlies all this, something that remains constant. That something is what spiritual seekers have been looking for for thousands of years. "Is there anything beyond the world of fluctuating forms? Is there anything beyond the fleeting existence of me as a form identity — psychological form, physical form?" If you look, the only thing that ever remains constant in your life is the fact that it's always this moment. One factor remains as your whole life unfolds within the Now. It's always Now. To say, "I am the Now," may seem to be a meaningless statement to the mind. When I say these words, they're not to be used as explanations, but as pointers. They point to an inner realization, rather than being an explanation. So when words are used spiritually, they are never an explanation because the words are never the Truth. They can only point; they can only be approximations to the Truth. So to say, "I am the Now" is a pointer to the Truth. And when you hear that statement, it's best to let it sink in for awhile. Become quiet and get a sense of what that means, a feeling of what that means... "I am the Now."

When one talks about the present moment, usually people think that the present moment is what appears. They think it is the external reality of this moment or the inner reality of thoughts and emotions that are occurring at this moment. Yet, that's not what the present moment is. Whatever happens in the present moment is the external appearance of the present moment. Something comes into the space of Now momentarily and then disappears. Then something else comes into the space of Now. What remains is an underlying field of stillness out of which everything comes and into which everything disappears. So, realize what the Now is — the field of pure consciousness that allows everything to be, that underlies everything, that enables everything to be. The Now is a vast field of stillness that enables the world to be.

An externalization of the Now would be the space that enables everything to be. Yet, what we perceive as external space and the Now have no concrete existence and cannot be grasped. We can only realize them as we enter the state of stillness. The realization of this comes when you become present to the Now. When your consciousness moves into the present moment, what arises is a state of great alertness and at the same time deep stillness. You could call this the unconditioned consciousness arising. Everything else is conditioned. All the baggage you carry in the mind, all the content of the mind, is the conditioned consciousness, and it takes on form as thought. Then consciousness takes on form as the universe. Prior to consciousness taking on form, consciousness is there in its undifferentiated or pure nonform, and that is who you are. That is the Now. That is the deepest meaning of what Now is.

So, in that still presence—from the point of view of mind and content of mind—you no longer know anything. People think self-realization or enlightenment is a state in which suddenly they know everything, or they know who they are. But in a way the opposite is true. In the state of self-realization, from the perspective of conceptual knowledge, that is relinquished. From the perspective of conceptual knowledge, you no longer know who you are, and you are happy with not knowing who you are. There is no longer a trying to interpret anything. Not only do you not know who you are, you no longer know who anybody or anything is. The world is no longer interpreted through the accumulated content in the mind. You no longer relate to the world through the conditioned consciousness that is the mind. So from the point of view of the mind, enlightenment is a state of ignorance or not knowing anything anymore.

JLW: *Yet, it is so profoundly satisfying, both for the person experiencing it and for everyone around them.*

ECKHART: Yes. The strange thing is that in that not knowing there is a deep knowing, but it's non-conceptual. And when you are the stillness, everything that you need to know at this moment comes out of the stillness. If there is anything vital that you need to know, then the knowledge is there suddenly. But it's only there when it is needed, and then it disappears. The wonderful thing is to relate to the world without the screen of conceptualization and interpretation. So, not relating to the world through mental noise, but through stillness.

JLW: *Is this what awakening or enlightenment means to you?*

ECKHART: Yes. Awakening is to know yourself to be the stillness, being the stillness. Then the world of forms including thoughts, the physical forms, galaxies, trees, blades of grass, no longer matters so much anymore. It doesn't have the heaviness about it and the seriousness about it that it does when it's the only world you know. When the world of form is the only world you know, then your mind is a serious matter, and the world is serious, and it's all there is. It holds great promise on one hand, because you believe it will take you to salvation some day; on the other hand, the world of form is continuously threatening. The psychological form of "me," which is a mental image of who I am, is in a constant state of fear and insecurity. And, of course, the physical form is short-lived and could disappear at any moment.

LML: *There is a continuous feeling of needing to defend and protect the physical and psychological "me."*

ECKHART: Yes, the "me" is a state of fearful, self-contraction. For most humans, this is so normal they don't even know it. If they haven't known anything else ever, a fearful self-contraction is normal. The "me" exists in a continuous state of unease because basically the "me" is a story in the head. It is simply mental content and emotions associated with the story of "me." The story of "me" up to this point is never quite satisfying. It hasn't reached a point of satisfaction or fullness. And so, the "me" is continuously looking to the future to fulfill itself. There is a deep longing for the fulfillment of being who you are. Even the bank robber is looking for that fulfillment. He believes that it will come through the money. In the state of the "little me," one is condemned to continuous seeking. *A Course in Miracles* says it beautifully, "The dictum of the ego is: seek but do not find." The ego is seeking in the future what can only be found in the present moment, which it always ignores.

The amazing thing is that time is obviously needed for almost everything in life. You need time for everything except one thing. You need time to accomplish a task, to learn a new skill; time is needed for all that. The one and most vital thing there is, which is knowing yourself at the deepest level, for that you don't need time. Not only do you not need time, but time is the greatest obstacle to that!

It is only when attention is withdrawn from mental noise that a state of alert presence arises; which is very, very still yet, vibrantly alive.

LML: *Eckhart, could you please tell us the story of how awakening occurred for you?*

ECKHART: The story which I describe briefly in the introduction to the book is that for many years I lived in a state of great fear and continuous fluctuation between states of depression and high anxiety. This was to the point of becoming almost unbearable. One night I woke up in the middle of the night, as I had many times before, in a state of even more intense dread and fear. The mind had lots of reasons why I was feeling fearful, and yet that state was continuous no matter what my external situation was. It became so unbearable that suddenly the thought occurred to me, "I cannot live with myself any longer." That thought was the trigger for a transformation. The thought kept repeating itself many times in my head and then suddenly there was a stepping back from the thought and a looking at the thought. I asked, "Who is the 'I' and who is the self that I cannot live with?"

In Zen they have koans, and it's almost as if a koan spontaneously appeared in my mind. A koan's purpose is to destroy conceptual thinking because it has no answer on a conceptual level. So, I asked, "Who is the self that I cannot live with? Are there one or two? If I cannot live with myself, who is that self?" Then, beyond thought, there was a recognition of the "unhappy me," as I later called it, as being something completely non-substantial and fictional. Then consciousness withdrew completely from identification with that "unhappy me." At that moment the whole structure of the "unhappy me" and its pain collapsed because the withdrawal of identification was so complete. What was left was simply beingness or presence. There was still a moment of fear. It felt like being drawn into a hole within myself, a vast whirlpool, and a realization arose in my chest, "Resist nothing." That was the key. Then resistance was relinquished, and I don't know what happened after that.

All I do know is that the next morning I woke up and even before opening my eyes I heard the sounds of birds and it was so precious. Everything was so precious. Then I opened my eyes and everything was alive and new and fresh as if I had never seen it before. And I walked around and picked up things and looked at them. I was amazed at everything. There was no understanding of it. I was not even trying to understand anything. It was just so beautiful. Then I walked around the city in the same state, even in the midst of traffic. I was in a state of amazement and it was all so beautiful.

LML: *Had you been seeking this?*

ECKHART: I had been seeking, but I had been seeking to find an answer through the intellect. The more I was seeking through the level of intellect through philosophy and reading books, the deeper the unhappiness became. I only later realized what I didn't realize at that point—that after this transformation the mind activity had been reduced by eighty to ninety percent. I was actually walking around in stillness, but I wouldn't have called it stillness. I simply knew it as peace. I knew there was deep peace, but I didn't yet realize that my mind was not very active anymore.

That went on with great intensity for several months. It never left me after that, but the intensity varies, even now. The stillness is always there. Sometimes it's in the background. And sometimes it fills everything. But it's always there, and I can see so clearly why some Indian sages said that the world is unreal. That statement doesn't really make much sense if one reads it in a book and makes it into a belief. But relative to the depths of stillness or beingness and aliveness that is there, the world of form seems very insubstantial. So, to me the whole world appears as though it is happening on the periphery of being, like ripples on the surface of being. There's the fullness of being, which is far greater than anything in the phenomenal world, and yet, the phenomenal world exists as part of that. The way I see it is like ripples, and no ripple actually exists as an independent entity. It's just a little wave movement.

JLW: *Some people who are reading this will be longing for freedom from the tyranny mind and want to know how to do this. What would you say to them?*

ECKHART: What I say is choose to step out of the mental noise. You can choose to be present. I wouldn't say this to anybody because it would not be true for everybody, but I am saying it to both of you. And anybody who reads your book will be able to choose to be present. To choose, to step out of mind, is simply to take attention away from mental noise and allow the alert stillness to arise. You will notice that the alert stillness affects the entire energy field of the body. It is not a head state. The alert stillness affects every cell of the body, and every cell of the body then partakes in the state of stillness.

So when I say you can choose, it is the truth, and yet the truth is beyond that. The question may arise, "Who is choosing?" The ultimate answer is, "Nobody is choosing to be present." It is simply a helpful perspective. The deeper truth is that when you believe that you are choosing to be present, presence is choosing to manifest through you at that moment. But it is a more helpful statement to say that you can choose than to say that there is nothing you can do. Ultimately, presence emerges when it wants to emerge.

JLW: *One of the things I enjoy about your teachings is how you include the physical body and the energy body. Can you talk about transformation through the body?*

LML: *. . . And how putting attention on the body can help people to remain present. It seems to be one thing to have a glimpse of the Now and another thing to live in the Now.*

ECKHART: The mind has such incredible momentum. It's been around for so many thousands of years, that even people who have a glimpse of Now, often cannot sustain it. The momentum of the mind is so powerful that the mental noise returns very quickly. So, it is helpful to have an anchor for staying present. The most powerful anchor for staying present is to inhabit the body. That means to have some of your attention in the inner energy field of the body—to sense, to feel the animating presence that gives life to the body, which ultimately is consciousness itself. The physical body is a temporary expression of that consciousness, but the essence of it is the consciousness itself. So to connect with the physical body, and even as you perceive the world and interact with the world, to have some attention in the inner energy field and to feel the aliveness that is there in every cell and every organ as a single feeling. You are then rooted in your body, which becomes the anchor for staying present and for staying out of the mental noise.

Then an amazing thing happens. You discover at first that when you enter the body and look around at the world, you perceive the world, and you are able to sustain perception without interpretation. That is the beginning of the state of freedom from the conditioned mind, freedom from the egoic "little me" entity.

When you perceive the world through the accumulated content in your mind and the egoic "little me," all you ever really encounter is the conditioning of your mind. The world will reflect back to you your mental content because that is the screen through which you interpret everything. So, wherever you go, you will only meet the conditioned "me." That's a dreadful state although it is normal. As you step out of that by taking attention into the body, you then realize for the first time that it is possible to perceive the world through stillness and not through the conditioned mind or through interpretations.

The stillness is highly conscious, and there is a knowing. You perceive everything, but there is no labeling. There is a deep knowing. You could call it unitive knowing, not a knowing that is conceptual, mental knowledge that separates you from that which is perceived. There's a knowing in which you know your oneness with that which is being perceived. But you know it beyond concepts. It starts with such a simple thing as sitting here, feeling the aliveness in your body, and then looking around the room. There's complete stillness and yet, you're highly awake.

JLW: *It's not as if the labels for the things that are seen are not available; it's just that they're not first.*

ECKHART: That's right. If a label should be needed, it will be there, but you will then not be lost in the labels. And you won't mistake the label for the thing itself. You could still say that you would be looking at what might be called a tree, but in the state of stillness, the depths of that which we call tree is so much more. To label something reduces it immediately—as if you knew what it is when you call it tree. You don't know anything; it's just a label. So, know that you don't know anything about it and stay with it. Then the essence of the tree reveals itself to you, which is one with your essence. You not only then relate to the tree through stillness, but love is also part of that because love is the recognition of the other as yourself. Then your very existence on the planet becomes a benediction. If a label should be needed, you still know that on a conceptual level it is called "tree," but the label won't obscure that beautiful field that we call tree. It won't obscure it anymore.

JLW: *It seems to both of us that there is a rapid increase in the number of people who are living more and more in just this way. There seems to be a spreading enlightenment. What is your perception of this?*

ECKHART: I happen to be at the epicenter of one particular wave of transformation of consciousness. So to me, it seems like everybody is going through that transformation, but that is not totally right. It simply means everybody that I meet is going through that transformation. Occasionally I switch on the TV and then realize, "Oh no, it's not yet happening to everybody!" But a collective transformation of consciousness is indeed happening. People sometimes ask, "Why is it happening now?" It's happening now because it has become a necessity for humans and the planet. The planet would not be able to sustain human life if human consciousness remained unchanged from the way it is now. Another hundred years of that would probably make it impossible for the planet to sustain human life. It's possible that the planet would eventually recover and perhaps produce a new expression of consciousness, but humans would probably disappear as an expression. It wouldn't matter ultimately, but there is a good chance that this won't happen. The transformation will occur because it is happening at this very moment, even as we sit here. In fact, this is part of it.

So, awakening has been a luxury for thousands of years, those few sages and teachers—Buddha, Jesus, and Lao Tzu and some we don't know about—they were rare flowerings of human consciousness here and there. I was told by someone who studied planetary evolution that the Earth was covered with plant life for millions of years before the first flower appeared. Then a day must have come when the first flower opened. Flowers could be seen as the enlightenment of plant life. The first flower opened, then probably thousands of years passed before another flower opened; then two or three. Then a day came when suddenly there was a profusion of flowers all over the planet. This is very similar to what I call the flowering of human consciousness now. Buddha, Jesus, and others were rare flowers, the first few flowers. And now we are about to experience a collective flowering of human consciousness.

Whether it will affect all humans on the planet, or only some humans, I don't know. Even to this day, plants exist that don't flower. That's okay too. But it does seem that this transformation of consciousness is so radical because it's not changing the content of our minds; it's going beyond all that. It's a completely new dimension of consciousness arising. It really is like the birth of a new species out of the old. And eventually, this will also transform the physical vehicle. But we don't need to speculate about that; the main thing is to be open to that transformation now.

LML: *It is now the dawn of this transformation of consciousness.*

ECKHART: Yes, yes, yes. And we don't need to make it happen, because it wants to happen; it is happening. Instead of believing that "I" need to do something about it, allow it to happen. Part of allowing it to happen is the simple thing that I call "allowing the present moment to be." That means open yourself up to the transformation. Allow whatever this moment contains. No matter what event or happening or situation, say "yes" to it. Allow it to be.

That allowing, that "yes" is saying "yes" to life itself which is Now and always Now. It requires no effort. In fact, it requires no time. But the mind says, "Okay that's wonderful news that there's a transformation of consciousness happening, now tell me what I have to do to get there." The mind is saying, "Tell me what to do and give me some time and I'll do it."

Of course, this doesn't work because that is the old consciousness speaking. There is no time. You step out of time. How do you step out of time? By allowing this moment to be instead of resisting it or running away from it or denying it, or making it a means to an end. Embrace it. That means you embrace life. That opens the floodgates, and then the new consciousness can move through you, the unconditioned consciousness can emerge.

The very structure of the self or the "little me" entity, as I sometimes call it, is based on saying "no" to what is. It cannot allow this moment. It needs to be in a fighting mode with what is. It must have some enemy to sustain the sense of separateness on which its identity depends, whether the enemy is a person or a situation or a condition. It must be fighting something. The "me" is always fighting the Now. The Now is the arch-enemy of the "little me." By opening yourself to Now, those structures dissolve and cannot operate anymore. So, the greatest spiritual practice is to say "yes" to what is, completely, because it is.

In that saying "yes," immediately a stillness arises. When you relinquish resistance to what is in this moment, suddenly a stillness arises. That stillness is the essence of the Now. That stillness is the essence of who you are. Then what happens in the Now becomes very much secondary. It doesn't matter that much anymore because you've gone beyond the appearance of Now—which is sometimes good, sometimes bad, sometimes indifferent—the external appearance of Now fluctuates continuously. But if you go beyond that, and a stillness arises which is the Now, that is the essence beyond the appearance. You can then allow whatever external appearance that happens to manifest in the Now to be. It doesn't matter that much anymore.

LML: *This allowing is bigger than what the mind can do. It's allowing the Now to be as it is regardless of the content. The mind can take this and think it means to accept the content or circumstances in the Now. The mind will say, "Okay, I need to accept this uncomfortable situation." But you are not talking about saying "yes" to situations.*

ECKHART: That's right. You focus away from the content to the underlying essence, the power that underlies all that—which is stillness, which is presence. It's simple, but words can only point to it. They can never contain that Truth.

LML: *In your book,* The Power of Now, *you speak of what you call the pain-body. We are both familiar with that personally and as psychotherapists. It is an enormous challenge for some people, particularly those who have had a difficult or traumatic childhood. Can you speak about how to become free of that?*

ECKHART: The pain body is what I call the accumulated pain that people carry inside from the past. Because of the human condition, every human being inherits pain, which is passed on genetically and in other ways. Every human already comes into this world with a certain amount of pain. That is added to by absorbing the pain body of parents during childhood. This is something that can easily obscure presence.

To explain briefly how the pain body operates... it's not continuously active. It has a dormant state and an active state. It cannot remain dormant for too long because it needs to feed. When it becomes active, it's looking for something to feed on, to add energy to its energy field, which is an energy field of contraction of either heaviness or agitation or intense fear or anger. That is the vibrational frequency of the pain-body. It is residues of past emotional pain, which are still alive in the body.

I look at the pain-body as almost an entity that lives in you. When it needs to feed, it will move into your mind and feed on your thinking. It will try to control your thoughts, and usually, it succeeds. At that point you become the pain-body. The pain-body becomes transformed from simple pain to a "self," an "unhappy me." Then it renews itself through one's thinking. Every negative thought feeds the pain-body—it loves that. This is one of the ways in which the pain-body feeds on you, on your thinking.

Another way the pain-body accumulates new energies is by provoking a reaction from somebody else. It says, "Please give me pain." In relationships it often happens between partners. The pain-body awakens in one partner and buttons are pushed in the other in order to get some feedback of pain. Then ideally for the pain-body, the other person's pain-body awakens also, and they can feed on each other. That is called drama in relationships. Pain-bodies love the drama. Once the pain-body has absorbed enough nourishment in the form of more pain, it will return to the dormant state. Then you feel, "Oh, it's over now." But of course, the cycle will start again.

To break the cycle of the pain-body becoming you, identifying with that, and making it into an "unhappy me" and then acting out and feeding it with your thinking, you bring presence to it. You observe it. You recognize it for what it is as it arises and then you stay there as the watcher, which is presence. Presence implies that you accept it and allow it to be. There is a stillness that comes with presence despite the agitation. In the background there is a silent watcher, a still presence. That frees you from identification with it. It doesn't become an "unhappy me." That also cuts the link between the pain-body and your thinking. It is vital to cut the link between the pain-body and your thought processes. Then the pain-body can not take in new energy. As you do this every time it arises, the pain-body will lose some of its energy charge.

In Eastern terms the pain-body is an important aspect of what they call karma. Karma is all the accumulated conditioning from the past that continuously renews itself and that you identify with as "me." That karma has no end until something arises that has nothing to do with that mental content—stillness, unconditioned consciousness, and presence.

As the unconditional consciousness arises, the ability to watch the mind increases, and you are no longer trapped in the content. You observe the content in operation. You also observe the pain-body, the emotional field; you are no longer it. There's a witnessing presence, and it grows and you realize that the presence is far greater than anything it witnesses. You are the presence more than that which is being witnessed. Increasingly, that which is being witnessed is a peripheral event, whereas before it filled your entire being. Even the pain-body, while it's still active, can become a peripheral event. "There's pain here, and yet, there's presence."

JLW: *The presence just becomes a lot more interesting.*
ECKHART: Yes, yes, and all the happenings of the world lose their fascinating attractiveness. You can enjoy the beauty in it, but it no longer draws you in. There is no self-seeking in those things anymore.

LML: *Some people have bio-chemical imbalances that cause a lot of disturbance in the mind. Would you consider that part of the pain-body or a result of the pain-body?*
ECKHART: It is a result of the pain-body. Whatever happens—any emotional state or mental state—will be reflected in some way in the

physiology of the body. People found that out for the first time in the 18th or 19th century when a man had a bullet hole in his stomach that never healed. So the doctors looked inside and saw that the moment he got angry the stomach lining changed color. Whatever state you are in is immediately reflected in the physiology, but that's not the cause. It's the reflection of the pain-body in the body.

JLW: *What do you see as the main obstacles to awakening for Westerners today?*

ECKHART: Well, the main obstacle is the mind and the momentum that is there, the incredible momentum of the incessant, compulsive thinking. This noise in the head and the pain-body, which is part of that, are the primary obstacles. The noise in the head and the pain-body are related because the identification with thought, which became a "me" entity, has created the pain-body; I call it the body reflecting a thought.

The emphasis seems to be for women to work with their pain-body. I explain this briefly in the book. The emphasis for men is the mental noise. It doesn't mean that men don't have a pain-body and that women don't have mental noise, but the focal point for women is to work with their pain-body. Many women are doing this very successfully now. Menstruation often brings up the collective female pain-body, which I mention in the book. Many women are now becoming very alert during that time instead of losing consciousness, and that's wonderful. They are using that to bring presence into it and transmuting the pain-body during that time.

So, there's the momentum of the mind and the force of human pain that is in the pain-body. They seem to be the obstacles. And yet, the unhappiness that arises out of that is also the motivating factor that moves people to get out of the dream they have become. So what seems like an obstacle is also a positive factor at the same time. This is why people with very dense pain-bodies are often able to become free more quickly than people with relatively light pain-bodies. The motivation to get out of a nightmare is greater than the motivation to get out of a dream that you can live with.

JLW: *Eckhart, I'd like to say that the whole idea of our book is that there is an awakening occurring among us, and we want to make it known. Through that, we want to make it much more available to people. So, perhaps in light of that, is there anything else you would like to add before we finish?*

ECKHART: Perhaps the most essential fact is that for the transformation to happen, you don't need time. Because time is part of the old consciousness. So many spiritual people are getting lost again in time; they are seeking for an answer in time. They are seeking for a method or a technique, "Tell me how to do it," which implies, "Please give me more time." The realization is that you do not need time for this transformation to happen; in fact, time prevents it from happening. Once you realize that, it's there. That is the essence.

What is emerging is a timeless state of consciousness. Once it has emerged, past and future are extremely peripheral to your life. They are only used for practical matters—like I know that I have to catch a plane in a few hours. But otherwise, past and future are no longer needed to give a sense of identity to who you are. The deepest realization is that I don't need time anymore.

LML: *The paradox is that it does not take time to be in the Now. It is immediately available. Yet it appears to take time to get to where you remain consciously in the Now.*
ECKHART: That's the paradox. You get drawn back into time and mind, and then you step out into the Now.

JLW: *Another piece is that the more we are in the Now, the more we stay in the Now. The longer the duration of times we stay, the more frequently we remember when we've become identified, "Oh, I've forgotten; I am here right now." Then we come back.*
ECKHART: Also the qualitative difference between the timeless state compared to the dream state of time is so vast...

LML: *So, the attention just becomes more drawn to the timeless state because it is more attractive, more deeply fulfilling.*
ECKHART: Yes, and it's emerging. It occasionally becomes obscured, but that's alright too. It becomes obscured and then it emerges more fully.

LML: *There seems to be another paradox in that there is nothing anyone can do, yet there is an intentionality that one can have that facilitates this.*
ECKHART: Yes. It's doing it. It might look as if there is someone who is choosing to do it, and yet it's happening. It's part of the totality. When it looks like I am choosing to step out of mind, presence is choosing to emerge.

JLW: *Thank you so much, Eckhart. It has been a great pleasure to be with you, to see the kind of impact you are having, and to share that with others.*

ECKHART: Yes, thank you.

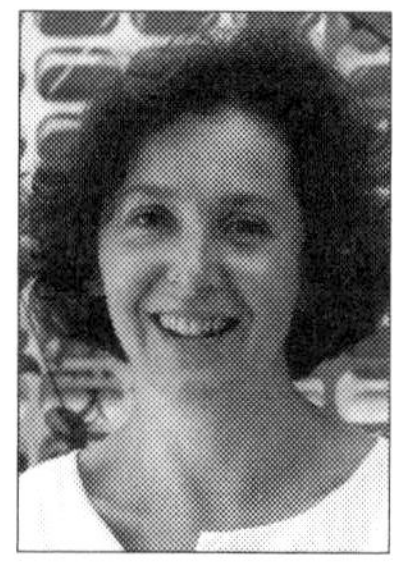

NEELAM

"AWAKENING IS WHO YOU ARE, AVAILABLE HERE EVERY MOMENT. DECIDE FOR THIS FREEDOM NOW. SURRENDER FULLY TO THE TRUTH — ABSOLUTELY, TOTALLY, AND REGARDLESS OF THE CIRCUMSTANCES. YOU ARE ALREADY FREE!"

Neelam had her first experiences of awakening as a young girl in Poland. These experiences were not understood by those around her. When she would report to her mother that we are all the same one, it was received with a negative response. But the interest in what is most real beyond what we know with our mind never left her. She moved to Germany when she was twenty years old where her quest for Truth began in earnest and led her first to America then to India in 1994. It was in India that she met her Master, Poonjaji. It was through her total trust in Poonjaji that she awakened to who she most essentially is.

Lynn Marie spent quite a lot of time with Neelam back in the days when she lived in Berkeley and gave satsangs two or three times a week and was available for private meetings at any time. Neelam now lives in Southern California and has given satsangs in the United States, Europe, Israel, and India. Many deepening experiences happened with Neelam. Lynn Marie's first trip to India was on a retreat with Neelam at the Phool Chatti ashram on the Ganges River where Poonjaji once stayed.

Neelam has a soft, loving presence that is uncompromising and caring. She is strong in her commitment to Truth. During the time we have known her, we have seen her go through a lot of changes as she continues to grow and deepen in her realization of Truth.

CONVERSATION *with* NEELAM

JLW: *At the core of the search for Truth are the questions "Who am I?" and "What is life's purpose?" In your own search, what have you found to be the answer to these questions?*
NEELAM: I am Being, Love, Peace—absolutely satisfying and fulfilling.

JLW: *So, the discovery of this is the purpose and meaning in life?*
NEELAM: Yes, of course. It's the only purpose and the answer to all of the questions.

LML: *Are you saying that you have no need to search anymore because there's an experience present that is completely fulfilling and satisfying?*
NEELAM: Right. It's simply what is, what is present.

LML: *So, simply what is is enough. It's that simple! Just coming home to what is here and now. You don't need to go anywhere else to find anything.*
NEELAM: You know, I thought I had to. I thought I had to go somewhere and find something. But in truth what I see now is that I never went anywhere or did anything to find this.

JLW: *Could you say more about that?*
NEELAM: You see, the Presence is always present. It always has been present and it's always going to be present. And every activity which takes place in that is just an activity that is being perceived with the mind. In that perception, yes there has been someone there who perceived themselves to be separate and who had to go on a search to find the Truth. But in truth, it has always been happening in that absolutely present Presence.

It's like waking up from a dream, you know. Suddenly you wake up and you realize, "Wow, I'm home!" And not only am I home, but I've always been home. I have never been anywhere else. All else has been just imagination, a perception of me not being home and searching for home and so on.

JLW: *Would you say that this waking up happens by grace?*
NEELAM: Yes, it happens by grace only! And it is so mysterious and incredible to see that nothing I did mattered. Even though it is necessary to search and to have the desire for Truth.

JLW: *How did the search begin for you?*
NEELAM: I have been consciously searching, maybe in the last ten years or so. Before that, I had an experience when I was seven or eight years old that I clearly see now as an awakening. And there was another experience when I was nine or ten, I don't remember, it's really difficult to put an experience of an absolute Presence in time. See, I always knew there was something; I always knew that. It wasn't like I didn't know it and I had to really make myself go on a search to find it. I remember speaking about it when I was a child and a teenager, but no one knew what I was saying. I would say, "Everyone is the same." And they would say, "No they aren't, what are you talking about!" I didn't know of anyone who understood that.

LML: *Often times it is a glimpse of Truth that begins the search, and once Truth is tasted, it's always with you and pulling you.*

NEELAM: Yes, it's something that is just simply present even though there are still a lot of other things that are present as well. But the knowing never goes away because it is not something that exists in time. And it is very precious.

LML: *Has Poonjaji been your only teacher?*
NEELAM: Yes, he is my Master. I remember first seeing him when I was young. In the awakening that happened when I was seven or eight there was a man wearing a hat. Then a couple of years after I met Papaji I had a dream where he came to me as this man that I remembered from that time. So, somehow the connection was already there when I was a child.

LML: *Did the recognition of the Truth of who you are occur in Papaji's presence?*
NEELAM: It occurred in his Presence, but not in his physical presence. It occurred moreover through the trust that I had gained being with him. I came to completely and fully trust what he speaks. I saw that what he speaks is absolute Truth.

There was a moment when the conditioning burned away. A fear of death arose and a desire to be close to my Master and then the whole world disappeared and everything, this body, and everything that ever existed disappeared.

JLW: *So, you had this visionary experience of the world and your body disappearing*
NEELAM: It actually happened! Everything disappeared, the world as I know it, the walls and the room and everything that was in it including this body, and still, in that, I remained.

JLW: *Do you think this is necessary for someone to awaken?*
NEELAM: For me this was the awakening.

JLW: *That is the form it took.*
NEELAM: Yes. Everything else before that was an experience. There was still someone there who was experiencing it. There were beautiful experiences, very powerful experiences, very expansive experiences, and bliss, you know, extreme bliss and all those experiences. And before that, there were a couple of years of incredible pain also. But still, until then, there was someone there who was experiencing all that. There was still a subtle separation. And only in the moment of this going beyond death was the separation finished. Since then there is simply no separation, no matter

what comes, no matter what happens, no matter what arises—and everything continues to arise in this—there is simply no separation.

LML: *The world disappeared, everything disappeared and you were still there?*
NEELAM: Everything that I knew disappeared.

LML: *And then, when it reappeared, it was never the same again?*
NEELAM: It was never the same. Of course, it reappeared; and after this experience, there was an incredible, tremendous bliss.

LML: *Could you say something about the process the bodymind goes through?*
NEELAM: There's is a continuous evolution, as I call it, of the individual bodymind stream, which is how Consciousness manifests itself here. That is the continuation of the realization, which is continuously evolving.

JLW: *Evolving from what to what?*
NEELAM: I can't say, I can only say that there is change.

JLW: *Are you referring to a deepening of the bodymind's acceptance of the realized state?*
NEELAM: I would call it penetration rather than deepening because everything that has been known before has to be absolutely penetrated by this recognition.

JLW: *So, the old habits of the bodymind occur and are transformed by the realization?*
NEELAM: Yes, they continue to arise and they are filled with That, they are penetrated, and in that there is a change in the relative perceptions. And, at the same time, nothing changes! As there is a clear and always present knowing of everything just is as it is.

LML: *Beautiful. . . Neelam, could you say that there is an "apparent" individual here on a relative level? Isn't it part of the manifestation of Consciousness to appear as an individual?*
NEELAM: Yes, absolutely. I call it the individual stream of Consciousness. There is simply no boundary between the individual and Being itself. And yet, it carries a certain amount of conditioning with it and that conditioning needs to be experienced. You could call it karma, or you can call it evolution, whatever term you use, that needs to be experienced. Everything that arises out of that conditioning needs to be experienced, but there's no longer a "someone" as there used to be. There is no longer someone who is separate from something. And yet, there has to be an

absolute ruthlessness about what arises. Because it arises from the conditioning and some identification and that needs to be ruthlessly looked at in the moment it arises, which means there has to be willingness to let it go along with everything else.

JLW: *How do you do that? How do you ruthlessly let go of conditioning?*
NEELAM: You just be quiet. Absolutely be quiet, which doesn't mean that you have to stop thinking in this moment. It just means that you are willing to stay with it as long as it takes to arrive at a recognition that there is no one there. Otherwise, somewhere on the relative level there is always some subtle identification. You have to be willing to stay with what arises until you know that it dissolves.

JLW: *And when it dissolves then you can see that there was no one there and it wasn't referring to anyone?*
NEELAM: Absolutely, because you are willing to go to the very core of it. And the very core of it is being dissolved in that moment. As its being looked at, as its being experienced, as you are willing to experience all the levels of this conditioning, with all of the involvement and everything until it disappears. And in that moment you recognize, of course, all there is is Being.

LML: *Yes, my experience is that if I stay with what arises without a movement towards it or away from it, then it naturally dissolves.*
NEELAM: And it reveals whatever it needs to reveal. Sometimes it just dissolves and sometimes it reveals something that needs to be witnessed, experienced, or an action that needs to be taken.

LML: *My experience shows me that the Presence is something that is very immediately available. No matter how engaged I am in thoughts and feelings they can instantaneously dissolve into Presence. And in that instant there is often an immediate bliss that deepens into a peace and silent resting as Being. Yet, when you speak of an absolute final recognition that no one is here. I notice that there is still a subtle sense of a someone who is experiencing what I just described.*
NEELAM: When I went to see Papaji I wrote him a letter about this. Because after being there two months I would have incredible experiences. I would experience times of an overwhelming bliss and then there would still be the engagement in everything. So I wrote to him and he said, "That's not

why you came here. You came here to discover whom you really are. You came here to experience the substratum of this experience."

LML: *Isn't the substratum the Presence that everything dissolves back into?*
NEELAM: The substratum is the very essence of everything.

LML: *And, right now there is an engagement happening of what does she mean? How is my experience different? And so on.*
NEELAM: So, let go of that!

LML: *I know Beingness, that Presence, and I know that is what I truly am. . .*
NEELAM: So, let go even of that, you see. Let go of everything and in that moment what is left?

LML: *When I let go there is an experience of what is left. It is not describable in words, but there is something.*
NEELAM: Yes, so you just stay with That, that's it. Where will you go?

LML: *This idea of a final experience that is constant—this is where a lot of confusion comes in for many people and me.*
NEELAM: You have to look at it directly. You can't understand it. You just have to look directly. You have to let go of everything, you see, and then look. And then you see if you are truly satisfied. And if you are really satisfied, there is no problem. It is only the engagement with it that makes it a problem.

LML: *In a moment of letting go and just Being, there is no problem. And yet I find that engagement occurs again and again habitually.*
NEELAM: Now at one point, for me, the distinction between engagement and everything else disappeared. I just realized that everything is absolutely included and nothing is separate. So, there's no problem. There is just this one Presence.

LML: *So I'm making the distinction.*
NEELAM: Yes, that's where the "I" comes in and says, "Am I still in the Presence?" Let go of that because that's just an idea that tries to divide your experience.

LML: *I see. I see that I am making distinctions between "I'm in the experience" and "I'm out of the experience." So. . . there can be recognition of the Presence even in the midst of engagement.*

NEELAM: Hold on! That has to be a direct experience right now, not an intellectual understanding. Let go!

LML: *[Letting go, laughter] I would like to acknowledge that you have been a teacher for me.*
NEELAM: Yes, and you for me too — same thing.

LML: *Each time I meet with you, something opens, more clarity comes. I am grateful for this.*
NEELAM: That happens spontaneously. That is the true meeting that we have. And it happens only if there is a true desire for Truth. That is why I say that you are a teacher to me also, because teaching happens only when there is a true desire, and then Truth can be spoken, then it can be manifested. When there is no need for it, it doesn't arise; the teacher arises because there is a student. But in Truth, no one is there, no student, no teacher, just the same recognition.

JLW: *Neelam, more and more people are experiencing a desire to awaken. There is a hunger for peace and freedom. Do you have any recommendations for these people? Is there anything that they can do to facilitate awakening?*
NEELAM: First of all, not to be so serious about it. You seem to be so serious about it! And in that seriousness you are giving it validity that makes it into a thing.

JLW: *Makes awakening into a thing?*
NEELAM: Yes. It makes it a process that we have to go through that is a big responsibility now. Somehow there is some kind of weight to it as you speak. First thing, let go of that. Let go of the seriousness of it. The seriousness makes it appear difficult. . . "Oh my God, now I have to awaken. What am I going to do!?" That has to go, you see.

JLW: *Okay. Then once that it gone, then what?*
NEELAM: Then be quiet for just a moment. We are so busy with those ideas. There's no quiet. I mean, look at the life we live. It's a life of running around like crazy trying to do so many things. I say, "Hey, just stop for awhile. Just allow yourself to be quiet." Settle into your Self because that's whom we are speaking about. Everything else is external — every book you read, every teacher you see, everything will be external until you are willing to just say, "Hey, it's about me!" It's me we are talking

about. It's not the search we are talking about. It's not a change we are talking about, it's Me, you see. Then what happens out of that I can't tell you because that is grace. Be it that the grace provides a teacher, then the teacher is there. Be that there is no need for a teacher, then there's no teacher. Be that there's recognition of a need to go somewhere, then you just follow that; this is pure grace.

JLW: *The quiet is the ground out of which what is next emerges?*
NEELAM: Absolutely. Otherwise it is just a search that is so removed from the object of responsibility, which is you. This would be a useless running around. . . "Let's do this practice and that practice and pray for peace and on and on." But where is this peace? It has to be known that it's here. And that's where things start. Then it really starts to unfold. And who knows what it will unfold into. It's a very, very mysterious unfolding. It happens very differently for everyone.

LML: *Neelam, what do you see as the main obstacle to awakening for Westerners today?*
NEELAM: I call it spiritual materialism.

JLW: *What do you mean by spiritual materialism?*
NEELAM: I mean making Truth into a "thing," something that you can own like anything else. Making enlightenment or peace into something you can own as you own your house or car. And no one can own that, it can only be surrendered to. That's God, that's Truth, that's Being, that's a mystery that is beyond what we can imagine.

I feel that surrender is so misunderstood in the West. It is feared and misunderstood. And surrender is at the core of all teaching, the core of all religions and traditions. And if surrender is not recognized as the most important, then it does not work. Here in the West there is such a strong feel of "me" and "I"; "I have rights to do that, and I don't want to do that, and I don't want you to talk to me like that," and so on. I'm not saying to push that away, and yet there exists a quality where everything is being surrendered. This idea of "me" is being surrendered to the being itself. When that happens then there's no question anymore.

LML: *A common misunderstanding is that if you surrender something will be lost.*
NEELAM: Yes, it's a perception. . . "If I surrender, I'm going to lose something and therefore I have to maintain a certain position because after all, I want to be equal."

JLW: *. . .or ahead.*

NEELAM: Or ahead, but at least equal. But in a moment of surrender there is an equality that is beyond any understanding. Everyone and everything is absolutely equal with no distinction whatsoever.

LML: *Another aspect of spiritual materialism is believing that you will be better or more or special if you get enlightened.*

NEELAM: And this "me" who thinks that is the problem itself!

JLW: *There is a belief that "I'm going to be enlightened" rather than enlightenment being the dissolution of the "I" and the recognition that there is no one to have it.*

NEELAM: Yes. So. . . it was a great pleasure being with you both.

JLW: *Yes, It was a pleasure to be with you also.*

NEELAM: Yes, thank you.

This interview took place in April of 1998 in Santa Monica, California.

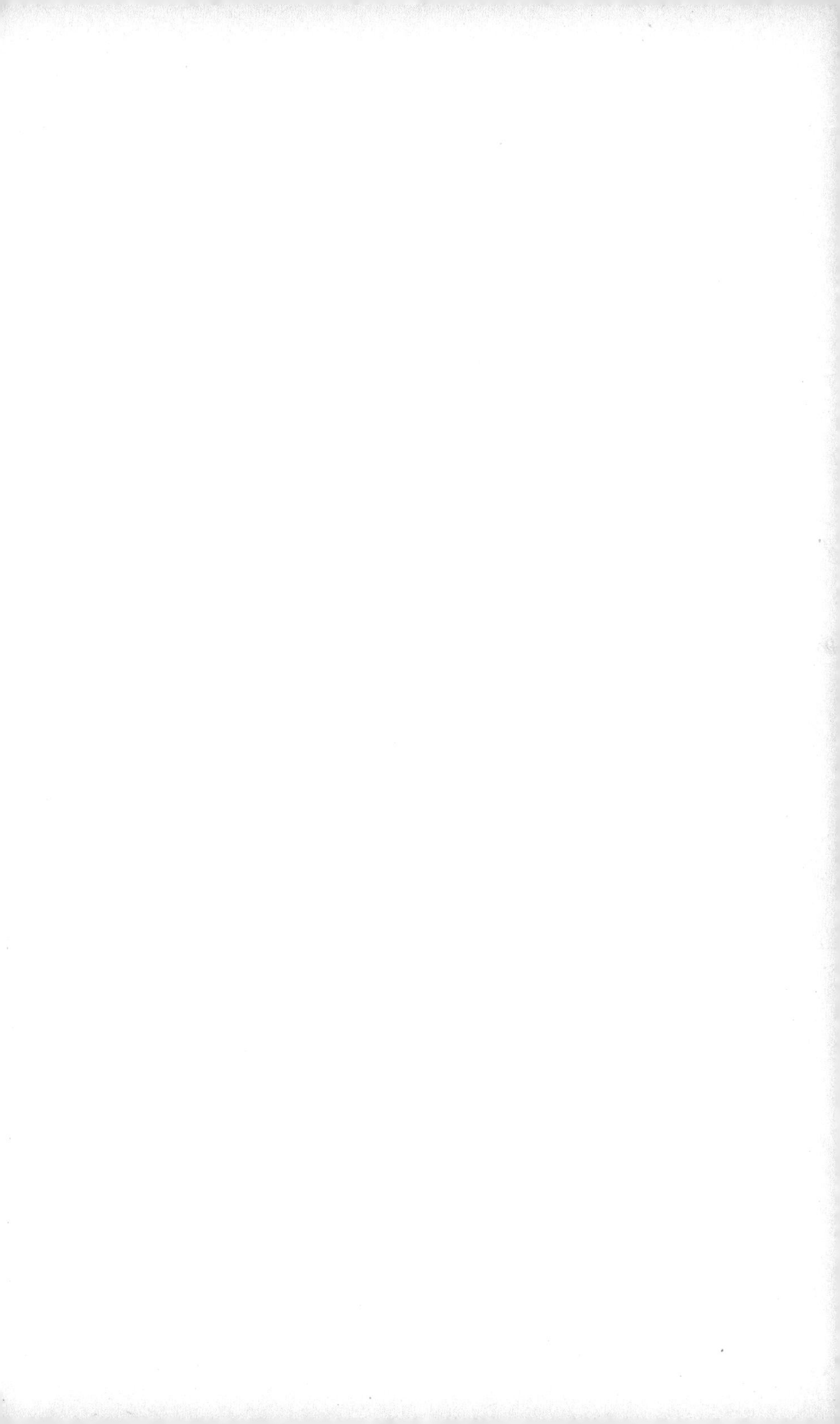

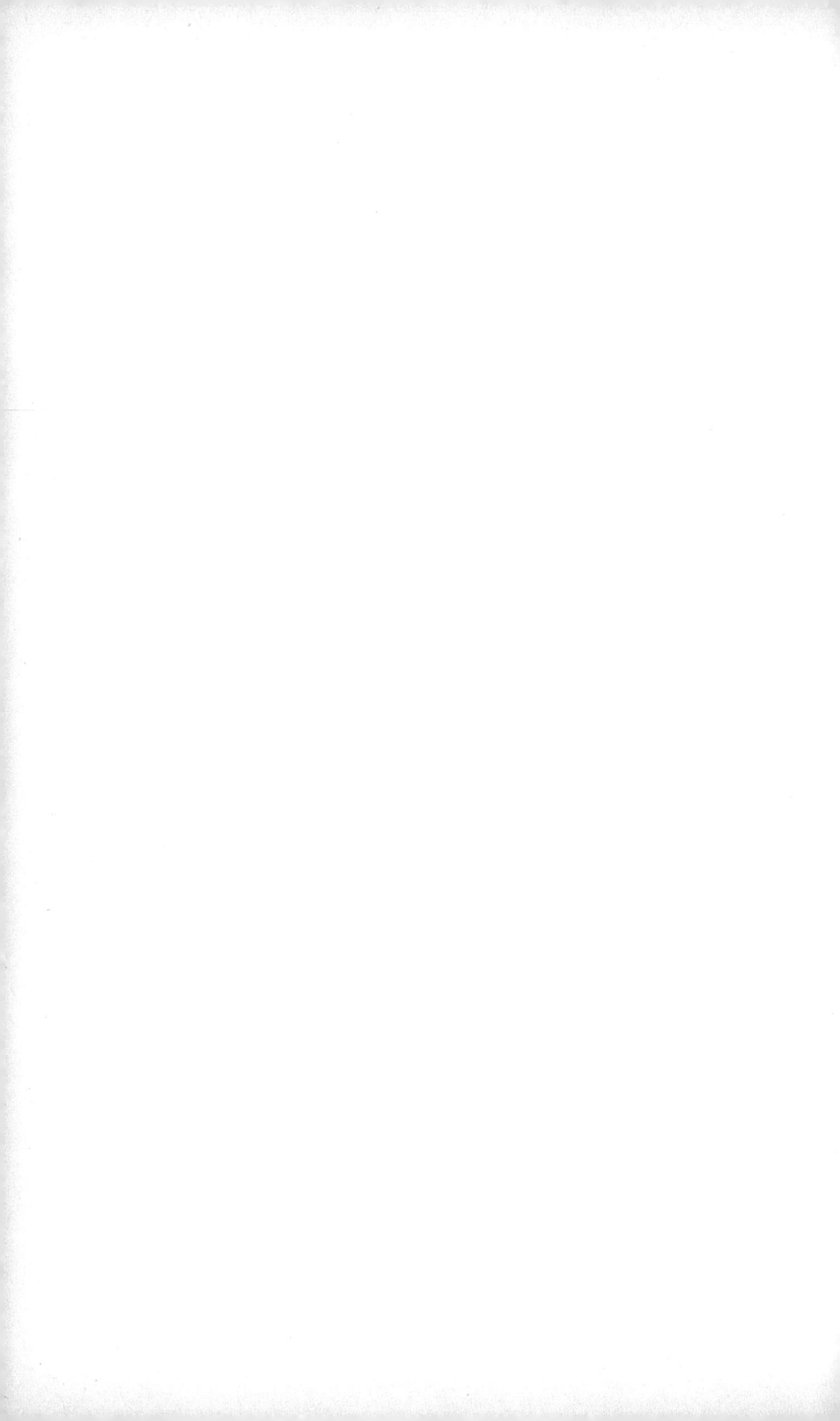

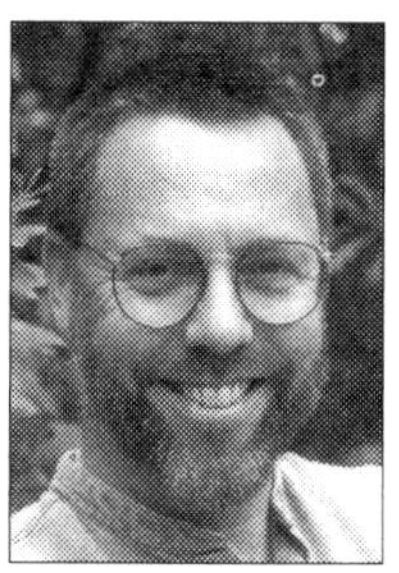

RABBI RAMI SHAPIRO

"WHETHER IT COMES FROM THE EAST OR THE WEST, ALL OF THE GREAT SPIRITUAL TRADITIONS OF THE WORLD ARISE FROM A SINGLE SOURCE... WE CAN HAVE A DIRECT EXPERIENCE OF THAT ONENESS, AND WE CAN WORK THROUGH OUR DIFFERENCES, BUT WE HAVE TO GO BACK TO THE ORIGINAL, CORE MESSAGE."

We had been searching for someone to interview from a Western spiritual tradition, such as Judaism or Christianity, and someone recommended Rabbi Shapiro. We didn't know who he was so we listened to an audiotape of a talk he gave at a conference on non-dual spirituality. We were both laughing out loud while listening to the tape. It was very humorous and entertaining, but what did he actually know about awakening? After all, we had our doubts about finding an enlightened being from the Western spiritual traditions since awakening is not generally supported in these traditions. In talking to Rabbi Shapiro, we saw that he was at the cutting edge of 21st century Judaism. Although by his own admittance he is not enlightened, Rabbi Shapiro is very beautifully pointing his congregation towards awakening to the essence of who they are and to the essence of Judaism.

Rami Shapiro has a passion for Judaism as a means to d'vehut or awaken to the divine identity of the Self. He draws from the Jewish tradition as well as mystical teachings including Buddhist meditations to create a non-denominational Judaism that provides a way back to it's original message. Rami has been a Rabbi for twenty years and a leadership coach and management consultant for fifteen years. He has published over a dozen books on poetry, philosophy, spirituality, liturgy, and guides to Jewish living. As we mentioned, he is an entertaining and much sought-after speaker and workshop and retreat leader.

In our interview with him, which had to be done by a three-way phone conversation because he was in Florida, his tone was not as humorous as we first experienced on the audiotape. He is serious about his commitment to help bring back the essential message of Judaism and in encouraging Jews to look there for the Truth in Judaism rather than leaving it to seek elsewhere.

CONVERSATION *with* RABBI RAMI SHAPIRO

LML: *This book is about awakening, and in the eastern traditions, it is taught that we can awaken to our true nature, which is divine. But the Western traditions of Judaism and Christianity are dualistic; it is believed that God is outside ourselves and we are not God. Awakening to our divine nature is not a part of the picture. Can you comment on this?*

RABBI: Well, let me start by saying that Judaism is so old and so diverse that you really can't say that Judaism says anything about anything. For every rabbi who says one thing, there are three who will disagree—not only with the first rabbi but also with each other! Every sage has an opinion and there is always one who says, "No, no that's not what it really says and that's not what it means." [Laughter] So, there's always going to be a difference of opinion.

Certainly, mainstream Judaism as it has been presented in the West for the last hundred years or so, has been highly dualistic. Theologically they posit God as "the other." Whatever we are, main steam theologians will argue, we aren't God. But dualistic thinking is really not the whole story. Judaism has a very strong non-dual thread running through it that can be found in its mystical literature going back thousands of years. This gives a different picture that is drawn right from the book of Genesis where God's breath in the form of speech is the power that brings the world into being. All things are a manifestation of God's thought and speech. Nothing is separate from God. Indeed the mystics of Judaism teach that creation takes place within God.

The Book of Genesis then tells us that we are created "in the image and likeness of God." Jewish mystics take this to mean that we are each a manifestation of God. Not the totality, of course. One cannot say: "I am God and you are not." But each of us is an expression of God in our particular time and place. It's like a hologram: even if you shatter the holographic plate, although each fragment contains the whole picture, it surely cannot be mistaken for the entire plate.

Saying that we are a manifestation of God means that our true nature is holy, pure, unsullied, and unsulliable. There is no room for original sin in Jewish thought. The actions of the body cannot stain the purity of the soul, for the soul is a manifestation of God. In traditional Judaism, one of the very first prayers you recite in the morning says: "My God, the soul which You have placed within me is pure. You have created it, You have formed it, You have breathed it into me." This prayer becomes an affirmation of our divine nature. This concept of the soul is much closer to the Atman of the Hindus than the separate inner self of more fundamentalist Christianity.

JLW: *I had the opportunity to record the first Judaism and Meditation Conference here in the Bay Area. This is the impression I got, that there was definitely a somewhat esoteric thread of non-dual wisdom running right through Judaism.*
RABBI: Yes, and you can trace it all the way back to the Bible. For example, the Psalmist uses the phrase, "kalta nafshi" which means "I obliterate my soul in my desire to become one with God." The idea is that the sense of separateness must be overcome if we are to awaken to the unity of all things in, with, and as God. The reason non-dual Judaism seems so strange is that it was a teaching reserved for the mystic elite and not shared openly with the general public.

JLW: *It's a much more of an esoteric tradition rather than a social or cultural tradition.*
RABBI: Exactly. Throughout most of Jewish history non-dual Judaism was limited to word-of-mouth—one master imparting the knowledge to one student or group of students more or less in secret. Even in those teachings that are written down we often find the authors refusing to reveal all they know and saying instead something equivalent to: "Those who know, know what I am talking about, those who don't will never know what I'm talking about."

The only way you can be sure that you have the whole teaching is to actually have a recognized master teacher, a rebbe. That in fact is one of the major crises and challenges that modern Jews are facing. The mass murder of six million Jews broke the chain of master and disciple. Those who might have brought the mystical tradition to us in a modern and much more accessible form were killed. And the Jewish people are still recovering from this huge deficit. It's a real challenge.

LML: *Yet, somehow the mystical traditions are making their way back.*
RABBI: Yes, I think they are making their way back because Jews have began to make serious explorations into other traditions, primarily Hinduism and Buddhism. What they find in these other faiths are non-dual teachings and authentic teachers who can impart the means for experiencing non-dual reality for oneself. For many this awakening is enough, they do not return to Judaism and their wisdom is lost to us. But there are others who venture into these non-dual traditions and then return to look at Judaism with fresh eyes, eyes opened to the oneness of all things in, with, and as God. Suddenly they see a depth to Judaism that was not previously

open to them. They say: "Now that I've had this experience of non-duality in Hinduism, I can see the same teaching in my own tradition."

JLW: *Is this what happened for you?*

RABBI: Yes, I guess it is, actually. I was raised in an Orthodox Jewish environment which I didn't find nourishing or satisfying, and discovered through the study of Zen Buddhism a much more insightful approach to reality. Then I came back to Judaism from that new perspective and saw things in Judaism that I hadn't seen before. But one of the things I am very careful about—and I think all of the people working in the field of Jewish spirituality and meditation have to be careful about—is not to not put a prayer shawl or tallith around the Buddha and say, "The Buddha is really Jewish." That isn't kosher. [Laughter] Having your eyes opened in another tradition allows you to go back and rediscover in an authentic manner the deeper, non-dual message of Judaism.

LML: *We would like to know more about your own experience of awakening. Has this occurred for you?*

RABBI: That's a loaded question! Let me say that I have had glimpses of the truth of who I am, starting when I was sixteen years old. But would I ever even whisper to myself that I have opened up widely to that? No, I wish I could say that, but I can't. I have had enough glimpses of it so that it's not a matter of faith for me anymore. It's not an intellectual exercise; it's an actual visceral experience, a palpable reality. I do not believe all is God, I know it. And I know it because I experience it.

LML: *So, you are saying that you have had glimpses that have given you a knowing of the Truth of who you are, but that you have not fully realized that?*

RABBI: Yeah, I'm not going to say that I am enlightened or that I am awakened. I don't think that's true of me at all. But, that I've had glimpses of that, yes, absolutely.

LML: *Could you please speak about those glimpses—what your experience is and how that came about?*

RABBI: Well, how it comes about is through meditation. I have my meditation practice which consists mainly of sitting quietly and chanting the Sh'ma, the Hebrew affirmation of the oneness of all things in God. I recite the Sh'ma very slowly, one word to one breath. Then at some point the Sh'ma fades from consciousness and as it does so, so do I. And that leads me to the problem of trying to explain what happens to me during meditation!

In effect, nothing happens to me, because the "me" is not longer present. The best I can do is reconstruct what happened as if looking backward through a rear view mirror. I come back to normal waking state consciousness and I sense lightness, an openness and joy that I didn't have prior to the meditation. I think that comes from having, at least temporarily, dropped the ego "I" and opened to the larger "I Am."

Torah tells us that when Moses asks God to reveal the true name of God, the one name that speaks to the core of what God is, God responds by saying "I Am." I think what God is saying here is that God is the deepest consciousness of all beings. God is the I AM that animates all existence. In Hebrew, the word "I"—first person singular—is "ani" and is made up of three letters: alef, nun, yud. The mystical name of God, Ain, the Infinite No-thingness, is made up of the same three letters in a different configuration: alef, yud, nun. So, when I'm referring to myself I say, "ani", and when I am referring to God, the Infinite, I say, "Ain."

JLW: *Doesn't that also refer to the nothingness or the emptiness?*
RABBI: Yes, exactly. So, "ani" and "Ain", "I" and God, are comprised of the same Hebrew letters. The difference is on the configuration. When the letter "i" is in the center of the word, you get God; when it is at the edge of the word you get "I." In Hebrew the "yud", the letter "i" in this case, stands for consciousness, or in Hebrew yadah. When your consciousness turns inward and is centered you get "Ain;" your sense of separate self is gone, your ego melts into God. When consciousness is focused outward, you get "ani," and that's when the individual self becomes apparent.

We have come a long way from your original question about what happens when I meditate, but it does get to it. When I meditate I turn inward and center my consciousness in a manner that erases my sense of self. The "me" disappears, the "I" disappears, and there is something else going on, but there is no me there to experience it. When the I returns, it returns lighter and more clear. It them projects backward and sees that the clarity is a by-product of the meditation.

JLW: *I understand. It's like a cleansing.*

RABBI: It's like a cleansing or a healing process. It's an opening. I think that most of us go through life with armor around our ego-self. Meditation pokes holes in that armor until it gets like Swiss cheese and eventually it collapses. Meditation cracks our armor until the "I" lets go and God is present. God is always present, but the defended ego blocks that knowing. Through meditation you become less defended, more open, more compassionate, more gentle. And that is the benefit of meditation—the emptying into God results in a more loving return to self. If meditation doesn't have any impact on your waking state, then what is the point of all this?

LML: *So there's a difference in perspective when you touch this greater consciousness and then go out and live your life.*

RABBI: Yes, an absolute difference in perspective—much nicer! It's no longer as egocentric.

LML: *Awakening has been described by many people as a shift in perspective or understanding. The ego self can still be here; it still operates—thoughts happen, feelings happen—but it is operating from a different perspective that is more loving.*

RABBI: That's exactly right. There is a story in the Talmud about four rabbis who experience enlightenment. The first one cannot integrate the experience with his daily life in the world and goes insane. The second one cannot understand what was experienced and rejects it, giving up on spiritual practice all together because the results don't fit his preconceived ideas of reality. The third dies; his ego collapses into God and cannot reconstitute itself. Without an ego to care for it, the body dies. Only the fourth rabbi, Rabbi Akiva, experiences awakening and returns whole and holy. The Talmud says of him: "He went up with 'shalom' and returned with 'shalom.' Shalom means both peace and wholeness. What the Talmud is saying is this: First, spiritual practice is hard work. Only one of the four made it, and these were highly accomplished sages. Second, we must generate a mindset of shalom before we awaken. That is to say we must cultivate peace and wholeness in our ego-centered lives as best we can so that when we achieve the ego-less wholeness of God it will expand our sense of peace. Of the four sages only Akiva was rooted in peace, in his connection with others. When he saw that this connection was even greater than his ego had imagined he was not threatened by the knowledge but blessed by it. Thus he returned just as he had left—at peace with self and others—only more so.

LML: *Many people have spoken of awakening as effortless and you are saying it is hard work. What do you mean by that?*

RABBI: I think it's both. The actual experience is effortless. It comes from grace. It isn't something you can guarantee. Meditation is not like a shovel; you can't just grab hold of it and dig until you find enlightenment. It isn't a recipe you can follow and be assured that a cake will result. Meditation is a vehicle for taking you to the edge, but crossing over into the world of God consciousness is not something you can willfully do. You can take yourself to the edge and then you must wait. God takes you the rest of the way. That last bit, the bit that God does is effortless from our standpoint. We do nothing, awakening just happens. But getting to the point where we do nothing is a lot of hard work. It requires discipline, time, and discomfort. Your mind starts to throw all kinds of garbage at you. There are so many distractions. The ego resists this with all its might. The ego sees awakening to God as the death of the self. And it is, albeit a temporary one. So the ego struggles to maintain its hold on things. Meditation is a struggle. A lot of people think that meditation is just a blissful experience and everything is wonderful, but that is not my experience. Indeed, when someone says to me: "Oh I love to meditate, it makes me feel so good," I cannot help but wonder if they are really meditating.

LML: *Are you saying that a meditation practice is necessary for awakening?*

RABBI: Theoretically, no. Rare individuals can experience it without meditation. But I think most people need to do meditation to "prime the pump," or to began to punch holes in that armor, which meditation does do, until it is holey enough that it can become holy. I think that meditation is necessary for most of us.

JLW: *In your work as a Rabbi, are you encountering many people who have a yearning for true freedom? Do you see this as a growing phenomenon?*

RABBI: Absolutely. I see it all the time. I see this not only in the small community with which I am involved daily, but also in the larger Jewish community. There were nine hundred people at the first Jewish meditation conference that you attended in San Francisco. A few weeks later, a similar conference was held on the East Coast and there were nine hundred people there also. They had to turn people away because they ran out of seats. There is a huge, huge ground swell of people looking for this this kind of thing.

I think everyone has that longing, but they are not all conscious of it. Jewish people who feel this longing are often very conflicted about it. They feel a desire for liberation and at the same time feel lost because they don't know how to get it within Judaism. Most often they find it elsewhere and then feel guilty for not finding it in the Jewish setting. The truth is, however, that most Jewish settings just don't offer an experiential, non-dual approach to Judaism.

LML: *What is it that you offer people who have this longing?*
RABBI: Luckily, I work with a congregation that is very open to the idea of non-dual Judaism and the whole notion of spiritual liberation. We actually have a meditation center here as part of our congregation. It is called the D'vekut Meditation Center. "D'vekut" is the Hebrew word for "oneness with God." It's a daily practice center that creates a place for meditation within a Jewish context. Ideally, if they follow our meditation program (which is outlined in my book, *Minyan*) and grace is on their side, people can experience d'vekut, oneness with God. They can bring their consciousness to the center instead of the periphery, and move from ani to ain, from self to selflessness, from I to I Am. So, when people come to me looking for spiritual guidance, I can say, "Yes, I understand your quest and you can achieve union with God in Judaism, and come and join us tomorrow morning and meditate."

Unfortunately my situation is not the norm. There aren't many Jewish meditation centers in the country and very few of these are associated with synagogues.

JLW: *Most people don't relate to awakening as something that is possible to experience, especially in the Western traditions of Judaism and Christianity.*
RABBI: Right, we have this idea that something is going to happen only after we die, if we were good little boys and girls.

Another one of the problems with Judaism as it is typically experienced is that people just go through the motions, say the right words, observe the right behaviors, and assume that this is all Judaism is—conformity to some external norm of practice. They rarely entertain the idea of actually experiencing a liberating moment or transforming spiritual encounter. For most Jews this is just not part of the Judaism they know, and they cannot imagine it as an alternative.

LML: *It's not experiential, which is also largely true for Christianity.*

RABBI: Yes, it's not experiential. I mean, it's there in Christianity; it's there in Judaism, but in most main stream synagogues or churches, you just don't run into it. What's happening is that Jewish people are saying, "It's got to be there and if it's not there, then I'll go where it is."

And, again, for Jews, this problem can be linked back to our recent history. Prior to the holocaust there were spiritual teachers and meditation masters with lineages going back hundreds of years. The Nazis murdered most of them. We cannot imagine what contemporary Jewish spirituality would be like if the students of these sages had lived and experienced the freedom and openness of the United States. Who knows what new forms of Jewish spiritual practice they would have created?

What mystics remain are often very hard to find and hidden from the main stream public. Which leads to another problem. Without recognized sages and teachers linked to an authentic Jewish lineage, it is hard to say who is a real Jewish meditation teacher and who is not; it is hard to judge what is authentic and what is not. Jewish people who are hungry for Jewish spirituality are vulnerable to con men and quacks who say, "This is Kabbalah, this is Hasidism" when in fact they are teaching nothing of the sort. It's very hard for the Jewish people to tell what is authentic and what isn't because there aren't enough of the true teachers left.

LML: *It's great that you are there to point them in the right direction and say, "This is possible. Freedom is possible."*

RABBI: Yes and luckily, I am not the only one doing it. There are some very fine Jewish teachers around the country doing this.

JLW: *It seems that inevitably it will grow.*

RABBI: It will if it is allowed to. The need is there, the hunger is there, and it will grow. It will just take a while. I'm hoping that people will be patient enough with the unfolding of this manifestation in Judaism and not simply say, "Well, Judaism doesn't have it", and go somewhere else. I think that's why we had the conferences on the two coasts—to help give these Jewish meditation teachers more visibility. And also to meet each other and talk about what we are doing and see that we're not alone. We're creating a whole new aspect of Judaism, and we're doing it almost out of whole cloth, from scratch.

JLW: *So, Rabbi, there is an incredible amount of suffering in the world. What can be done to eliminate this suffering?*

RABBI: I think that the root of all of the kinds suffering you see—the self-inflicted suffering and the person to person suffering that we inflict on each other—all of this comes from the same place. It comes from the conflict that we have inside of ourselves.

Each of us carries a heavily defended ego that we have invested with the illusion of permanency. We drape this ego with all sorts of identities and allegiances that require a conflictive "us versus them" mentality. And the only way to defend our identities is to say, "We're right and you're wrong." All of this leads to the violence that we see. It's the false ego struggling to maintain itself and the only way it can do that is through violence.

The solution to this on a very practical level is meditation. Meditation reveals that the ego has no clothes. It reveals the emptiness of that small self, and allows us to peer beyond it. And when we do, we see that we are all manifestations of one reality. With that insight into unity, the violence disappears. We see that we are all limbs of one being, or waves on a singular ocean. When that realization comes, we don't have all that conflict.

It's a challenge though, because we are labeled from the moment we are born. "I'm a Jew and you're not." "I'm a Muslim and you are a Christian." And then we are told that certain labels are in conflict with other labels. The violence is programmed into us. We need to be able to break that programming and I think meditation is one way to do it.

LML: *Here we are in the 21st century and there is still so much fighting and killing over differences on this planet.*

JLW: *And the ironic thing is that all of the different traditions come from the same essential root. Of course, there is only one Source.*

RABBI: I don't think you would ever see Mohammed and the Buddha duking it out in a boxing ring! They would see each other as kindred spirits.

JLW: *Absolutely, when you read their writings, it's obvious.*

RABBI: Right. Prior to the writings, they all had the same experience, the total dropping of the individual self and awakening to the divine as everything.

But there is another thing going on here that is also true. I tend to be optimistic. We are actually living in an amazing time in history. In 1969 when the American astronauts beamed video footage of the earth floating in space the entire planet received what I believe to be a divine revelation for the 21st century and beyond. For the first time in human history we could see the singularity of the planet. We didn't see in that photograph nice, neat, black lines separating nations. We saw that it is really just one world. We saw that we really are on space ship earth.

Whenever I teach this new revelation I articulate it this way: One God, one world, one race—justice and compassion for all. That to me is the core of any true spirituality, and various religions and teachings, if they are true, must ultimately lead to that unifying fact: One God, one world, one race—the human race—and one moral code. I would even go further and include all beings, animate and inanimate in this. This world is whole and we must be holy.

There is a movement towards becoming more globally integrated. And at the same time, those who are really invested in a fractured planet have to perpetuate violence in order to keep that integration from happening. I think that it's good to act politically if you can. We can't just sit back on our meditation cushions and wait for the unification to happen. We should do what we can to reduce the violence on a physical level. But I also think that part of a person's peace work ought to be self-transformation. You cannot unify the world if you cannot also unify yourself.

LML: *That's were it needs to start, with the individual. And yet, the more individuals who are awakening, the more the consciousness is growing, and those who are invested in maintaining separation are also intensifying.*

RABBI: Yes, because unity is frightening to many people. I deal with Jewish people, obviously, and one of the concerns that I hear is, "If everything is one, then what happens to our Jewish identity?" My prime response is that when you have that awakening moment, you don't have it as a Jewish person. All labels drop off, for there is no separate self on which to hang them.

LML: *You don't have it as a person period.*

RABBI: Exactly. When you enter into that level of consciousness your individual label that you invested so much of your energy in is gone. God is without labels and conditions; God is the unlabeled and unconditioned. And when we empty ourselves into God, when we awaken to our essential oneness with, in, and as God, then we too are without labels and conditions.

JLW: *And that doesn't detract from the beauty of the diversity. It actually allows us to appreciate all of it and deepens our intimacy with it.*

RABBI: Precisely. Our spiritual practice does not end with our emptying into God. We come back to the world of separate selves, but we do so without the illusion that diversity is fundamental or permanent. We come back knowing that God is playing all the roles, wearing all the masks and labels. We can enjoy the display without having to defend one mask against another. We can choose one mask to wear over the others because for whatever reason it seems to suit us best, but we know that it is a mask and that beneath all masks is the shared face of God.

JLW: *But it doesn't actually work that way.*

RABBI: Definitely not. When you get to a point in meditation practice when the ego is screaming, "Stop!" "Don't do this to me!" I don't want to see this, many people quit in order to maintain their loyalty to the label of their birth, or even the more primal loyalty to the label "me." This is something that ultimately has to be surrendered.

LML: *It seems that there needs to be a ripeness or readiness first and that is growing in people.*

RABBI: Like I said, I tend to be optimistic, even with all of the violence that we are seeing. It's the birth pangs of the Messiah. We are moving in the right direction. The question is, can we do it fast enough before we blow ourselves into oblivion?

LML: *You have spoken of many obstacles that Jews have to awakening. What do you think the obstacles are that we all have as Westerners?*

RABBI: In the West we are really locked into a fundamental dualism that is supported by what Albert Einstein called the "optical delusion." We look around and cannot help but see things as being separate. So when spiritual teachers talk about a non-dual reality that our eyes can't actually see, we just say its bunk.

In the West it seems to be science that is moving us beyond duality. This is going to allow us, as good, hard thinking, rational Westerners to see that dualism is wrong. Science will show us there is no split between mind and body. Science will uncover the truth that reality is of a singular nature. Physics has been the most spiritual science of the last two decades. Biology is the next science to take off in this direction. Biologists already know that biologically there is only one living system. They are already speaking of the web of life. So science in the West is going to bring us to the nondual worldview that meditation has revealed in the East. But that is not to say we do not need meditation in the West. Science is not a replacement for spirituality in the West; it only sets the groundwork for it to be more widely accepted. Meditation will allow us to apply the unity revealed by science to the subtle realms of psyche and morality. Science reveals the wholeness of life. Meditation reveals its holiness.

JLW: *In closing, is there anything else you would like to add?*

RABBI: Whether it comes from the East or the West, all of the great spiritual traditions of the world arise from a single Source. And the great wisdom teachers that have carried on that original message are really beyond labels such as East and West. They really are all pointing in the same direction. Whatever the tradition, if you look deeply enough into it and go back to the original message—not the sidetrack ramblings of professional clergy or the paranoid politics of religious bureaucrats—but if you go back to the core teaching and explore it with the same kind of openness that says: "Let me see, let me test the hypothesis of this one God, one world, one race, one moral code idea." If you test it for yourself through meditation, then, as the Bible says, "You taste and see that God is good." We can have a direct experience of that oneness, and we can work through our differences, but we have to go back to the original, core message.

JLW: *Then it's not a conceptual overlay, then it's a direct experience that becomes the root of its expression.*

RABBI: Right, we need that direct experience. For too many of us religion is a vicarious experience, we get our God second hand, we worship ideas as idols, and let labels determine the worth of people. We need to get beyond all of this. We need that direct experience that will free us from the garbage that surrounds so much that passes as religion today. We need to hear the original message of one God, one world, one race, and one moral code. We need to meditate and see for ourselves what is true.

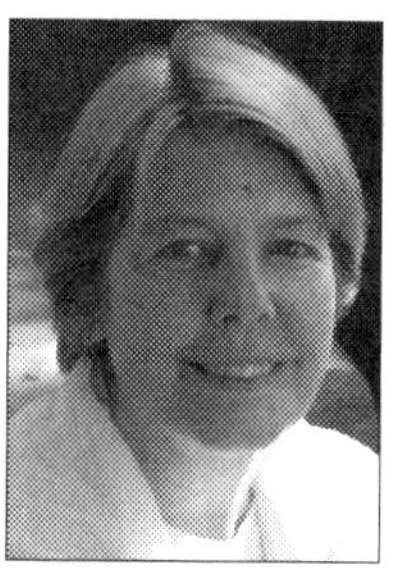

SHANTIMAYI

"MANY, MANY PEOPLE ARE REALIZING THEMSELVES, EVEN IF THEY HAVEN'T CROSSED THAT LAST THRESHOLD... AND I FEEL THAT THIS COULD BE THE BEGINNING OF A QUANTUM AWAKENING ON THE PLANET. IT IS POSSIBLE NOW."

At this time in our process we had become involved in a large and growing community of people in the San Francisco Bay Area who are dedicated to the truth and to awakening. This has been a group of people who we would run into again and again at the satsangs or teachings of the growing number of teachers who either lived in or came to the Bay Area. A friend in the community told us about the pending arrival of ShantiMayi about whom we had heard favorable things from friends who were present when she and Gangaji met in India in 1994.

Lynn Marie was scheduled to be on retreat during ShantiMayi's visit and so John did this interview while ShantiMayi was staying at the home of a friend of ours. We met on the carpet in the den as we sipped a fragrant green tea and spoke of awakening. ShantiMayi shares some of the story of her awakening in the course of our conversation.

In spending some time with ShantiMayi on several occasions since this interview took place, it became apparent that, of the people we have interviewed, she is one of the more traditional teachers. In other words, even though she is a Westerner, ShantiMayi is a lineage holder in the Hindu, Sacha lineage and she presents herself very much like an East Indian guru. And she is likewise responded to in a devotional manner by many of her followers. At first we did not think she would be appropriate for our book because we were looking for Western expressions of awakening, not Westerners with an Eastern expression. But, we came to see that this is just another flavor of the vast number of ways that Consciousness is manifesting itself in awakening among westerners at this time.

ShantiMayi grew up in a Russian Orthodox church. Her master, Maharaji, is a traditional Hindu. ShantiMayi has been given quarters in her Maharaji's ashram for her work. She believes that she is both traditional and not traditional at the same time. She teaches Mahayana Buddhism, the path of dedicating oneself to awakening for the sake of all beings. ShantiMayi says, "If Ch'an, or Zen, could be taught, that is what I would teach."

She lives at her ashrams in India and Europe and travels the world extensively, sharing her expression of the traditions she is drawing from.

CONVERSATION *with* SHANTIMAYI

JLW: *So, firstly, I'd just like to thank you for speaking with me today. We have been starting our dialogues with the question, "Who are you?" Who are you in the most essential sense?*

SHANTIMAYI: In that sense it cannot be answered. Whatever the essence is, it must to a large degree, be understood. It is better to say nothing because nothing can be said. Spiritual language is often not understood in its profundity, yet it is repeated and repeated and repeated like a parrot. It is very difficult to speak in verbal language to That which I am, and all are. We hear so many times; I am not a body; I am not a mind; I am not my bundle of ideas or my idea about my history. This is precisely accurate; still the language is over used and misunderstood. The deeper meaning is often missed altogether.

JLW: *Yes, there is a way that any languaging rapidly becomes jargon and pretty soon it will be commercialized and used to sell cars and hair spray.*

SHANTIMAYI: Yes, and also Babylon. This is a great danger. You must come to realize the deeper meaning or the teaching itself is conceptualized and remains superficial and misunderstood.

JLW: *And yet there is something that occurs that is called awakening, or realization or enlightenment.*

SHANTIMAYI: Yes; yes.

JLW: *What do these words mean for you?*

SHANTIMAYI: Enlightenment may mean pure unobstructed awareness piercing through the appearance of duality and through an apparent unity as well. Neither objective nor subjective it is undivided emptiness in the deepest, unimaginable sense; it is your nature. Of course, enlightenment is not describable. Yet, enlightenment, its meaning and incomprehensibility has been described in infinite ways.

JLW: *One can also have "glimpses" of enlightenment.*

SHANTIMAYI: Yes, and glimpses are very important. Glimpses come and go as all experiences do. Glimpses reveal a depth of insight that was not reached before the glimpse. However, when the wisdom of insight remains without dwindling, when it stays with you forever, when you no longer can see double, no matter what the senses report—this is not a glimpse. You realize that all that is experienced is indeed the total and undivided essence. This is an opening to enlightenment; little can be spoken beyond this.

JLW: *And Awakening?*

SHANTIMAYI: Awakening is a little bit different. Awakening may be what appears to be the process in time; as in the sequence of glimpses leading to enlightenment. Finally, when the psyche is ready, one will realize enlightenment. Enlightenment is radiant and like the sun's rays, never cease illuminating all that is. And does it get deeper and deeper? In someway, yes; in someway, no. Its like floating in space—this is just an analogy, it is not really like this—like floating in a marvelous spaciousness and pushing yourself, like a space shuttle. Does it go deeper in space or is that all relative?

JLW: *Yes and no.*

SHANTIMAYI: Exactly. So relatively, it is not that you actually go further or deeper or more, but this is never ending. It's as far as the imagination can imagine, and this is just the beginning.

JLW: *There is a continuous unfolding.*

SHANTIMAYI: Indeed. There are not really levels of enlightenment. Either you are enlightened or you are not. Essentially, all are enlightened. This is absolutely the way it is. Buddhists say that there are levels of enlightenment. I would say there are levels of awakening. Enlightenment itself is when you come to realize existence for what it is and that is it. This is no small matter. Whether you can remember past lives or whether you have siddhis or not or whether you just end up a monk sitting on a cushion or an executive; whether you turn the beads for ever and ever for the great awakening of the planet or you forget it; it is still the very same totality and unobstructed emptiness; it is still the very same spacious Awareness. It is the very same.

JLW: *So these words that you are using now, "this spacious Awareness". . . What I notice is there is nothing here and there is Awareness, there is a presence of Awareness. Those words really point very directly to what it is for me.*

SHANTIMAYI: Yes. That is absolutely accurate. What it is for you, it is for all—presence, absence, totality, all things, no thing. Awareness is also a conceptual word that is very difficult to intuit because the moment you intuit nothingness it becomes something.

JLW: *Awareness is rapidly conceptualized as nothing.*
SHANTIMAYI: That is right. And that conceived nothing is something. So therefore, you are in a paradox; which is great. If you are in the center of a paradox, your mind is at ease; it is not a problem. Thinking is silenced. If you are trying to balance the paradox, then a struggle arises. The greatest insights are realized without conceptual inference.

JLW: *The presence of Awareness is not nothing in the sense of a dead void; there is a clarity and a presence.*
SHANTIMAYI: The void is not dead or alive, it is empty and potent and beyond description. Awareness is present and absent. One must be aware of absence as well as presence. The void is clearer than diamonds. Awareness is the permeating quality, so to speak, of every experience. It never fades, it never wavers, it never comes when arriving and never goes with departure.

JLW: *Yes. The Buddhists say that this, which we are, is neither enhanced by enlightenment nor tarnished by samsara.*

Now, my next question. You have spoken of what we call glimpses and a final cut after which there is never a wavering from the intuitive perception of totality. Is this what occurred for you?
SHANTIMAYI: Yes. However, the term "final cut" may be misleading. There is unexcelled enlightenment and unwavering totality is realized, final is a distance I can not measure. As far as glimpses go, it was like this: many bubbles of insight came up. The insights delivered wisdom and were then "pop"—gone. Again, like all experiences, gone.

JLW: *So you had had many glimpses.*
SHANTIMAYI: A lot; a lot. I mean, I spent my life very intensely focused spiritually—not that it has to be like that at all. I spent my life very intensely with my Master and very focused with my guru. I stayed in his ashram six months a year, cloistered actually. He wouldn't even let me out of the gate. He said, "Stay here" and I did. I was living in solitary to a

great extent. And every six months I went into the world, returning to the United States to earn the money to go back to India. A friend gave me her storage room to live in year after year. It was packed with her things and a mattress for me. I worked very hard and lived very simple for many years. This was such a great blessing. I stayed with my Master and it was by his grace that my eyes were cleared and my heart was opened. It was by his grace that I matured. I swear by it. The Guru was everywhere for me. The tree was my Guru, my boss was my Guru, everything was my teacher. Many insights came with great wisdom and compassion. Heavy delusions were lifted off my shoulders. Encrustations of ignorance were broken away from my heart.

Enlightenment is your very nature. You attain to what is present in you always. You gain the Truth which you always are. You cannot really become: you realize the ever present reality. Understand?

There was one moment in time that doubt could not enter. Not like ever before, this time nothing could enter. There was no language for doubt or validity. I could see all that my Guru had ever transmitted to me in silence. In that moment, enlightenment removed that which could be enlightened. There was no longer a question, nor an answer. There was no need, no one, nor nothingness. The mirage of myself and what I thought the world to be, vanished, leaving no trace. Ego and ego-less-ness could not arise as concerns. Everything that seemed to be disappeared. Now all would be as it is. As I has always been; not less, not more.

At the time I was at work in a cannery, a factory where vegetables from the summer crops are put into cans. There, alone, in an isolated area at the back of the cannery, a sensation ever so slight, ever so delicate, consumed me. It was like a needle piercing a soap bubble. The entire universe, as I knew it, disappeared with a very subtle pop of that delicate tiny bubble. I stood very still for about an hour. I could only look into the emptiness. There was no I or not I. Emptiness in emptiness. Impossible to describe. Nothing had changed but, oh, what a relief.

No one could guess that the lady wearing the yellow rain gear, a hard hat, and boots had just been crowned by a line of Perfected Masters. No one would care. Then at 2:45 I just took my time card and clocked out of the cannery; nobody knew; nobody had any idea. Then I went home only to return the next day. Identity had awakened to the immutable perfection unruffled by perception. Since that day, change has no grip in the same way that a day never passes in a dream.

As for mastery, my Guru entrusted his work to me. Along time ago I had promised my life to him, and this is part of it. It is by his grace that I have realized my nature. It is by his grace that my life has come to this, that I grace others to awaken. The Master bestows grace, transmitting the Truth in silence and inspiring a deep commitment to realize the Truth.

It is by the grace of the cliff that the river becomes a waterfall. It is by the grace of the water that the basin fills. The Master is the waterfall, the disciple is the basin, grace is the flowing of a higher power which opens the way beyond consciousness.

My guru was intent in me taking a lot of time for settling without saying a word about what had happened to anyone. When I went back to him, I told him and asked him, "What do you think?" And he said, "Wait." I said, "Okay." So the next year I came again and I said again, "What do you think, Maharaji?" And he said, "Wait." And I said, "Okay." And then, when he knew and I knew he knew, we didn't even speak about it. He never ever said, "Go tell the world." He just said, "You just sit here and when the rose begins to waft its own scent, people will come and enjoy; until they do, be still." I said, "yes." It happened like that. People began to come into the ashram some four years later. From there the teaching began.

JLW: *So beautiful; so wise.*

SHANTIMAYI: He is very wise; he's very simple. And he taught me in a way that he doesn't teach his own Indian people. He is Vedic and he teaches ritual and the Scriptures and the Vedas. And he taught me silence and self-realization by heart and surrender. This was my way; I had never heard of self-inquiry.

I also tell people not to go out and tell others right away. Don't promote yourself at all. And ironically, one day a lady came, and then another, and from then on people came through the gate by the hundreds. In India, usually I see about seventy to a hundred people a day. It is not much, but I never went out to see them; they came through the gate. I love my guru very much.

JLW: *It's very clean for it to come about in that way; I like it.*

SHANTIMAYI: Me too.

JLW: *Can you say a little more about that last satori?*
SHANTIMAYI: I can tell you that for awhile after, I was very shaky. The sight or understanding didn't change; but in maya, I was very wobbly. There was something completely centered and completely monolithic in every wavering and wobble. It was completely still, unchangeable, hard, and undeniable. And recently someone asked me if there has been any shifts in the Awareness. And I said, "No. I've not had any shifts in the Awareness. There is no movement in it." There is nothing to shift; there is not deeper or higher or anything like that. Even though, again, you go across that threshold forever. And yet there is an unending, empty radiance; maturity blossoms and blossoms and blossoms. It is very difficult to speak of.

JLW: *Yes. In the Avadhuta Gita it speaks of the homogeneity of it; homogeneous, it is all one thing.*
SHANTIMAYI: The essence does not change but the experience does; the two are actually one. Still the essential nature does not change or transform. It cannot change.

JLW: *How could it? There is nothing to change and there is not time during which it could.*
SHANTIMAYI: This is realized amid limits and changes; it is a very common sight; people see it all the time.

JLW: *Yes. And there is something really amazing that some of us are graced with recognizing the significance of this which is stable through change. I have known people who have seen it and they dismiss it as nothing.*
SHANTIMAYI: Or run away from it because there is nothing there and it is a little scary. Now imagine this: you are afraid of nothing. This is amazing isn't it? I always say to people, "If I had a sense to be fearful, I would be much more afraid of the ignorance than the silence."

JLW: *In a sense the fear is the reaction of the so-called "ego" to its imminent demise.*
SHANTIMAYI: Of course.

JLW: *Because, when the individuality opens into totality...*
SHANTIMAYI: Then it is no more.

JLW: *ShantiMayi, you give satsangs and I notice that you do make some suggestions for people. In fact, I have noticed that sometimes you highly recommend self-inquiry.*

SHANTIMAYI: Yes. I have read a lot of Nisargadatta and recognized inquiry's value. In fact, in reading his words , I felt my guru was working in it all the time. In fact, in everything, all that was shown to me, I felt Maharaji was at the center of it.

JLW: *This is the blessing of having a guru.*
SHANTIMAYI: Yes, indeed. He has also given to me the shakti of our lineage. The power of our lineage supports whatever I may do in service to this world and awakening the hearts of people everywhere. He has entrusted me with his work, after some time.

JLW: *What I have noticed is that many of us have had a recognition and then there is a process or an unfolding, like the peeling of an onion, which leads to stabilization of the recognition. Some people began to teach before this stabilization occurs. The way your guru had you wait shows his wisdom, verifying stabilization first.*
SHANTIMAYI: Absolutely. Look at what the fifth Zen Patriarch did to the sixth Patriarch—thirteen years in exile, "Go to the kitchen. Don't tell anyone; keep quiet. I am not going to even look at you." Great Zen Masters were tested again and again by their Masters. Even Master to Master the tests were welcomed, as long as the body remained. I too welcome the challenge and the turning and polishing of the Buddha gem.

JLW: *In the Zen tradition, you don't teach until you have been realized for seven or ten years.*
SHANTIMAYI: That's smart. I actually don't know why we are being put out so fast now.

JLW: *Many of us are. I can't say I am fully realized; I have had the insight and I come back to it almost instantaneously when it seems to waver...*
SHANTIMAYI: That satori will come to you.

JLW: *I assume it will.*
SHANTIMAYI: Yes. It will.

JLW: *It seems that it will and like everything else about this, it has its own timing, and that's fine.*
SHANTIMAYI: Exactly; it is by your own grace that this occurs.

JLW: *Well, yes, if you mean by the grace of That which I am.*
SHANTIMAYI: Exactly! Isn't it exciting?

JLW: *Yeah. It is beautiful and yet, I know that I am already being used. There is an old woman in the Berkeley hills who is a friend of mine. She's ninety-four years old and getting close to her death and one day she spontaneously asked me to teach her to meditate. So I sit with her regularly and I point, "...No that's a concept; come back to what is aware of that concept." That kind of thing happens to me often now. This comes to the whole thrust of this book which is that something seems to be happening. Many of us seem to be awakening—I don't know but I assume it is global; it is certainly in the West.*

SHANTIMAYI: It is global.

JLW: *I don't know if it's because somehow astrologically it is time, or because of emerging ecological calamities, or because of the superficial confusion of western corporate hegemony being spread around the world.*

SHANTIMAYI: It is all of it and beyond reason or need for reason. It is always possible for the world to awaken and now is always the right time.

JLW: *Well, this is the vision and prayer of every Bodhisattva, every master, "May all beings recognize this easily, effortlessly, and now."*

SHANTIMAYI: Exactly. This is my heart, our way. Let it shine, let it shine, let it shine; let everyone realize its own significance and its true essential nature.

JLW: *So be it!*

In your satsangs, I have heard you mention several forms of self-inquiry, and chanting as a way of balancing, catharsis, and letting the mind come to rest here. Is there anything else you recommend, or would you like to elaborate on why you recommend these things?

SHANTIMAYI: Chanting has the quality of exulting the heart, hmm? It has the quality of catharsis; it lets all of the energies that are penned up out, particularly when you just let yourself go into the song, listening or singing. And it also has the quality of something having a beginning, a middle, and an end and you are sitting, mindless in the center of it, in presence without thinking. So, chanting has many good qualities.

JLW: *I know what you mean. When I first heard bhajans being sung, before I knew what a word of it meant, I had learned fifteen of them. It just touched me so deeply; I just loved the heart and the spirit of it. So beautiful.*

SHANTIMAYI: That's right. The heart and the spirit are very important to the chant. Chanting opens the heart and uplifts the spirit. Another quality of the chant is that all of these voices become one sound and one song like universe, eh?

JLW: *And the catharsis, is that for clearing what is blocked?*
SHANTIMAYI: Yes, because even though from the view of the Truth, nothing is there, people are always feeling hurt or wounded or angry. They tell all the time that they have these feelings. So, singing or chanting is really good for transforming the energies really deep inside oneself.

JLW: *What about self-inquiry? Self-inquiry seems to be very direct, to me.*
SHANTIMAYI: Self-inquiry is very direct; a very direct route because you are face with boundless, nameless silence. That silence eventually reveals the incomprehensible truth in all.

JLW: *Do you think a teacher or a guru necessary for awakening?*
SHANTIMAYI: Yes. A true Master is a gem, a rich experience, a bath in the Ganga; a complete resolution, a totality, a giant of emptiness, a giver, a reliever. A master brings out the Master in the disciple and dissolves the sense of ego. A true resonance.

JLW: *Well, certainly in the sense of sympathetic vibration and resonance, if a guru is living as the qualityless quality, then there is a way that over time you cannot help but come into resonance with him or her, if you are open.*
SHANTIMAYI: Yes. And the totality of the love and the totality of the compassion are the only expressions that can come from that.

JLW: *ShantiMayi, as you awakened, your sense of a personal self was put into a much different perspective. Did these effect relationships and your responsibilities?*
SHANTIMAYI: Absolutely. I was always kind of reclusive, anyhow. And in my guru's ashram, I was learning unconditional love. All relationships were drenched in the mists of unconditional love. The one was all and that became very obvious. There were great challenges in this life. All the cuts and scrapes led again and again to the essential one.

JLW: *Well, perhaps it could be said that what happened was that something didn't continue to happen — there wasn't a return again to a sense of duality.*
SHANTIMAYI: Yes, exactly. I couldn't express it better. There was never a sense of duality again; either for or against. And yet, here I am doing this Gayatri Mantra for the world, huh?

JLW : *You are doing the Gayatri Mantra for the world because there is a lot of suffering in the world?*
SHANTIMAYI: There is a lot of apparent suffering.

JLW: *Exactly; there appears to be a lot of suffering in the world. And one of the things you are doing in relation to that is chanting for the awakening of the world, which is the solution to suffering.*

SHANTIMAYI: Yes, the solution to the suffering of the world is a mass awakening. Just between you and I, the only thing that I can see helping would really be a mass awakening. Because, when you are awake or aware of the possibility of being your true nature, when you really have your "I" rooted in that emptiness, then of course, the "I" is no more.

Yet, you have to remember that Ramana died of cancer. And though he had his sweet, sweet smile on his face, the pain was in the body. He wasn't attached to this body, this illusion, but it was there. Nisargadatta was screaming but he wouldn't own it for himself; he said it was just an experience, it was not who he is. Suffering is a potential that lies in this "I." Any subtle or tremendous suffering is rooted in believing "I am this experience." Suffering will only cease when one realizes that they are not; but the pain may still go on.

JLW: *Some of the pain will go on, and if the mass awakening we are envisioning does occur, a lot of the needless suffering will be eliminated because people will be much more compassionate with each other. They will recognize that this is me, I cannot let me suffer like this.*

SHANTIMAYI: That's already happening, isn't it?

JLW: *Well, yes, and no.*

SHANTIMAYI: Yes, but you say you see, and I see also, that many people are indeed awakening. Many, many people are realizing themselves. Isn't it true? And I feel that this could be the seeds scattering of a quantum awakening on the planet. It is possible now.

JLW: *There certainly is a lively vision of it in our hearts right now, and in many others' hearts as well.*

SHANTIMAYI: Yes, and it opens up in interesting and surprising ways. One time I was working in the cannery, cleaning with one of these pressure washers with 2,000 pounds of pressure and this biker—in the cannery you get such a diverse mix of characters—this biker came into my stream and I just avoided him but got some other people wet. He was really sorry and apologized and said, "I bet you think I am an ass." And I said,

"I can't perceive of you like that at all. It never went through my mind. Not possible." He was so touched by that; and I was also.

JLW: *Well, it has been a great pleasure to be with you, thank you very much. Is there anything you would like to add?*

SHANTIMAYI: Yes, there is. John, I would like to add before we depart a bit about the teachings. I am most moved by Ch'an and convey the teachings of great Masters such as Bodhidharma and Huang Po. There has been an endless succession of Great Ones. Also we chant the Gayatri Mantra and meditate in the way of the Bodhisatvas for
world awakening.

This is an inheritance of our Sacha lineage. We support impersonal, universal awakening for all beings. We hold the lineage in our hearts and they live in us as our breath and blood flow. Therefore we wish to live in spiritual excellence every moment of our lives. We feel that the Master and disciple relationship is precious and is of great importance.

Buddha (enlightenment), Sangha (the spiritual family as well as the world family as well as the lineage), and Dharma (the way to realization) are the three jewels in our treasury. Our life is the dharma as long as our priority is awakening. We are not confined to anything and are free to awaken in all ways. Diminishing concepts and piercing through delusion is our concern — totality and emptiness in the truest sense; this is our diamond-cutter heart and concern. That pretty much sums it up. I deeply bow to you, John, and to all who read your book.

JLW: *And I to you. Thank you.*

SHANTIMAYI: Yes, thank you also. Namaste.

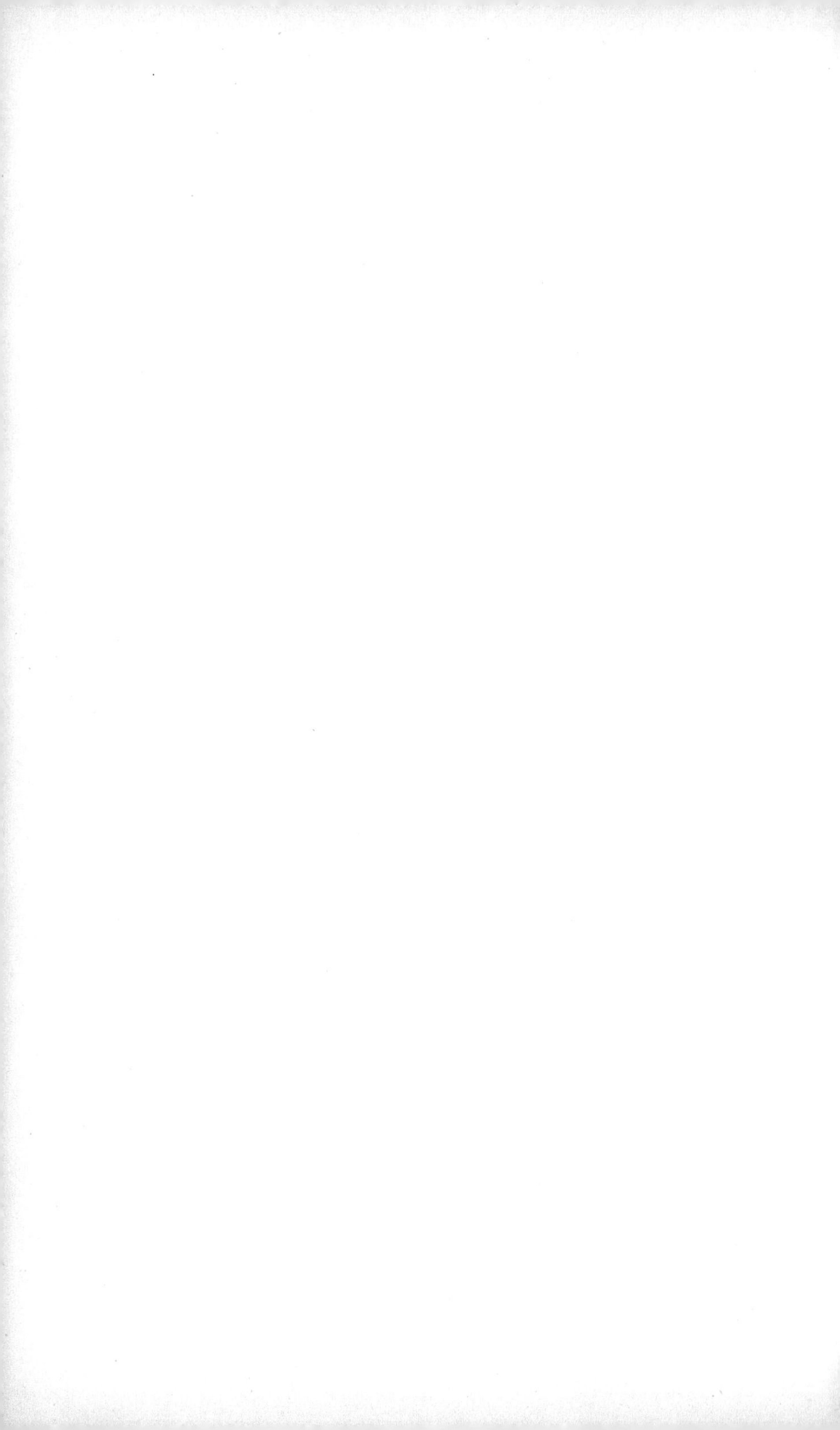

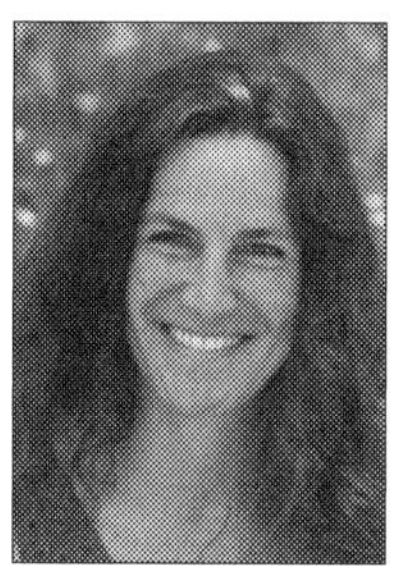

SUZANNE SEGAL

"THESE EYES SEE THE INCREDIBLE BENEVOLENCE OF THE UNIVERSE, WHICH IS COMPLETELY TRUSTWORTHY IN ALL RESPECTS. THERE IS NOTHING TO FEAR. EVERYTHING IN EACH MOMENT IS COMPLETELY TAKEN CARE OF — AND ALWAYS HAS BEEN."

from Collision with the Infinite

Suzanne referred to the body-mind as "circuitry" that has been created so that the Vastness can experience the ecstasy of Itself in a way it could not without it. Suzanne exuded this ecstasy with a child-like delight and wonder, full of exclamations such as, "It's so Awesome!" The circuitry called Suzanne Segal shined radiant with the love and beauty of the Vastness we all are. As she could only see others as That, and nothing else, this Vastness was often brought foreground in the awareness of those who were fortunate enough to be in her presence.

We are two of those fortunate few who were able to be with Suzanne during the six months of her life when she was such a powerful expression of this Vastness. She was like a blazing comet that shone so brightly for this short period of time, then was gone. This interview was done in 1996 and Suzanne left her body on April 1, 1997, April Fools' Day. It was important to her that the messages her powerful life experience was meant to convey become known. She told her story in her book, *Collision With The Infinite*, and we are happy to share her message further here.

Suzanne referred to herself as a "describer," rather than a teacher, and related to others as her buddies. Calling us her "buddies in the Vastness," she emphasized that we are all in this together as "co-describers" of the incredible miracle of life and its unfolding awakening. Suzanne offered no teaching, no practice, only descriptions of her remarkable seeing of the Truth of what is.

Suzanne's life is an example of how an awakening can occur spontaneously, and without even understanding what had happened for as long as ten years. She often told us that she wanted her experience to give the Western world an important message that the mind can have an extremely strong reaction to that which it cannot understand. And that those reactions, such as fear, do not mean for an instant that we are not the Vastness. She wanted her life to convey that everything is here in this Vastness, nothing is excluded, and that everything is as it is.

We will always fondly remember the blissful walks on the beach we had with Suzanne, and weekly group meetings where she shared her experience. Lynn Marie shaped several paragraphs of this introduction at her memorial, which took place at Stinson Beach, north of San Francisco, where her ashes were returned to the ocean she loved so much.

CONVERSATION *with* SUZANNE SEGAL

JLW: *Suzanne, we'd like to begin by asking how you see yourself; who are you?*

SUZANNE: I'll give you the straight answer here. There is only one answer that I can give you. I am the Infinite—no personal reference point—the substance of everything; I am the Vastness that is everyone and everything. And, I must add here, never for a moment does the awareness of that infinite substance that is everything ever move out of the foreground of awareness whether there is waking, dreaming, or sleeping states of consciousness occurring in the circuitry. There is no where for it to go. Where could it go? It is constant, every moment experience.

JLW: *That is a powerful answer. . . How did this experience come about for you?*

SUZANNE: Fourteen years ago, when I was four months pregnant with my daughter, I was standing at a bus stop in Paris, France. In one moment, everything that I had ever taken to be my personal self completely disappeared. It was just gone. As I waited for the bus to approach, something in consciousness was loosening somehow. And when it got there—I am sure it had nothing to do with the bus driving up—this reference point of an "I," a someone that everything was about and that everything that occurred in life was structured around, was gone. It was like a switch had been turned off. And it was never to turn on again.

The first response that the mind had to this completely ungraspable experience was absolute terror; but that terror never changed the experience for a moment. In other words that terror never got the reference point back again. There was no personal self, but nothing stopped; the functions continued to function just as before. In fact, better than before. Speaking was still speaking and walking was still walking. I even went to graduate school and got a Ph.D.

I experienced this fear for ten years. During this time, I consulted a lot of psychotherapists because it seemed like something I needed to be cured of. Every single one of these therapists considered this to be a problem. And they all had a diagnosis for it. They couldn't quite understand how it could be that there was such great functioning occurring, but they took the fact that there was a lot of fear to be a sign that this was a problem.

Towards the end of the ten years, there was a clear awareness that this was not something that was going to go away. It was time to start investigating other possible descriptions of what this was. It was time to investigate it with people who maybe knew more about it than Western psychotherapists. I started reading spiritual books and I came across a description of something that was exactly what I had been experiencing. It was an interview with Jean Klein, an Advaita teacher, and he was saying that there is no personal I, that it doesn't exist. He was saying that there is nothing wrong with this; it is the naturally occurring human state.

I also found a Zen teacher up in Northern California who told me that I was seeing with the eyes of the ancients; his assurances that the fear reaction was just a season and that spring would come were very helpful. In talking to him, it became very clear that everything is there, too. I saw that the presence of fear meant only one thing—it meant that fear was present. And that was it.

Shortly after realizing this, I had the experience while driving that I was driving through myself to get to someplace that I already was, because in fact I was everywhere. I wasn't going any place because I was already everywhere. There was a shift from no personal self, no "me," to seeing that this experience of no personal self was actually the substance of everything. That is when the springtime began with the quality of joyfulness to it.

What I can describe about what is being experienced currently, is residing in the Infinite within which the Infinite resides. There is no end point in all this. We are talking about the Vastness. It is very large. It continues to show Itself and show Itself.

JLW: *Initially, you thought something was wrong and now you have discovered that what you are experiencing could be called enlightenment or awakening. Is this how you see it now?*

SUZANNE: I have tended not to call this enlightenment and to call it only the "naturally occurring human state," because this is who everyone is. The most obvious thing to this view of the Vastness is that it is who everyone is. And so to call IT something like "enlightenment" or "awakening" . . . well, maybe. The Infinite does become something that is forefront in the awareness, so I guess you could call it a "waking up" to That. But it is not like you become something else once you see That. It is who you are. It is always who you have been. So, it is the seeing of what you have always been.

JLW: *Could you say then that awakening is a shift from not seeing who we have always been to recognizing That?*
SUZANNE: Okay, but that recognition doesn't change who you really are, ever. You have always been That. And yes, there is a way that the Vastness Itself can perceive Itself so directly, without any fogging or shading or taking anything else to be who you are. I guess you could call it a waking up, but what seems most important to convey is that this is who everyone is all the time, whether the direct awareness of it is there or not.

JLW: *Do you have any suggestions or recommendations for others who are experiencing the desire for this recognition? What can one do in order to have this experience?*
SUZANNE: These "doing" questions are the ones that I have wanted to address the most, particularly in this Western culture which is so strongly based on doing in order to accomplish something. From the point of view of the Vastness, doing something is slightly absurd. First of all, who would be doing the doing? And secondly, That which is doing has always been doing, and will spontaneously continue to do. The only answer the Vastness has been able to come up with in terms of anything resembling an answer to this question would be to see things for what they are.

JLW: *Could you please elaborate what that means?*
SUZANNE: Seeing things for what they are means purely that. The Vastness that we all are is like an ocean that exists in relation to everything—as the Infinite notice of everything being just what it is—Itself included. It sees thoughts for thoughts and feelings for feelings and sensations for sensations. There is never a desire or request that anything be anything but what it is. The Vastness knows that everything is there just as it is, so the desire for something to go away, or be something different doesn't occur.

Let me get real specific in terms of what we were talking about. A few minutes before we started taping, we spoke about the "I" construct that passes itself off as who you are, as your reference point. From the view of the Infinite, of the Vastness, that construct is seen for what it is—a construct, an idea. And an idea can only be what it is; it can only be an idea. When an idea is seen for what it is, there is a way that it empties itself of what it appeared to be full of—some defining determinant of who you are. And when the perception is emptied and seen as what it is—just a concept, a construct, an idea—it ceases to act as any sort of compelling screening of this Infinite Presence which you actually are. This seeing things for what they are is occurring all the time. That's another thing that doesn't just start at some point.

JLW: *There is a shift in identity though, or a dropping of this "I" construct. . . Something happened for you.*

SUZANNE: Something happens. It seems like most of this occurs within the mind. In the Western culture, which I am most familiar with, the mind is trained to adopt a personal construct as the reference point. It just believes that there is a personal doer. It's made to believe that you have to "make something of yourself." The Western mind believes that you have to be a certain way and you have to figure out how your life is going to go in order for it to be successful, in order for it to happen the way you want it to. Everything that you hear in the culture, in Western psychology in particular, is all based on the assumption that there is a personal doer that has to be the best one it could possibly be. So there is all this work that is brought to bear on it. It is like the work on the mind that is asked to happen within the mind. The mind has to go in and look at itself and try to see how it needs to be changed around, how the furniture needs to be moved around in the house of itself.

JLW: *And instead of trying to change the mind, your recommendation is to just notice, "Oh, it's the mind." Something like this?*

SUZANNE: That is what the mind says, "Oh, it's the mind." The view of the eyes of the Vastness is hard to describe as it is brought to bear on anything because it isn't perceived through the mind. And it isn't perceived through the perceptual apparatus of the circuitry. The view of the Vastness, the eyes of the Vastness, exist within the Vastness Itself. It has its own sense organ that permeates it and exists at every point in it that is always seeing things for being what they are and seeing Itself for what it is. And yet, it does seem that what happened when I was standing at that bus stop included the mind, and its circuitry became a participating portion of that sense organ of the Vastness. It's like the mind and circuitry joined into the sphere of the Vastness. Another way to describe this is that the way the mind and circuitry are always permeated with the sense organ of the Vastness must have come foreground and then that took over as the main perceptual stance or position, a position of placeless origin.

JLW: *Suzanne, does it seem to you that more human beings are awakening to this Vastness at this time in the Western world?*
SUZANNE: Yes. Isn't it great! It seems that a large amount of folks now are opening to this. You have to remember though that we're talking about the San Francisco Bay Area here, which seems to have a higher concentration of folks who have this interest. The Vastness does carry a very strong, non-personal desire to know Itself. It does appear to be the real purpose of human life, for the human circuitry to participate in the sense organ of the Vastness. And that does seem to be happening. There are people who have come to talk with me who have spoken about their lives joining into that sense organ of the Vastness in a conscious way.

LML: *It does seem like there is more interest in this. I know that in the seventies when I first studied transpersonal psychology and meditation, enlightenment was something that wasn't even being considered. Now, people are seeking and experiencing this.*
SUZANNE: Yeah, it's really wonderful. I can't possibly convey how totally, ecstatically, joyful it is for the Vastness to move in Itself like this, when awareness of Itself is carried through the human circuitry. It is just amazing!

LML: *Are you saying there is a joy in it moving unobstructed, consciously?*
SUZANNE: Well, it is always moving unobstructed. The joy is when this is expressed and received in the foreground of the Vastness. It really is amazing. And, sometimes people say to me, "I don't want to give up the personal because I really feel attached to the personal. It really seems that that is where I feel the most feeling, and depth and falling in love, etc. How could I give that up?" The folks that are very involved in studying with Hamid Almaass are very big on deepening and developing the personal. They are the ones that have said to me most directly, "I don't want to give up the personal. I don't know what you are talking about. Why would I want to give it up?"

What I tell them is that it was never there to begin with. And anything that feels like a personal kind of joy pales in comparison to the joy that is experienced when the eyes of the Vastness are the only thing that is being seen through all the time. These eyes exist in the Infinite, at every point in it. There is a joy that is not personal—you almost have to find another word for it because it transcends the category of personal joy—it is so constant and so extreme. It is in everything, everything; it doesn't have to be just certain things that reveal this joy, it's everything.

JLW: *It's just the innate delight of being.*

LML: *And outside of that awareness there is suffering. Identification with the personal always involves suffering, even with what people call happiness.*
SUZANNE: Identification and taking something to be other than what it is—seeing it as something that is not the Vastness, or as something that is not good, or not desirable. There is one way to end suffering and that is for everything to be seen for what it is, because then we don't ask that something be different in order for suffering to stop.

JLW: *So, seeing something for what it is implies seeing with the eyes of the Vastness.*
SUZANNE: That is correct.

JLW: *Thus, the way to end suffering is to. . .*
SUZANNE: ...see with the eyes of the Vastness.

JLW: *People are going to read this and out of their deep yearning, they may try to apply it and wonder, "How...*
SUZANNE: "...How am I going to do this?"

JLW: *Yes, how does one shift from seeing through the personal eyes to seeing through the eyes of the Vastness?*
SUZANNE: Your question is contrary to how the Vastness actually exists, which is that it is always perceiving things for what they are from within Itself. The implication that one should figure out what to do in order to see with the eyes of the Vastness implies that that isn't already constantly occurring, and you have to do something to connect with that. I have always hesitated to say, "do this or do that." I say only "see with the eyes of the Vastness," which is already happening, because this leaves the mind confounded about what to do.

JLW: *When the mind is confounded, it is stopped, and there is an openness.*
SUZANNE: I am not necessarily aiming for the mind to be stopped. I guess the aim would be for the mind to recognize that it doesn't know. The mind needs to see that there is nothing for it to do. It is not the doer and it doesn't have to find the correct position. It's like, That which has been

happening all the time and which has always been the doer, finally shows Itself to Itself for what it is.

LML: *So, that showing Itself to Itself just happens?*
SUZANNE: It just happens and it is always happening. There is this wave of constancy of the Vastness perceiving Itself that is always going on and the mind can say, "How am I going to do that? How am I going to perceive that? How am I going to perceive that wave of perception that is always perceiving itself? How am I going to connect with it? What can I do in order to see with those eyes that are seeing all the time?"

LML: *All of those questions are just thoughts in the mind.*
SUZANNE: Exactly! So there, you just saw it for what it is—just thoughts. In seeing things for what they are, the Vastness is doing the very thing that the mind tries to figure out how to do.

LML: *The mind didn't see that? Something beyond the mind saw that?*
SUZANNE: Yeah! The mind didn't see that. So, how do you try to explain this in a practice, right? If I gave a practice, it would be colluding with that same construct that passes itself off as the doer.

LML: *Are you saying that spiritual practices can perpetuate the construct of a doer?*
SUZANNE: Spiritual practices imply that something has to be done in order to become the Vastness or in order to see that the Vastness has always been the doer. That is part of what I think this life of Suzanne has just been trained to convey—that this is always who everyone is, nothing changes. This is always who the doer has been. It is seeing itself all the time, in every moment.

JLW: *I am having a reaction to what you are saying. For myself, and for many others, life has been so difficult at times. There is a lot of suffering in this world. So, I'm thinking, "Yeah, so the Vastness is having a great time perceiving Itself as the Vastness, but what about the tumult of suffering that is occurring in the mind and is identified as 'me' by the mind?" I look at the world and I see that so much of the suffering is a result of the ignorance, fear, and greed that this confusion perpetuates.*
SUZANNE: The truth of this life is interested in showing everyone that things are what they are and that is the relieving of suffering. You don't have to make something look different in the world in order for suffering to be relieved. It is that which everyone is, seeing everything for what it

is, that makes it impossible for anything to be seen as suffering. It is simply and completely what it is; it is going on all the time, John.

JLW: *It's as if I get it and I don't get it. . . maybe it is just the mind reacting in the face of something it can't understand.*
SUZANNE: As you have heard me say many times, the mind has a very strong reaction to this which it can't grasp, and which is basically structured in a mystery that is so completely confounding.

JLW: *Yes, the mind exists within the Vastness, so how could the mind comprehend it? This, I understand. There is that understanding. All I can do is surrender and see that here I am actually knowing nothing.*
SUZANNE: This culture is really not hot on knowing nothing. It wants everybody to know as much as possible. The highest accomplishment in this culture is knowing, "I know this, I know that." You get tested on all of it too!

I want to comment on what you said about both knowing and not knowing simultaneously. You know that you don't know and you know that the Vastness is experiencing Itself. These two experiences are going on simultaneously, seeing the construct of the "I," the personal reference point, and seeing that it is empty of what it was taken to be full of. Simultaneity is very much the experience of the Vastness perceiving Itself, by the way, because that is what is always occurring.

JLW: *There is the arising of appearances, which actually do appear, and there is also the recognition that there is nothing really there. The emptiness I am is what they are made of.*
SUZANNE: Exactly. That's it! That is a description of it. You come to know that this apparent duality doesn't exist, but there is also the simultaneity of diverse things appearing that are all made of the same substance. This does not imply duality; everything is there too.

JLW: *Suzanne, we'd like to address one of the main fears people have about awakening to the Vastness they are, which is that they will not be able to function well in the world.*
SUZANNE: Oh I know. That is the main fear. That was the main fear that I had for ten years. "How am I going to get anything done when there is no one here to do it?" "If there is no one here to do, how is anything going to get accomplished?" Then it became so clear that that which had always been doing had always been taking care of everything. So, nothing

really changed. [laughter] There is the appearance of, "Oh, this is the next thing to do, and the next thing to do," and it is not like somebody has to be brought to bear to accomplish any doing or any decision. There is never anything that looks like weighing pros and cons, or figuring out the best way to go because this all comes out of that which tries to imagine, or construct how things should be. The real doer is so unimaginable, so completely mysterious. Everything that has been calculated as the next thing to happen is calculated in that mystery. If it waited for the mind to figure out what the next thing to do was, then, well, I don't think we would have what is naturally occurring as the planet and its seasons. If everything waited for the mind, do you think that we would have all these trees and sky and planets and stars and human bodies? It would really be a bummer if it waited for the mind to imagine it, in order for it to be there. So, doing and accomplishing continues as before, and as a matter of fact, is even more fully accomplished, even more fully doing. There is not ever a screen or a question of how things are going to happen; they just happen.

JLW: *From the perspective of no personal "I," how do you experience relationship with others.*

SUZANNE: Relationship with others, of course, we have to talk about that, right? Everything that arises, arises for a completely non-personal purpose. So, relationship is no longer something that we can call "personal." I don't ever experience myself relating to another, and what I am always relating to is the Vastness that everybody is. It is just obvious for me that everyone is that Vastness. It is relating to Itself. Now, there happen to be different flavors of relationship with different people. I just have to say that it is calculated in the mystery to be whatever is necessary to serve that non-personal desire of the Vastness to know Itself.

JLW: *Is it true that relationships are always serving that non-personal desire of the Vastness to know Itself?*

SUZANNE: Yes. Just as it is true that there has never been a personal doer, that has always been true.

JLW: *Well, this issue of a personal doer leads into the next question. . . Do spiritual practices assist in recognizing this natural state of every human being?*

SUZANNE: I haven't found one yet! There are people who have been pretty upset about my saying that I don't see any techniques or practices to do. They believe that I am saying it is equal if somebody goes out and murders fifty people or they sit and meditate. I am not saying that at all. I know That which every one is, and the Vastness is completely trustworthy in what it does.

I don't know how this happened to me; I was standing at a bus stop. Yes, I did eight years of transcendental meditation, from the time I was seventeen. But I also did this practice when I was a child of sitting and saying my name until I saw that that name didn't refer to anyone and the personal self disappeared. I would do that when I was five, six, seven years old. I don't know if these practices did something or not. I don't know if there is a technique to bring this about. The implication is that a technique is needed to bring about something that wouldn't be brought about unless you did that technique. That is just not how I see things. I see this as always occurring, that no one changes when what is, is seen to be what it is. I also think that meditation is fine, but who is it that would stop the mind? And, stopping the mind is something that is not required, because the Vastness doesn't use the mind to perceive itself. Also, the "I" that would be brought to bear to try to make the mind stop doesn't really exist.

If it is obvious to meditate, then that is what you are going to be doing. If it is obvious to not do that, then it is obvious to not do that. Again, I see how trustworthy the Vastness is, and it shows Itself in this obviousness all the time. You don't need any reasons for living by what is obvious. This is just what you do. You meditate, you don't meditate. If you are doing your personal growth work, you are doing that. Of course, seeing it for what it is would be kind of nice.

LML: *It seems that the non-personal desire for the Vastness to know Itself would just make it obvious to each person to do certain things that somehow are part of the unfolding — and it could be anything.*

SUZANNE: That's right. It can be anything, and it can be different for different people.

LML: *In the West, many people do psychotherapy when they are suffering. I am interested in your work as a therapist from this awakened perspective.*

SUZANNE: I've actually started a couple of groups for psychotherapists to try to convey the view of the Vastness, and that freedom is what every person who comes in to see me is after. Psychotherapy has traditionally formed very rigid views about how people are supposed to be if they are healthy. People have been pathologized because certain things happen to arise, and the smallness of the acceptable range is so unhelpful that many people end up feeling worse about themselves after engaging in therapy than they did before they started. Therapy in the traditional sense is structured around an idea of an "I" that has to be presented in the best possible way. So, I do a lot of investigating with people about who they take themselves to be; how they got those ideas about themselves; which ideas end up passing themselves off the most compellingly for the Truth; recognizing fear for what it is; and really pulling the plug on this whole campaign to have people live by ideas and ending up with the belief that those ideas are who they are. What's naturally occurring is helping people to see these ideas that have made up their identity for what they are—ideas.

JLW: *Are there any other questions you are frequently asked that should be included here?*

SUZANNE: Well, there is one thing that I think people hesitate to ask. They want to ask, but they don't. It was contained, perhaps in your question about relationships. There are many ideas about what relationships look like or are supposed to look like once the Vastness is constantly being seen for what it is in everything. Nothing goes according to any ideas about how anything is supposed to look. There are many spiritual systems and traditions that say you should only live like this, you should only eat these things, you should dress like this, you should be celibate, you should this and this and this. They're saying that if you are seeing with the eyes of the Vastness this is what your life will look like. One of the most important things that I think my life has been put here to convey to the West is that it doesn't look a certain way, that everything is there, too. Most of the spiritual traditions say, "If there is fear there, then she doesn't have it or this is not the Vastness because fear is there." The presence of the fear never for a minute brought back a personal reference point. It never for a minute obstructed the view of the Vastness for Itself.

LML: *What a statement that is making!*

SUZANNE: That seems to be what this life is meant to convey. That everything is there too, and it is what it is. This means that looking for life to be a certain way comes completely out of the mind and its ideas of how things are supposed to be. That ten years of fear that I went through actually was the most important time for what this life is trying to convey to people in the West.

LML: *Because the fear didn't change the recognition that there was no personal reference point.*
SUZANNE: That's right. From that bus stop time onward it was clear that there had never been a personal reference point—absolutely no personal reference point at any moment.

LML: *Could you say that you were believing the fear, and not seeing it for what it was?*
SUZANNE: Yeah, okay, and that was the training in seeing the sphere of the mind and how things are taken for something else within the mind. It still didn't create a reference point. When I say, everything is there, too, I mean everything is there, too. Mind is there doing its interpretations, doing its fear about what something means, and trying to understand what it all is.

LML: *So, you are saying that all of that was there, but still there was no "me," no reference point.*
SUZANNE: No reference point. And there were so many years of that. Who knows what would have happened if there had been more years without somebody saying, "Yes, I know what this experience is." A big part of that change of season came from mind realizing that it couldn't grasp what was occurring, it was too mysterious.

LML: *The mind just went to the end of its road where there was nowhere else for it to go.*
SUZANNE: Yes. And the mind couldn't actually gather any evidence for the fear being justified. Functioning was going on just fine, everything was happening, it was all unfolding, one thing would happen then the next thing would happen, then the next thing. The mind wasn't required to make decisions about how things were going to be.

LML: *So, the mind wasn't needed for what it previously thought it was necessary for. It was seen to not be the central doer.*
SUZANNE: Yes. I think that is the most important thing that this life is conveying. There has never been a personal doer. The seeing that there is no personal doer is not when it starts that there is no personal doer.

This gets into something that I actually want to convey. This is the kind of thing you want to mention, that seeing everything is being done by a non-personal doer is not the same as nothing being done. The obvious will still always be showing itself. It is really ultimately unavoidable to live by the obvious because it is always showing itself.

JLW: *I think we are complete; this has been wonderful.*
SUZANNE: It was nice.

JLW: *It was fun being with you.*
SUZANNE: That's another one of those things that this life is to convey—this is fun! It's not all serious and it doesn't have to be a certain way. That is just not so. I'll say it again and again; everything is there too. It always has been. You cannot say that because something is arising it means that the Vastness isn't vast, or it means that it is not made of the Vastness.

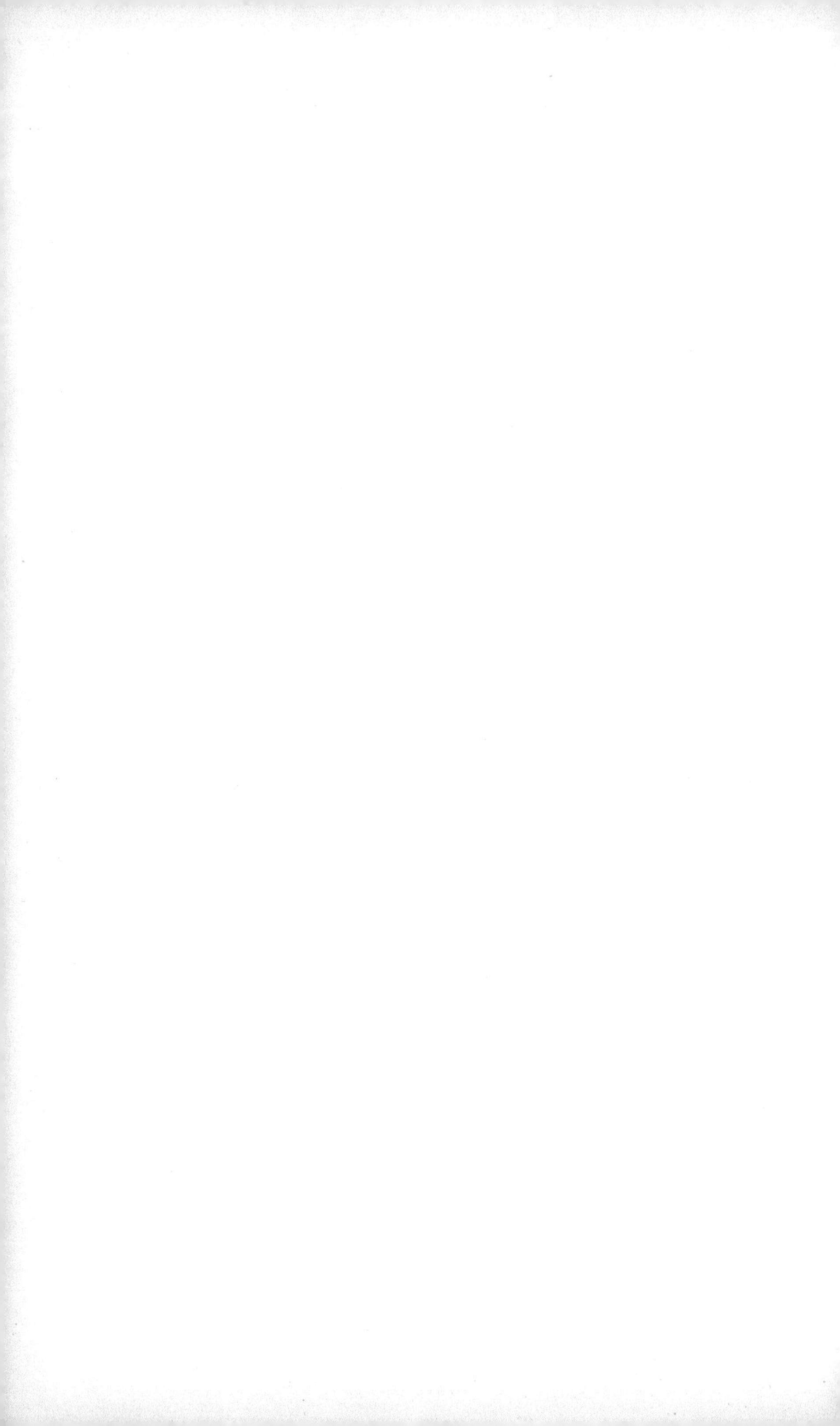

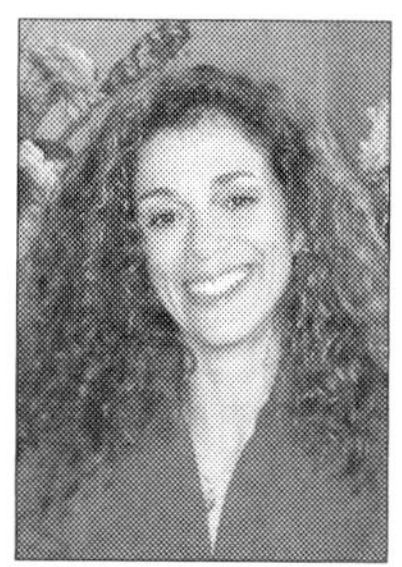

VALERIE VENER

"IT COMES DOWN TO THE TRUTH WE HAVE HEARD FOR CENTURIES THAT NO ONE UNDERSTOOD BECAUSE IT'S A SECRET UNTIL YOU TACITLY UNDERSTAND IT. I AM THAT VERY ONE THAT LIVES ME. I AM THAT THAT'S LIVING YOU. I AM IN THAT THAT'S LIVING YOU."

Valerie's expression of herself is so lively and so animated in her body that a written transcript of her words is missing a significant component of her communication. She is in almost constant motion while she talks, utilizing her entire body to articulate her experience. You could say that she "dances her talk." Valerie is a highly creative person who has been a dancer and choreographer as well as an actress, musician, poet, and artist. The continuous flow of energy and movement through her being visually demonstrates what she teaches: an allowing of all energies—physical, mental, and emotional—to be, fully as they are.

One aspect of her expression that does come across in words is her grounded earthiness. Valerie gets down into the "nitty-gritty" with people; into the grit of life in the body with all it's functions, its desires, aversions and pains. There's nothing that she's uncomfortable talking about. We noticed that this made us comfortable talking about aspects of ourselves and our lives that we usually don't discuss with "spiritual teachers." With Valerie, there is an unusual aura of ordinariness, not being anything special or particularly spiritual—just another human being. One might even say that she leans the other way and expresses herself in a way that is contrary to what one would think of as spiritual. But this does not appear to be intentional. It seems that she is just being naturally who she is. Also, we should note that Valerie's dialogue is more circular than linear and takes you on a journey that sometimes seems to go off the point, but always comes back on target.

In 1981, when Valerie was twenty years old, she was caught in a house fire and had a profound near-death experience that was a significant part of her awakening journey. At one point she surrendered completely to her death and everything was transformed; the fire which had been terrifying a moment before was now fascinatingly beautiful. She became absorbed in a realm of brilliant light that left nothing to fear and nothing to be desired; there was nothing left to reach for. She saw that this brilliance was her own true Self and realized that the Valerie who had been identified with the body was not in control, never was, and never could be. It was during this near-death experience that her spiritual teacher, Da Free John, appeared to her expressing eternal love and two choices: to return to her present body, or take on a new one. Either way, he said, she was his. Valerie knew nothing of Da Free John before this experience and after her recovery found him and became his student. What she considers her true awakening experience occurred ten years after the fire and is described in this interview.

CONVERSATION *with* VALERIE VENER

JLW: *Probably the most essential question that all of us ask at some point is, "Who am I?" What comes up for you when you ask, "Who am I?"*

VALERIE: This is essentially what I am talking about all the time with everyone I meet. For me, answering that question had to do with being able to sit in a place in myself, or rest in a place in myself. And for a long time, "Who am I?" became how to get to that resting-place. The one "I" was was always trying to get to the resting-place. This became very funny to me at some point—that I was trying to get to the resting-place by doing something that wasn't resting. Then it just became obvious who I am.

I am that very One that lives my body, that lives your body, and I am absolutely energetic; I am in energy, I am as energy. And, I am absolutely delightful, delightful in my trillions and billions of modifications, and "how wondrous it is to be me!" [Laughter] All that exists outside of me is a modification of me, and all that exists inside of me is also a modification of me. Simultaneously, I am all of that modification, and this one that I am. Now, if That can be expressed clearly in writing, I'll be happy!

LML: *Can you say something about what that one thing that lives you and lives all things is?*

VALERIE: The best way I can express that with words is to say that there is a stillness and then there's a wave and then there's a stillness and then there's a wave, and I am That which is the stillness and the wave. This sounds ridiculously intellectualized, but that's the best way I know how to say it. In motion, or in discussion, in love-making, or in shit-taking, or birth giving, or even in sitting at the bottom of the breath, just sitting and waiting for a breath to come in, I experience my being as the One who observes the waves, allows the waves, feels the waves and is the waves.

JLW: *Nice description.*

LML: *Valerie, what does "awakening" or "enlightenment" mean to you?*

VALERIE: I hate this question. I am especially hesitant to answer this question because after the fire experience, it was very important for me to get back to that experience of my Self that I remembered. That was the beginning of what I would call my conscious spiritual life. Before that "spiritual life" was just very natural as a child, I would stand on my head and put my legs in a full lotus position because it felt good and my body would be involved with energies that would now be called clairsentient. I was experiencing life from an energetic point of view. After the fire, it became apparent that the one who was experiencing life from an energetic point of view was suffering and was unhappy. I had always known I was unhappy, but now I knew that this unhappiness was a sense of individuated self. From that point on, I considered the "awakening" to be relaxing past the sense of "I" that was suffering and identifying again with the sense of "I" that was not suffering.

So, the reason that I hesitate to answer that question is that as soon as I start talking about enlightenment people imagine that it's something that they don't already have. And they have that same sense of wanting to get back to themselves. Now, at this time in my life, I do not have any sense of wanting to get back to myself anymore, anywhere, anyhow. The whole quest to get back awake was recognized as the mistake. This was seen as what was causing the feeling in my body and mind of unhappiness. So, I don't know how to describe awakening because from one point of view it's a ridiculous quest that is actually the cause of the sense of "I" and its suffering in the first place.

JLW: *It creates an "I" and the discomfort of the one who is not awake.*

VALERIE: That's correct. When I wasn't fully rested in this simplicity, for whatever mysterious reasons of my unfoldment, "I want to be enlightened" was very, very important. We all experience this in some way—"I want to be a fantastic artist, free in my expression. I want to be able to play racquetball where there's no mind. I want to be in relationship where I can to be absolutely fully free and able to love and be loved."—All of these things are associated with this yearning, burning place of wanting to be other than who we now are. And from my point of view, enlightenment is the natural ability to sit in that yearn, burn place and allow even the yearn, burn to exist without contracting or pushing away from it. But from the point of view of the physical, seemingly separate self, that is a very painful thing to allow.

So, before my fire experience, I found myself always wanting to avoid feeling that pain. It was very scary to feel my separation, my mortality, my isolation, my intense, burning sorrow of "not good enoughness." From the point of view of my body, that still exists, but without interference. In that freedom, it makes so much sense that it's my joy to allow it. It's joyful because I'm not trying to go anywhere to get out of it, so it's freely allowed. When a wave—any emotion, or anything—is freely allowed, it quite naturally works itself out. When it's resisted, it stays in place in a way that feels uncomfortable. So, if a wave is going to move through anyway, you might as well relax and enjoy it.

JLW: *Could you tell us the story of how awakening occurred for you?*
VALERIE: Again, this question assumes the point of view that I was "unawakened" and an "awakening experience" occurred. So now we're going to talk about my unenlightened, unfulfilled self, and how it finally, perfectly became fulfilled. This is were I get frustrated because I can talk about that and in talking about that I am going to have to paradoxically, simultaneously, symptomatically disagree with myself—disagree with that perspective altogether! I would say that my awakening has always, already occurred and that I feel sort of tumbled through it almost like a drop in an ocean. It's something that is always occurring. We have one essential Self-occurring.

LML: *Did awareness of this awakening that's always occurring begin with the fire experience?*
VALERIE: No, I couldn't say that the fire was the beginning. I could say that because there was a profound, near-death experience, there was a Self understanding that was not yet full and perfect, but very, very close. But that experience was itself a result of a prior Self-understanding. And self-understanding allows natural, true, and human behavior.

I guess the answer is that it's been coming in waves, this awakening experience. It has certain moments. It has great big moments. It has great deep moments. But, if I were to say when my actual awakening experience occurred, it was not until ten years after the fire. In the fire there was a very dramatic understanding of my brain core in relation to how it perceives energy, how it interprets energy, how it relates to energy and how it contracts upon energy and locks itself in place. That occurred in the fire, and then from that point on my experience of self was very, very different.

But the actual awakening, where there was no longer a search for awakening, happened in a very simple moment. For me, my practices have always involved the body and what tends to happen is that I just freely let go into myself whether I'm in a tub of water, on the floor, or even leaping through the air. When I was trying to get "enlightened," it was about letting go so that the Divine could teach me or awaken me. At a certain point there was about a three-day period where I called in sick to work and I was alone in my house. I felt a lot of energies moving, but very simple, ordinary energies. I was spontaneously doing yogic movement and there was a lot of crying and emotional/bodily releasing, but this was very normal for me. I felt very happy, very, very happy and free and ordinary. I wasn't even thinking about spiritual practice at the time.

At a certain point I found myself grasping my left hand with my right hand, a very spontaneous movement. I remember cellularly realizing that my right hand was squeezing my left hand literally out of love. I was crying and weeping and holding myself and allowing energy to move through me and there was just a moment of looking at it. Really, that simple. Looking at it and realizing that I was squeezing myself because I loved myself—and something simply and finally relaxed. The squeeze stopped, not just in my hands, but from way, way inside my brain. And my body also relaxed in a very simple, very ordinary moment.

From that moment on, because of that change in asana, a tacit experience in my body, seeking for enlightenment was an impossibility, there was nobody left to seek. My unenlightened experience had been resistance to feeling the waves of me, especially the distasteful ones. Now I was freely able to experience the things that I had thought were my unenlightenment before. I would say that that was the experience that really was "the one."

JLW: *One of the many things that is really a treat about the interviews we have done is the spectrum of experiences that people share with us. It's amazing. It's really amazing.*

VALERIE: Yeah, yeah. And they're really all saying the same exact thing. We're all doing our best to say the same exact thing which is a description of our Self. Now, when you are identified with the Self who lives all things and all beings, describing yourself becomes difficult for many people to understand. This difficulty can be seen using our shared human body as a metaphor. "I want to see myself perfectly," "I want to understand myself perfectly." But there are places in my body that I can't see as easily, like up inside my ass hole. Yet I keep trying to and trying to and trying to. Once you realize that you can never see yourself perfectly and then somebody asks, "Well, who are you perfectly?" it's kind of a funny joke. Who I am perfectly is the one who is relaxed about finding itself. This gives me the simplicity that allows the asana for perceiving things a little bit more as they are than I used to be able to see them.

JLW: *When you say asana, do you mean the positioning within yourself?*
VALERIE: Yes, I use the word asana because for me it's a very physical experience. Hatha yoga is when you are moving the body into very simple, yet demanding positions or "asanas" that allow the energy to move freely through it. In order to do that, you must go beyond your restricted capacity. So, you're moving the body into shapes, integrating the breath, integrating the being, to literally move beyond itself to find more freedom, more space. Each asana represents a very different vessel for receiving energy, and therefore offers a different perspective. Imagine how someone standing on her head would have a very different perspective than someone standing on her feet, even if they are both looking at a painting on the wall. From each asana the painting looks different, even though it's the same painting. Unenlightenment is a particular asana, and it provides a distinct perspective. Once this position is released, a different perspective is just naturally so. And from that perspective, there is a different way of relating to self that people notice is more free. But the actual picture is the same damn picture. The picture hasn't changed.

JLW: *Yeah, it's more or less the same world, it's just that your frame of reference is different.*
VALERIE: Yes, your perspective for reception is different.

LML: *You said that for you it's a very physical experience. Could you talk about the body in relationship to awakening?*
VALERIE: I'm going to do a little metaphoric shift here for you. We have all these shared human, cultural, archetypal systems. We are attracted to, and comfortable with certain archetypes and not others. Yet, they all represent different kinds of essential conversations with ourself. "Let's look at ourself and understand ourself through astrology or science or through

gardening," whatever. We have a set of ways of picturing ourself. But from my point of view, we all have the same deck of cards in some very systematically essential way. We are human bodies. We want to have a language then, that we somehow share and feel comfortable with.

When I was very young, I realized that my language, my way of sharing, had to do more with energy than other people did. For example, I have been deaf in one ear since I was three months old due to a viral infection. So certain parts of my nervous system have become more sensitized to make up for that. I needed to open the best I could to get the communication from someone speaking to me, especially in a crowded room. I noticed that a bodily practice was required for opening in this way. My body had to relax. My body had to go beyond its fixed state of being. Somehow it had to let go. This practice of letting go made things much, much easier and became my way. People call me a risk taker. My energy archetypally represents a kind of risk taker energy. It demands a bodily understanding of itself. All of my passions and attractions were about that, as a dancer from a young age, an actress, a musician, and I love to talk, I love interpersonal relating.

JLW: *You dance when you speak. You are never not dancing.*

VALERIE: [Laughter] It's very difficult for me to communicate without movement, that is a natural expression of my energy. Dance is a way of speaking energetically, without words, or in this case, to enhance words. The freedom that I represent in certain body movements would offend some cultures and other cultures would not be offended. So then it became even more, "How do I communicate even when my energy is being rejected?" All of these things have always been very passionately exciting to me. It was just very clear to me that relationship to Self included understanding what I was as this bodily vessel—related to itself, to others, and to the energy that was living it.

The question is funny to me in a way. I have friends who are awakened and they look very "intellectual" to me. They're speaking about these things very articulately, sometimes, you may have noticed, more articulately than I! But for me, there's a dryness in it because all the waves and the energy are happening from the heart to the brain and above the brain. The body is still living and functioning, but I don't see the same electricity moving all the way down, fully down into the whole body. I have seen very few where the electricity is moving freely throughout the body, where there is a whole being existing there without much interference.

LML: *To me, this appears to be what's happening with you.*
VALERIE: Oh? That's nice! [Laughter]

LML: *There is a difference we experience in you that we have commented on and noticed and maybe that's a description of it. At first I thought, "Well, maybe she's just comfortable in her own skin."*
VALERIE: I'm actually very uncomfortable in the skin. If I'm going to be honest with you, it looks comfortable, but I'm allowing the uncomfortableness of what it is to be fully human. It's not necessary always fun to feel those waves moving through certain areas; in order to feel them one must relax and expand and essentially increase capacity for more. And when you let in more, you realize, "Wow, there's more still!" It's never ending. There's always more than this capacity can seemingly hold.

For me from very early in life it's been about surrendering, which was archetypally demonstrated in the fire experience. It was always wiser to let go. I was always letting go beyond my limited capacity because I was attracted to what would happen when I did. "Relax, you understand the teacher more." "Let go and the argument even becomes more real." "Run very quickly down a mountain, letting go completely, and marvel as you are moved down the mountain." "Let go as the fear moves through." This has always been very pleasurable for me. But it has been harder to let go on the emotional level than on the physical level. It is difficult to allow that incredible wound that you feel in the emotional body when you let go there. That place, for me, was more risky and took a lot longer to allow in my human body.

LML: *Yes, most people have such deep emotional wounds.*
VALERIE: It's just one universal emotional wound—individuated sense of self. It's a horrible, painful experience. But you don't get to "non-individuated" consciousness without having individuated consciousness. You're a human being. [Touching Lynn's leg] I feel your skin is hotter than mine is right now. We are separate as we sit here, gazing into each other's eyes. That's painful when you really feel it. Because that means that you're going to die and I'm going to die. So, I have to allow that, not disengage from that.

I allow that in every given moment, and then it's obvious that there's no one else but me sitting here. But I'm still me sitting here feeling the pain of loving you. And the pain of seemingly being separate. It has to be a bodily practice for me. Emotionally, I can't get past that.

LML: *Are you saying that for you the only way it works is to work through the body?*
VALERIE: No, for me it works as the body. It is the body. It is the mind. It is the emotion. But for me, the body itself was such a teacher. "Relax your legs and oh wow, you feel different." "When you're fighting with someone, let a breath come and go and you see it differently." It's just so instantaneous. You don't have to figure anything out. It's just so simply true. Now I'll get all philosophical and guru-like on you. When you see a flower grow, the flower is simply growing. It doesn't have a consciousness in which it's figuring out how it's supposed to grow more correctly. It doesn't have a sense of looking at its dying leaf and thinking it's fucking up, that it must do something to fix this leaf. You know what I'm saying? There's a freedom in just allowing the flower to grow. And that was always a bodily practice for me. I am simply "being the flower." [Laughter]

JLW: *Valerie, if someone comes along who has this yearning, burning desire for freedom and asks you, "What can I do?" what would you say to them?*
VALERIE: Actually, that is one of my favorite, favorite questions and I have to say that that is the only question that people ask me, once they understand me enough. When people come to me at this point in my life, when they're coming to me as a spiritual teacher, they're coming to me with that question essentially. But first they come with, "Let me see if this bitch is someone I can feel safe enough with to trust."

JLW: *And also, "Is it real?"*
VALERIE: Yes, but "is it real?" is really about "can I trust this person?" And I've been there, believe me. I met my spiritual teacher, thank god, in an archetypal death experience within my own brain. So, that relationship was never a question for me. It was never a question of, "Is he enlightened?" It was more a question of, "How am I going to do it?" "How am I going to surrender to this?" "How am I going to surrender to this seeming separate being when I know it's me?" "How am I going to do that?"

But when people come to me, I'm not presenting a guru-devotee relationship, I'm just here to discuss whatever the hell they want to talk about. And they want to be out of this wound that we just discussed, this individuated consciousness. They want to be—especially those who have studied a lot, they want non-duality, I think is what they call it. They want oneness, sense of Self. They want what I wanted. They want to not be feeling the suffering of their life.

So, what I do is point out in whatever humorous way I can how they are trying to relax. And trying to relax and relaxing are two very different things. I joke, I laugh, I essentially use my whole body. I do my best to allow people to know how much I feel that wound that they're trying to get out of. I let myself feel it fully with them, as them. It's like, "Look, I know your whole quest for sense of Self is about avoiding self. So let me just sit there with you. And then the question really doesn't come up as much. It's always burning there, but what comes up now is the want to ask the question and then the realization that the question itself is coming from an asana that must be let go of—then the question doesn't exist anymore.

So, when people ask me, "What can I do?" I go, "Yeah!" Cuz now we can really talk about it. You can't do anything is the answer to that question. There is nothing to do, nothing to do. And yet, when I die in forty years or so, I'm sure there will be people who will talk about me and say, "She said to do this and that." But I'm just allowing my being to be choreographed; I'm freely allowing it to be lived. There's nothing I'm doing.

JLW: *It's not so much the content as the demonstration.*

VALERIE: Yeah, but see once you really tacitly get it—I mean tacit with a capital "T"—once it's not just a belief system. . .

JLW: *You mean kinesthetically?*

VALERIE: Kinesthetically, but tacit also has to do with the mind. My cells understand, and my asana is naturally and forever switched. It's like when babies first start to walk. They haven't yet incorporated bending their knees so they walk with their knees straight and it gives them this kind of waddle, hip walking hiddle-wiggle thing. And it's very fun to watch cuz they're cute as hell. But once they've learned to bend their knees, it becomes a whole new thing for them. Now they have an all-new capacity.

You would have to go back through dance or mime or clowning, or whatever, to re-learn how not to bend your knees because it is so natural to do when you walk. It's the same for in my awakened body. Once I identified with myself differently and there was no longer the struggle to identify with myself, my knees bent in a different way. [Laughter] Just seeing someone "easily walking with their knees bending," you don't have to do a whole lot of work. The teaching process becomes a demonstration of a much easier way to walk. People realize that they're walking with their knees straight and naturally something relaxes. That can only be taught and learned through tacit understanding within yourself. Then, it's not even a thought anymore.

So, my answer to the question of what to do is, "NOTHING!" Sit in that yearning, burning to do something, anything to get out of the wound. Just allow the yearn, burn to exist without avoidance. That requires a new and very different asana and will provide a new perspective. That would be my greatest advice.

LML: *Okay. Could you talk about how the experience of awakening has affected your relationships?*

VALERIE: There was this passion for relationship early in life; a passion for allowing energy flow between people; being disturbed if it didn't flow correctly; feeling responsible if it didn't flow correctly; and having to deal with a sense of self-hatred about not being able to make it flow correctly. And this still buzzes through my being.

But how has awakening made a difference in my life? Because I'm walking differently within myself, I'm capable of relationship in a way that I wasn't before. A lot of what I was afraid of in terms of just being in myself was essential relationship. Because relating to "others" means I am individuated consciousness. "If I love you, we're in trouble."

JLW: *Because we're separate.*

VALERIE: Because you're separate and I'm going to get fucked! I'm going to lose you either by betrayal or death. So to love you fully means great risk. Now it is not a possibility for me not to take that risk. Now there is no separation between you and me so love will exist. How is this paradox so delightful that I sit separately and yet I am One? That does not erase the burn of individuated consciousness or the fear of love, it actually allows them fully. Love, bliss, and that yearn, burn place are like the same pitch of music. When you relax into the yearn, burn, the love is there too—same. Allowing separated, individuated sense of self was what finally allowed fully integrated sense of Oneness. That changes everything. And it changed nothing. I'm still the idiot that was living before that. The body is still animated, only more so now that there's no holding back. I still like to watch *Matlock* on TV. [Laughter] You know what I'm saying? Nothing changed. There used to be this universal, "running to try to find herself" woman and now she still exists but she's the universal "found her Self" woman. It's amazing to me. Because nothing changed except my sense of self. So, did I answer that question?

LML: *Yes, you did.*

JLW: *You're doing fine. So far you're passing! [Laughter]*
VALERIE: Oh good, my Jewish parents would be very happy. "I'm gettin' an 'A'!" [Laughter]. You guys are obviously not Jews or you would have laughed at that.

JLW: *So, many of our friends, many of the people we have encountered are having glimpses of recognition of who they truly are.*
VALERIE: Isn't that awesome?!

JLW: *It's wonderful . . .*
VALERIE: You know what, I have to interrupt your question for a second... You've had glimpses of that since you were suckin' on your mother' breast, if you had the opportunity to do that. Sometimes when you're taking a shit, sometimes when you're watching a beautiful sunrise, sometimes when you love your son or daughter, you've always had glimpses of yourself beyond the contraction. Yes? Somehow, something mysteriously allowed you to relax more than you usually do. The fact is that people are now somehow being able to allow that more and more and more. So, back to your question . . .

JLW: *As I was saying, many of us had glimpses or profound recognition and our experience is that our conditioned identity comes back and seems to obscure the recognition again. There is a desire to stabilize and this seems to be what has occurred for you. You had a series of glimpses then.*
VALERIE: I'm going to interrupt you again . . . From my unenlightened asana I very much want to be enlightened. In some way I'm not liking some of the energies moving through me. I feel that the only reason they are moving through me is because I am in some way constricting energy. I am in trouble and I want to stabilize the moments when I felt like I wasn't in trouble. And I'm saying to you that that is in itself the difficulty.

If I were to think of the perfect place to hang out as a body maybe it would be like a tropical island, a place with great weather always, a community of loving people, a system of trade and support that did not dishonor my being, where my art was allowed and honored, where true freedom was allowed, my natural relaxations were allowed and I had fresh water and healthy food, lots of culture, and so on. All these things could allow for an easier sense of self in the body. But the fact of the matter is that I live in Oakland, California in 2000! There is pollution going on here, emotional and physical pollution. There are chemicals moving through my body that may be called "toxic." We are receiving chemicals in the nervous system at all times. Thus, surrendering to myself isn't always "pretty."

People want these glimpses of freedom, these "bliss moments" to be their constant state of consciousness. And you imagine that freedom would be void of the senses of self that you're trying to fix, trying to get out of. Now the allowing in my body is such, that even that idiot you're trying to get rid of, is free to be here as it is. And when I allow that idiot, when Valerie just is herself completely—even the parts that are frustrated, or don't want to be here, or are jealous, or say stupid things, whatever the hell it is—when I allow it all freely, then I see how universal and how perfect it truly is. When you're a jerk, be a jerk. It's trying not to be the jerk that makes you an asshole! [Laughter]

From the point of view that "Valerie is in charge," there is self-consciousness. Nobody really likes feeling self-consciousness. But, the chemicals of self-consciousness don't go away by avoidance. If I'm sitting in a room and somebody says, "Answer a question about enlightenment." My body goes, "Oh fuck, now I'm going to have to say something great. What the hell is enlightenment from Valerie's point of view?" If I'm trying not to be a jerk while that's occurring, then I'm not going to allow Valerie to actually express what enlightenment is. There is an assumption that I would sit here and not feel self-consciousness. And I'm saying that self-consciousness exists and I exist, and I house self-consciousness. I don't avoid self-consciousness. That's the only difference. In your question, you're saying that you've glimpsed this sense of Self, and then you seem to go back to the self you dislike, and so you try to get back to Self again. I'm saying, that no matter what comes up, I'm fine. I'm not going anywhere, or trying to get back to anything.

We are born through a system of contraction and release. When giving birth, we are sacrificed to a system of contraction and release. We know intuitively, that relaxing into the process as much as possible and participating as fully as possible, makes the whole thing easier. When you're giving birth, your capacity is being stretched and stretched and believe-you-me stretched beyond it's seeming capacity. This process of contraction and release (and the demand for increased capacity) is always occurring, at all times whether giving birth or not. How perfect that our way of coming into this world is a dramatic and tacit experience of what it is to be lived in this world. That same contraction, release, inhale, exhale, expansion, sacrifice—that is what you are.

So, if you are resisting this process, or see it as distasteful, you might seek enlightenment with the hope that you wouldn't have to experience this sacrifice anymore. Your question is "How can I maintain this sense of Self that I find more pleasurable than the "me" I usually identify with?" And I say to you, I am doing what I do in every occasion at all times—naturally surrendering. I'm not saying that waves of self-consciousness, or waves of whatever, no longer come and go through my being. Enlightened or not, waves come and go. The relationship to the waves is what changes. I'm fully allowing them. I am a conscious sacrifice to the Self. And that sacrifice is my pleasure.

In my near-death experience, it became evident that the more blissful states of Self, those less identified with the human body, were much more pleasurable, and therefore, harder to let go of. But it's always the same, whether I'm experiencing seeming pain or seeming blissfulness. It's the same practice. This is why I get all grounded and earthy and talk about taking a shit. Because whether you're taking a shit or sitting on a high mountain in the most blissful, contented state, you're still the same receptor/releaser. And you're an integral part of a larger, much larger process of reception/release. When you believe you are supposed to be different, in any given moment—different than you are perfectly being lived—you have just made your small "s" self the center of the universe.

JLW: *Everything would be different. I understand . . .*

LML: *Here's another question . . . Most people in the West don't relate to awakening as something that's possible for them to experience. Do you see it as something that is available to everyone and not just a rare few?*

VALERIE: I love this question, I really do, because when "I" was trying to become enlightened, it was impossible . . .

LML: *That's what I'm finding out!*

VALERIE: Yes. And then when I realized that I already was enlightened, but I wasn't particularly fond of what that meant as a sacrifice. We are one functioning being, so of course, every single being has the capacity. And every single being is required to feel very specific energies moving through it. So, if I am one point in a geometric circle and I decide that from my little point of view I'm not happy with the way things seem and I would like it to be different from what it is. I'm being silly because I'm just a point in a much larger circle. The unenlightened asana believes that point over there is a better point of view. But from the point of view of literally being the circle then all points are obviously perfect, and thus, perfectly allowed. All of us are enlightened simultaneously. Not all of us are experiencing the pleasure point of that. Some of us are holding up different ends of ourselves.

JLW: *What about those that carry evil for the world? Some people seem to embody it archetypally.*

VALERIE: They certainly do. And it's a great sacrifice.

JLW: *In a way they sacrifice their whole life to show it to everybody.*

VALERIE: That's correct. We're holding ourselves full. These ends that are extremes have to be held. And I swear, when you're at either end, you're at the same place. So, the most truly evil and the most truly good are doing the same practice. They may have their attention in different places, but they're doing the same practice.

The point for me is not, do people have the capacity for enlightenment, it's are we willing to be that vulnerable? We may get hit over the head with a bat at any given moment; we are not in control of any of it!

LML: *We don't have any control over stopping pain from happening.*

VALERIE: That's correct. And how many people are even capable of relaxing past the want to stop the pain from happening? Everybody thinks that enlightenment means that they wouldn't feel the things that they don't like feeling. However, fully human manifestation—as the body—allows extreme energies to move through without interference, even those that are distasteful. Self-consciousness is most distasteful! But if I didn't allow it, then I wouldn't be able to help you allow it.

So, how many people are capable of my ridiculous, seemingly heroic, vulnerability? I think literally every single human being has that capacity and is doing that perfectly, already, in a larger system in which we exist. So whether you're enlightened or not, you are absolutely perfectly living as the vibration that you are.

JLW: *In the Buddhist teaching of Prajnaparamita, it speaks about the Bodhisattva, the one who is dedicated to the awakening of others, praying that all beings experience conscious enlightenment. It's recognizing that everyone is already that, but it's not conscious. And because it's not conscious, there is a lot of suffering.*

VALERIE: Yes, but even here, it's about getting to enlightenment and getting out of "suffering"—it's still the same asana. Saving the world is very noble, very heart felt. But praying for everyone's enlightenment is still an avoidance, still seeking. When you die, really die, completely die, capital "D" die, the whole conversation changes.

LML: *Are you noticing that more people are receptive to what you are saying than earlier in your life, like at the time of the fire?*

VALERIE: I don't know, either people are more receptive or I'm meeting more people who are receptive. I know that my ability to speak it has changed. I've been honed by the people who didn't understand me. Let me tell you honey, I have been honed! It comes down to the Truth we have heard for centuries, yet hardly anyone seems to understand, because it's a secret until you tacitly understand it. I am that very One that lives me. I am That that's living you. I am in That that's living you and me.

JLW: *What do you see as the main obstacle to awakening for Westerners?*

VALERIE: The belief that they are unawakened.

JLW: *Is there anything else you would like to add here?*

VALERIE: Yes, as an aside. . . vulnerability and surrender, we seem to put those two things together. If I surrender, I'm vulnerable. In my experience, surrender meant strength, literally so. Vulnerability meant strength. But then whenever something vulnerable occurs, and I have to feel the chemicals of vulnerability happening in my body, I can see why people don't like to be vulnerable. For example, you're interviewing me and asking me about my enlightenment experiences, and it's hard to describe these things. So, I feel vulnerable. This is really a confession of my own vulnerability and my own strength.

I want to embrace John's question of how do I maintain the remembrance of who I am to the point where I can allow myself to be fully, without encumbrance? Be simple. Take it to the most simple place in your being. Relax and notice that when you are trying to get to anything great stress is occurring, because it means that where you are is not okay. I've heard that forever, right? So, I thought, "Oh, I've got to try not to try." Now the chemicals of "trying not to try" are going to move through my system. There they are. "Oh now I'm being interviewed and there are chemicals of vulnerability going through." "Oh look, there's my voice getting higher and talking faster." If I added to that, "Jesus, I'm not enlightened because if I was I would transcend those chemicals and I wouldn't be vulnerable." Horrible!! What's fun for me this time around, in this body, is being the monkey that hangs in front of you and says, "Look! You can speak any fuckin' way you want!" If my voice gets high it's because it's embarrassed; it's because the chemicals of embarrassment went through my body. So I'm the jerk that got embarrassed.

JLW: *And fundamentally, so what.*
VALERIE: Yes, and fundamentally, how fun! [Looking at Lynn Marie] If I get to be a jerk then you get to be this jerk that you're holding back, which I find exquisitely beautiful, exquisitely beautiful. You know this one that you're afraid of? Let her in! Let her in. She's so exquisite.

LML: *It seems that what you are saying is that you are not identifying with anything that's moving through your body. It's not "me" that's embarrassed, or "me" that's a jerk; it's just embarrassed or jerk energy moving through—not personal.*
VALERIE: If I say what is paradoxically true, you're right, I'm not identified. I'm able to show my asshole to anybody because, you know what, we all got one! [Laughter] But it still doesn't keep me from having the asshole. Those are two very different things.

LML: *Well, do we want to end on that note?*
VALERIE: Sure, why not!

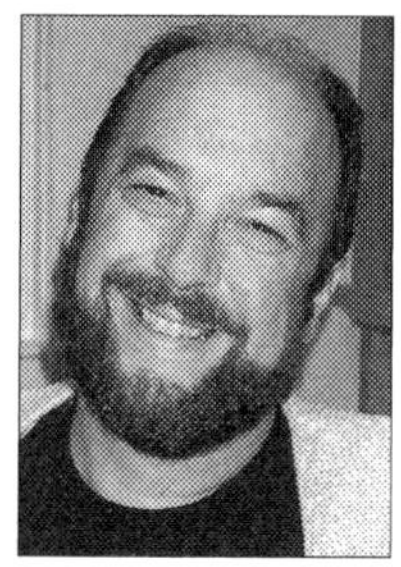

WAYNE LIQUORMAN

"RAM TZU KNOWS THIS... WHEN A GLIMMER OF UNDERSTANDING APPEARS, YOU HAVE CANCER. IT WILL GROW... RELENTLESSLY REPLACING YOU WITH ITSELF. UNTIL YOU ARE GONE."

from No Way for the Spiritually Advanced

Wayne Liquorman is also known as Ram Tzu. Even though Ram Tzu and Wayne Liquorman are two aspects of the same consciousness, he makes a distinction between that which appears to be an individual, Wayne, and Infinite Consciousness, which is Ram Tzu. We interviewed Ram Tzu since Wayne says Ram Tzu is in a much better position to talk about "these things."

We approached Wayne with some trepidation. After reading his book, *No Way For the Spiritually Advanced*, we knew that he had a sense of humor, but also that he could be iconoclastic and quite intolerant of the spiritual games people play. He skillfully exposes the absurdities and arrogance of spiritual efforts made in the pursuit of enlightenment. Some might even say that Wayne is irreverent. He is definitely direct and to the point, and certainly does not seem care what others may think of him.

It is an interesting twist of fate that Wayne's family name is Liquorman, a name he says he tried hard to live up to. He refers to his nineteen years of alcoholism and substance abuse as his sadhana. He says that it prepared him to open up to something larger than himself, and to ultimately find his teacher. This former alcoholic and his teacher, Ramesh Balsekar, a banker from Bombay, are as unlikely a pair as one could imagine. Yet the deep love and respect Wayne has for his teacher was palpable.

Wayne is a clear example of someone who would not fit anyone's "picture" of what a person who awakens should be like. Certainly alcoholism is not in the picture books of most people's minds as a preparation for enlightenment. His life is an example of how there truly are no definite standards for how one must live, or what one must do in order for awakening to occur.

At the time we met with him, Wayne told us that he does not have any desire to become a guru. To quote Ram Tzu, "I don't want a bunch of miserable seekers cluttering up my living room." However, during a visit with Ramesh in July 1996, Wayne was given direct instructions to teach Advaita and has begun to do so. He also writes poems when they come forth. Wayne runs Advaita Press in Redondo Beach, California which publishes Ram Tzu's books as well as books by Ramesh Balsekar and others.

CONVERSATION *with* WAYNE LIQUORMAN

LML: *Who is Ram Tzu?*
WAYNE: Ram Tzu is consciousness, pure and simple. This is where it gets interesting because Ram Tzu and Wayne Liquorman are essentially two aspects of the same consciousness, but Ram Tzu doesn't have a body, doesn't have a family, doesn't have any of those qualities that identify us as individuals. So, Ram Tzu is in a much easier position to talk about this stuff, realistically.

JLW: *Wayne Liquorman is the publisher and Ram Tzu is pure Consciousness?*
WAYNE: Yes. I make the distinction between Wayne Liquorman and Ram Tzu because we are talking about the identified consciousness and infinite consciousness. I find it useful to make the distinction to say Wayne Liquorman is not enlightened; Wayne Liquorman is not enlightened because no individual can possibly be enlightened. And Wayne Liquorman goes about his daily routine just like everybody else does and for all intents and purposes he's just another guy, just an ordinary guy making his way through the day. Whereas Ram Tzu is in fact enlightened. And in fact there is a line in a Ram Tzu poem which says, "If you find Ram Tzu, kill him!" Because Ram Tzu does not exist in phenomenality.

JLW: *He doesn't exist as a separate individual in phenomenality.*
WAYNE: Correct.

JLW: *Phenomenality exists within Ram Tzu.*
WAYNE: Ram Tzu is consciousness without any of the meddlesome properties of ego and personality that is what confuses the issue when you are talking with someone who is "enlightened." It appears as though you are talking to an individual. And no matter how many times in the course of a conversation that that person said, "there is no such thing as an enlightened individual, enlightenment is the absence of the individual." You can't help but supply, in between the lines, an individual.

JLW: *You can't help but notice that it appears that somebody is speaking to you.*
WAYNE: Absolutely, and that is the rub. There are various ways of reconciling that but the problem remains.

JLW: *So, in your experience—and I'm not sure to whom I speaking—[Laughter] are these two separate experiences, or are they two aspects of the same one?*
WAYNE: Well obviously, when consciousness identifies itself with a body mechanism which has certain characteristics it is born with, such as gender, temperament, and all of the influences it has on its life, that all serves to effect the perceptions that go through that mechanism. So, the way the mechanism articulates is determined by all those factors. More specifically, the way the organism responds is determined by its nature. If you have a consciousness that is not identified with the body then it is much freer than one that is. Even though there may be understanding here, the understanding is tempered by the fact that it exists within a body-mind mechanism. The reason we say that there is no such thing as an enlightened individual is because by its very nature a body-mind mechanism cannot be enlightened. It is a limited quantum.

LML: *And what we truly are is and always was enlightened.*
WAYNE: All there is consciousness. All there is is enlightenment, fundamentally.

LML: *So, what does enlightenment mean to you?*
WAYNE: Not much! [Laughter] Within the context of the phenomenal manifestation, it is another event. The mistaken assumption is that that event happens to an individual, and it doesn't. The occurrence of enlightenment is the falling away of the veil of identification as a separate body-mind organism. Yet, the body-mind organism stays around and functions, usually in much the same way it functioned previously. How could it not? It is still determined by all the same things that it was determined by previously. The myth is that when there is enlightenment, all of a sudden there's this unbelievable sense of bliss. The word "bliss" has been taken to mean some kind of ecstatic personal state. And it's not a personal experience at all.

LML: *There are many ideas of how an enlightened person should appear—holy, blissful, serene, never getting angry, and so on.*
WAYNE: Absolutely. You can hang around in certain spiritual camps and see the people who have very clear perceptions of how enlightened people, or people close to enlightenment, are supposed to look. You see these beatific looks on their faces, and these kinds of "seeing into the ethers" look in the eyes. It's really comical. But, it couldn't be any other way!

LML: *Could you tell us about this occurrence of enlightenment that happened here? What is the story?*

WAYNE: Well it happened right there in the chair John is sitting in, as a matter of fact.

The story is that I was essentially in love with two women and in the same week, each of them decided to clear the field for the other. One of them came here to tell me this and I experienced an incredible wave of sadness come over me. It got deeper and deeper until a deep emotional pain started to envelop me. I had never experienced anything of this dimension before. It kept growing and finally there was this huge blackness, everything blanked, and I had this sensation of being sucked into a pit of unbelievable pain. The perception was one of falling into a pit of all the suffering that has ever been. I was racked with huge sobs of excruciating, emotional pain. And it was obvious that it was not in any way related to the fact that my girlfriend was breaking up with me.

So, I'm having this experience and something in me broke or let go, and I let myself go into it. All of the fear and resistance to the pain and suffering I was experiencing went away. I opened to it entirely and essentially merged with it until there was no longer any separation between it and me.

JLW: *You weren't experiencing it, you were it.*

WAYNE: Correct. And that was it. After that, in that complete acceptance, if you will . . . this is where it gets real tricky because we have to speak in personal terms—the language is designed this way. The acceptance is simultaneous with enlightenment, oneness, understanding, whatever you want to call it, they are undifferentiated. The minute you start talking about it, you start breaking it back up again. To say that it's an experience is not precisely correct, because an experience always presupposes an experiencer. In That, there is no one to experience anything.

LML: *Did that sense of a one who experiences things ever come back again?*

WAYNE: Of course it did, but not as the doer. The one who is responding to your questions, who articulates, that's all very much there. I still yell at my son when he doesn't do his homework; all of the mechanisms for functioning within the phenomenal manifestation still exist.

JLW: *So what is different?*

WAYNE: Not much! [Laughter] There is an underlying understanding.

But that underlying understanding is not part of the functioning of the mechanism.

JLW: *They are independent of one another. The functioning will happen with or without the understanding.*
WAYNE: Correct.

LML: *Is there any way at all that this understanding has changed the quality of your life?*
WAYNE: Not really! My teacher, Ramesh Balsekar, used to say that if you are given the choice between having a million dollars and enlightenment take the million bucks because at least there's someone there to enjoy it! [Laughter] In enlightenment there is not a "one" to enjoy enlightenment.

LML: *I'd like to back up a little here and ask if you could tell more of your story leading up to the understanding that occurred when your girlfriend was breaking up with you—your nineteen years of alcoholism, and meeting Ramesh.*
WAYNE: Well, there were nineteen years of alcoholism and drug addiction that got progressively worse as those years went on. I had alcoholic edema in my ankles and wrists, and was all puffed up. I was drinking a quart of hard liquor a day and snorting a gram of cocaine everyday, just to keep going. I was dying. And I was absolutely dead inside; there was no spiritual connection at all.

I had thought that I was the master of my destiny, and that anything I set my mind to do I could do. If I were going to have any chance of being successful, I'd have to use my native intelligence, quickness, and wits to outwit the other guy because he was out to get me. I just had to be smarter, quicker, faster, slicker than he was if I was going to survive. That's an incredibly painful way to live your life—to be fighting the entire world all of the time. My solution to that problem was to medicate myself. And it got a little out of hand!

So, at the end of one weekend binge I was laying in bed all coked up and trying to pass myself out with alcohol and pot so I could sleep. I was sweating and miserable, incomprehensibly demoralized. Then I had a moment of absolute clarity when I felt my entire being change and knew intuitively in my soul that I couldn't do this anymore.

After that, I found a group of other alcoholics who had a way of living without alcohol. They had a program of recovery that was about finding some kind of spiritual power to live by. When I told Ramesh many years later about this, his comment was that the alcoholism had been my sadhana. Other people go do charity work and meditate and I got to do alcohol and drugs. That's what it took to bring me to a point of sweet reasonableness, if you will. It broke down the ego at least enough so that I could admit to some quality in the universe, other than myself, that might have some source of power. In that moment my entire world shifted.

I then started reading the *Tao Te Ching*, doing Tai Chi, went to hear Ram Dass. I spent a couple of years checking out all kinds of things, various meditations, reading Rajneesh and this and that. When I went to hear Ramesh for the first time, the whole thing was just beyond me. It didn't click with me at all. I didn't understand the language, but I felt there was something there. So I went back and this time it was more intimate, in someone's home.

It was a beautiful house in the Hollywood hills and the whole scene was completely enchanting. Ramesh walked in, there were about eight of us, and I sat at his feet. From that time on I was just hooked. I started going up there every day. I was doing everything I could to be in his presence. I was as hopelessly in love with this guy as I had ever been with anyone. I just wanted to be with him every minute if I could. It was horrible because I was always scheming ways to get in there to see him.

JLW: *It's really beautiful though. When that spark is ignited and you just can't not be with somebody like that-that's rich.*

WAYNE: Oh yes, it was very rich. It is as vibrant an experience as one can have, I think. That experience led to a time when Ramesh was leaving and we were at the airport discussing turning the tapes of his talks into a book. And someone asked me if I had ever been in the publishing business. I said no, then Ramesh, who had been out of this conversation entirely, said, "Not yet." It was as profound an experience as that night when I got struck sober. There was that intensity and quality of knowing that something irrevocable had just happened in my life. Without doubt, deep in my guts, there was an intuitive knowledge that something had happened again. So, I then went to Bombay a couple months later to work on a manuscript with Ramesh. That was 1988.

Then he came back to the United States again and I was in charge of the tour. My relationship with Ramesh deepened to a point where he told me I was his spiritual son. This was one of the most special moments of my life. When the relationship between guru and disciple reaches that kind of intensity, there is no other kind of relationship that can match it. It has a dimension beyond a relationship with a lover or your child, because it goes into the realm of consciousness. It transcends the purely phenomenal in which all the other relationships exist.

LML: *Could you say something about the guru-disciple relationship in terms of non-duality. There is no other, yet there is this beautiful relationship.*
WAYNE: It's one of those really sweet paradoxes. There is this underlying ambiguity and paradox that all there is is consciousness. All there is is the oneness. In the ultimate understanding when the disciple realizes the Truth completely, the distinction between the guru and the disciple evaporates. And yet, there is at the phenomenal level, an incredibly intense continuation of the original relationship. When I go to Bombay and visit with Ramesh we don't talk about any of this shit anymore. [Laughter] What's the point? It's all a load of crap. To talk about the Truth is like a mere child's finger painting representation of Yosemite Valley. But we still genuinely enjoy being with one another.

LML: *There are people who are seekers of enlightenment, they have a longing for this. Do you have anything to say to these people? Is there anything they can do to have this occur?*
WAYNE: Who is there to do it? That is the question. That which thinks that it's functioning, that which thinks that it is the operating center of the universe that can do something is an illusion. It has no independent power. It can't do squat. So, it does all kinds of things as part of the functioning of the totality, but it has no more volition about what it does than the light bulb has about turning on when it's switched on. The only difference is that when we do something we think it's our own idea.

LML: *So what to do? Here in the West people are very much into self-improvement. There's therapy, meditation, many spiritual practices. What value does all this have if any?*
WAYNE: The problem is all you get is an improved self! But all of it can have value. You've got huge ashrams full of people getting up at 3:00 in the morning and doing all kinds of bizarre shit. That's all happening, and

in some cases benefit is derived from it. In a few cases it is a stepping stone to some kind of ultimate understanding, but you have to understand that it's not causative. Ram Tzu says that he believes in cause and effect, but he's just not sure which is which! [Laughter]

JLW: *You mean whether it is teleological or sequential?*
WAYNE: Right. Which is the cause and which is the effect; what causes what? The example Ramesh uses, because he likes to go to the racetrack [Laughter] is, do you win money on a horse race because the horse wins or does the horse win, because in order for you to win money, it has to. And therefore, what seems to be the effect of the cause—that the horse won and you got the money—it may actually be that the cause for the horse winning was that you needed the money.

JLW: *Cause and effect is based in a sequential idea of order and that's an idea.*

LML: *So someone can do twenty years of meditation and then have ultimate understanding but there is no direct cause and effect that understanding happened because of meditation.*
WAYNE: Obviously, because there are a lot of cases like Ram Tzu.

LML: *Would you say that more people are having this ultimate understanding in the West? Do you feel that there is a quickening of this Consciousness occurring at this time?*
WAYNE: I haven't a clue. I certainly see a lot of people who have spiritual experiences which they believe are enlightenment, but regrettably aren't. I think the whole question of enlightenment is really kind of funny to begin with. The notion that this is something that some one desires—I promise you that if they knew . . . I mean there is nothing to want. It is not an experience worth having, it is just not! [Laughter]

LML: *What do you mean by that?*
WAYNE: It is not an experience possible to have. It is not an experience period.

JLW: *But it is a realization that alleviates the kinds of suffering we go through because we are identified with our ideas of who we are.*

LML: *Yes, doesn't awakening bring freedom from suffering?*
WAYNE: Yes, there is freedom from suffering. But I'll make a distinction, it is a freedom from suffering, it is not the freedom from pain. Suffering comes about as a result of the identification with the apparent individual.

And yet, the pain, be it emotional or physical, is felt as profoundly by the organism, maybe more so, because there isn't quite the resistance to it that there was . . . There is a guy who lives by Santa Cruz or someplace, he writes on a chalkboard.

JLW: *Baba Hari Das, at the Mount Madonna Center.*

WAYNE: Yes. I never met him but whenever I start getting into the depths of this subject, I often think what a great idea it is just to have a chalkboard on which to write a couple of words. It keeps it much simpler. As we get involved in each of these concepts of suffering, and the difference between pain and suffering, we can bring in the thinking mind and the working mind. The thinking mind is mitigating the experience of the working mind, "blah, blah, blah, blah, blah, blah." All of which doesn't go to answer any questions; it goes to create more. And it is endless. So, there you have it.

LML: *You did say that there is a freedom from suffering that results from this understanding—not from pain, but from identification as one who is in pain.*

WAYNE: Yes. But I'm not even comfortable with that concept. Because where you go with it is, "Okay, now we have established that enlightenment does, in fact, improve you and is now, in fact, a desirable state because you have these benefits. It's not really so.

LML: *You make it sound like there aren't really any benefits.*

WAYNE: There are not really benefits, [Laughter] to the individual concerned.

LML: *So the individual concerned is not more peaceful or happier?*

WAYNE: Maybe, depends on the day. [Laughter]

JLW: *I'd like to pursue this a little bit too, because I think what I'm hearing is that the individual who is seeking enlightenment, is blindly, or perhaps not so blindly, moving to his own demise. So, in that sense, there is no benefit to the individual. But, after there has been a realization, it's not that the individual realizes, it is that Totality realizes Itself in a particular locus of individuation of Itself. It is hard to say it in words, but there is something very rich in this, and very satisfying, in an impersonal way.*

It's like being a dirty piece of glass or a clean piece of glass. I mean ultimately there is no difference, the dirt is part of the same thing, the individual ego is part of the same thing. Yet, when it is realized, there is clarity, there is presence, there is an openness, an acceptance of what comes and a release of what goes. There is fullness and a freedom and a flow and an ease that wasn't there as much before. Isn't this so for you?

WAYNE: Yes, but that came about gradually. For me the step from identification to dis-identification was barely noticeable. There was that dramatic event which is spiffy to point at and say, "Okay, that was it." But for me, the changes which had been taking place in me over the intervening years, had brought about already a tremendous amount of acceptance and intellectual understanding that all this is a dream and that it is just unfolding as it is supposed to. And in fact, I would say that subsequent to the understanding being complete, the external perception of my life, of my friends and others—it probably looked as though I was more involved in my life afterwards. Because there wasn't that last vestige of intellectual bullshit of, "Oh this is all just a dream; this isn't real," which is an intellectual thought.

JLW: *And a subsequent pulling back from being with. . .*

WAYNE: From being with whatever the actual experience was.

JLW: *So you knew simultaneously that you were with whatever the experience was and also, you were none of it—is this correct?*

WAYNE: Well, what I am saying is that prior to the final understanding, there was still that mentation going on in which there was the evaluation of the experience based on the Truth. Now there is none of that. I mean, this all just is. The whole question of it being real or not real—it all goes away. It is moot.

LML: *In your case then it wasn't a dramatic shift; it was subtle.*

WAYNE: Very subtle.

JLW: *Because the organism had made a significant adaptation to the non-dual perspective already?*

WAYNE: Absolutely. Because I was living with Ramesh, three months at a crack, and almost every waking hour was spent with him. Lord knows how many hours of talks I sat through!

LML: *We would like to ask how you experience relationships since the shift in identification.*

WAYNE: Let's define the ego as the operating center, the thing that responds when its name is called, that which was born with certain qualities and characteristics. Its subsequent development elaborated certain qualities and diminished others until, on a given date, it has a certain set of characteristics. Those characteristics respond to a situation according to its nature and that is the thing that has relationships. That ego, if you will, continues to interrelate with people and the world according to the way this script is written.

And so when two people fly down from Oakland and set up a tape recorder in its living room and ask it questions, it responds according to its nature and according to its perspective and according to its background. And the relationship that evolves between these two mechanisms and this one has to do with the dynamics of all of those mechanisms and it couldn't be any other way. That is the understanding. Did I answer your question?

JLW: *Yes, you did for me. So, if I understand, relationships exist for you as they always have with a kind of ground of understanding that they are the way they are because they just happen to be that way.*
WAYNE: Yes.

LML: *Another question we hear people ask a lot is, "How do things get done?" How do decisions get made if you don't function as an individual, separate "I"?*
WAYNE: This is an outgrowth of the same question and it has essentially the same answer, which is that there is an operating center here, without it this body is a vegetable, it doesn't function. There has to be something that enables the mechanism of the body and the mind to function.

LML: *And what is that? Who is that doer?*
WAYNE: Ultimately, the doer is consciousness. There is only one operating center and it functions through a variety of mechanisms. The analogy that Ramesh uses all the time is that of electricity operating through a variety of devices. The devices are established in such a way to perform certain tasks—when the electricity goes through the microwave it heats up your food. And the light bulb, when the electricity goes through it, illuminates the room. All these various devices had particular functions. They are all animated by the same energy and the only thing that determines the output is the nature of the device.

This particular device, the Wayne unit, if you will, on this given day is sitting and answering questions posed to it, because that is what is happening. It is what is supposed to happen and in order for it to happen, this Wayne unit had to exist and these two units had to exist in order for this moment to occur and whatever flows out of this—for that to happen, this had to happen. And on and on and on and on.

JLW: *So the doing just happens.*
WAYNE: Doing happens, clearly. But where we get screwed up is in the notion that enlightenment somehow transforms the individual into some kind of super man, creature, thing that has all these extremely desirable qualities and various powers and various capabilities. Let's face it, as egos, what we want is control, we want power, we want to be able to make things happen because that is how the ego is constructed. There is this notion of enlightenment being this state of supreme power, because you are now identified with God, rather than being identified with this puny, rotten, little body that is going to get sick and hurt and feel bad and vomit and do all kinds of lousy shit and die— its just not going to be pleasant. So we believe that the obvious solution is to be God because that's going to be a lot better.

LML: *Yes, the ego likes to believe that you will be better than every one else and you won't hurt...*
WAYNE: ...And you won't die. So what could be better than that?

LML: *That's the ego's idea of enlightenment.*
WAYNE: Un-huh. And it's all true!

LML: *You mean it's true that you don't hurt and you don't die...*
WAYNE: Uh-huh, and that you are God. That is all absolutely true. That is exactly what enlightenment is. But it is not happening to an individual body-mind mechanism. That's the rub. [Laughter]

LML: *Anything else you want to add that we haven't covered here?*
WAYNE: I can't imagine what it would be!

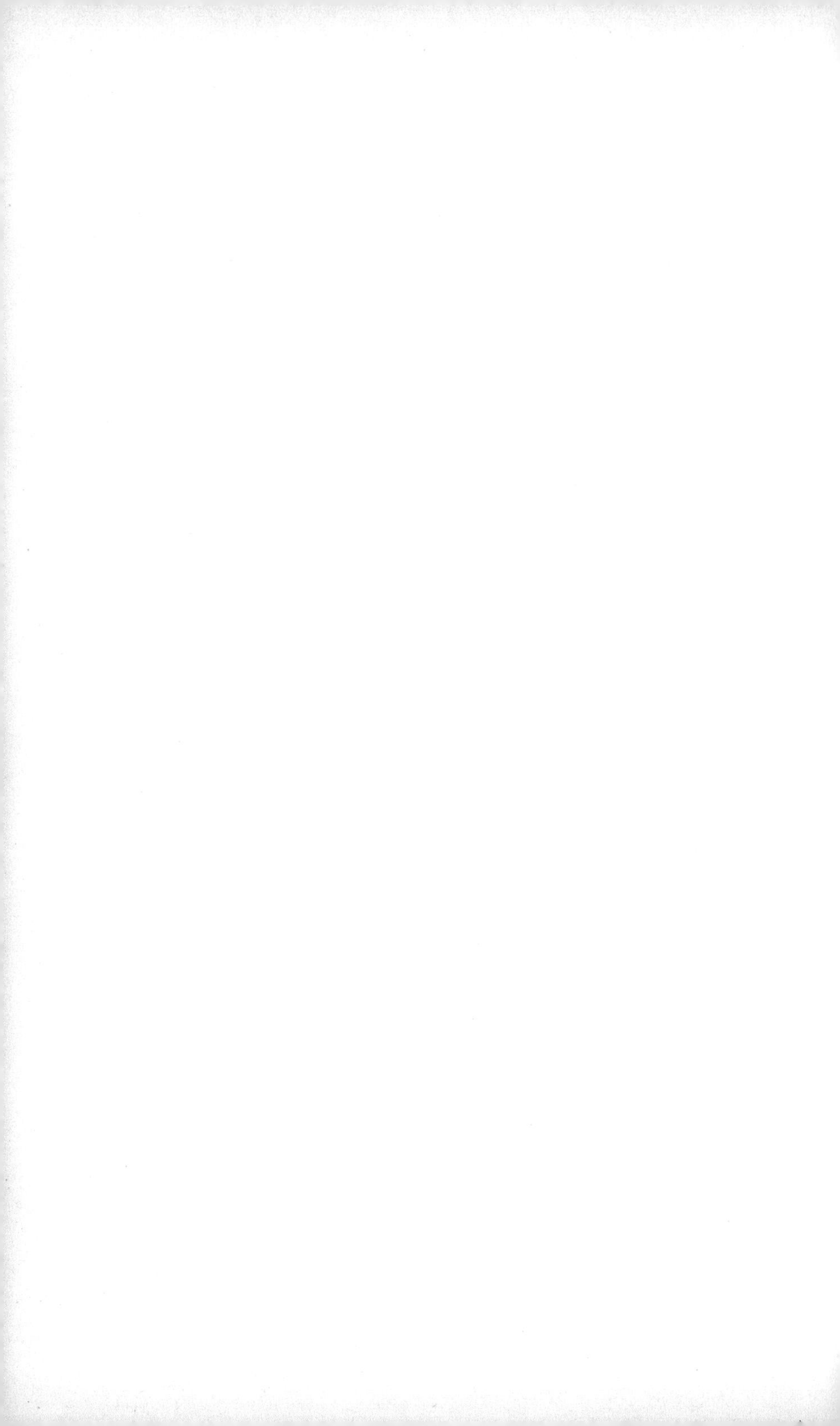

APPENDIX I

WAYS *of* CONTACTING PEOPLE *in the* BOOK

ADYASHANTI	Open Gate Sangha P.O. Box 782 Los Gatos, CA 95031-0782 Information Line: 408-236-2220 Web site: zen-satsang.org
PETER FENNER	Timeless Wisdom P.O. Box 302 555 Bryant Street Palo Alto, CA 94301 Phone: 888-772-4452 E-mail: peter@fenner.org Web site: nondualtherapy.com
GANGAJI	The Gangaji Foundation 505A San Marin Drive, Suite 120 Novato, CA 94945 Phone: 800-267-9205 E-mail: info@gangaji.org Web site: gangaji.org
DOUGLAS HARDING	Douglas Harding Shollond Hill Nacton, Ipswich Suffolk, IP10 OEW England Phone: 0044-1473-659-558 Web site: headless.org

CATHERINE INGRAM	Living Dharma P.O. Box 10431 Portland, OR 97210 Phone: 503-246-4235 Web site: dharmadialogues.org
KENNY JOHNSON	Kenneth Johnson 4431 Montgall Avenue Kansas City, MO 64130 E-mail: johnsonkenneth@hotmail.com
FRANCIS LUCILLE	Truespeech Productions 19303 Stonegate Road Middletown, CA 95461 Phone: 707-987-2276 E-mail: lucille@telis.org Web site: francislucille.com
MIRA PAGAL	Mira Pagal Decoux 54, Rue E. Oliver 1170 Bruxelles, Belguque E-mail: mira_pagal@skynet.be or mira_pagal@hotmail.com
SATYAM NADEEN	New Freedom Press P.O. Box 1496 Conyers, GA 30012 E-mail: info@satyamnadeen.com Web site: satyamnadeen.com
ROBERT RABBIN	20 Sunnyside Avenue, Suite A-118 Mill Valley, CA 94941-1928 Voicemail: 415-705-0807 E-mail: robrabbin@robrabbin.com Web site: robrabbin.com

ISAAC SHAPIRO

Isaac Shapiro c/o Deva Stadler
HutbergstraBe 14B PO Box 213
85256 Pasenbach, Germany
E-mail: premram@aol.com
or
Isaac Shapiro
Prashant, Greys Lane, Tyagarah,
N.S.W., 2481 Australia
E-mail: namaskar@ozemail.com.au
Phone: 61-266-847-519
Web site: isaacshapiro.de

LAMA SURYA DAS

Dzogchen Foundation
P.O. Box 734
Cambridge, MA 02140
E-mail: foundation@dzogchen.org
Web site: dzogchen.org, surya.org

CHRISTOPHER TITMUSS

Gaia House
West Ogwell, Newton Abbott
Devon TQ12-6EN
England
E-mail: enquiries@gaiahouse.co.uk
Web site: insightmeditation.org

ECKHART TOLLE

c/o Namaste Publishing, Inc.
P.O. Box 62084
Vancouver, British Columbia
V6J 1Z1 Canada
Web site: eckharttolle.com

NEELAM	Fire of Truth Satsanga 451 Sky High Drive Ventura, CA 93001 Phone: 805-649-2272 E-mail: FireOfTruth@compuserve.com Web site: neelam.org
RABBI RAMI SHAPIRO	E-mail: rabbirami@simplyjewish.com Web site: simplyjewish.com
SHANTIMAYI	E-mail: shantimayi@shantimayi.com Web site: ShantiMayi.com
VALERIE VENER	Phone: 510-869-2680 Web site: valerievener.com
WAYNE LIQUORMAN	Advaita Fellowship P.O. Box 911-WS Redondo Beach, CA 90277 Phone: 310-376-9636 Web site: advaita.com

APPENDIX II

BOOKS *by* THOSE INTERVIEWED *in* *THE AWAKENING WEST*

ADYASHANTI

The Impact of Awakening

My Secret is Silence

PETER FENNER

Intrinsic Freedom, with Penny Fenner

Reasoning Into Reality

The Ontology of the Middle Way

GANGAJI

You are That! Volume I and II

DOUGLAS HARDING

On Having No Head: Zen and the Rediscovery of the Obvious

Head off Stress

The Little Book of Life and Death

The Trial of the Man Who Said He Was God

The Spectre in the Robe: A Modern Pilgrim's Progress

The Hierarchy of Heaven and Earth

The Science of the First Person

Look for Yourself: The Science and Art of Self-Realization

To Be and Not to Be, That is the Answer

FRANCIS LUCILLE

Eternity Now, Dialogues on Awareness

SATYAM NADEEN

From Onions to Pearls

From Seekers to Finders

ISAAC SHAPIRO

An Outbreak of Peace

It Happens by Itself

ROBERT RABBIN

Echoes in Silence: Awakening the Meditative Spirit
Invisible Leadership: Igniting the Soul at Work
The Sacred Hub: Living in Your Real Self
The Value Workbook: Creating Personal Truth at Work
Igniting the Soul at Work

LAMA SURYA DAS

The Snow Lion's Turquoise Mane: Wisdom Tales from Tibet
Natural Great Perfection with Nyoshul Khenpo Rinpoche
Awakening the Buddha Within: Tibetan Wisdom for Today
Awakening to the Sacred: Creating a Spiritual Life from Scratch
Awakening the Buddhist Heart

CHRISTOPHER TITMUSS

An Awakened Life: Uncommon Wisdom from Everyday Experience
Fire Dance and other Poems
Freedom of the Spirit: More Voices of Hope for a World Crisis
The Green Buddha
Spirit for Change: Voices of Hope for a World in Crisis
The Profound and the Profane: An Inquiry into Spiritual Awakening
Light on Enlightenment: Revolutionary Teachings on the Inner Life

ECKHART TOLLE

The Power of Now: A Guide to Spiritual Enlightenment

RABBI RAMI SHAPIRO

Open Secrets: The Letters of Reb Yerachmiel
Gefite Fishing: A Guide to Spiritual Awakening
The Simply Jewish Manifesto
The Eleven Irreducible Laws of Rabbinic Leadership
The Five Worlds Journal
The Simply Jewish Billboard Project
(and others)

WAYNE LIQUORMAN

Acceptance of What Is: A Book About Nothing
No Way: For the Spiritually Advanced

GLOSSARY OF TERMS

ADAMS, ROBERT

An American spiritual teacher and jnani (q.v.) who passed away in 1997. (He was interviewed for this book in late 1996 but his estate did not give permission to publish the interview.)

ADVAITA

"Not two." Non-duality or absolute unity; a subdivision of Vedanta, one of the six orthodox schools of Indian philosophy; the non-dual approach.

ALLAH

Arabic word used in the Islamic tradition for the Source and Substance of All That Is.

ASANA

Physical postures that are regularly performed as a standard feature of many yoga practices.

ASHRAM

Residence of a guru, saint or sage; place where a community of disciples live and gather.

ASHTAVAKRA GITA

An ancient Advaita teaching on non-dual realization from an anonymous source told in a narrative form.

ATMA VICHARA

See Self-inquiry.

ATMAN

In Hinduism, the Self, the seed of perfection in all beings, the Divine within, which is recognized in Self-Realization.

AVATAR

God incarnate in a physical form who comes to earth for the purpose of restoring moral order, such as Jesus Christ in the Christian tradition and Krishna in the Hindu tradition.

AVIDYA
Ignorance; fundamentally, the belief that one is a separate entity.

AVUDHUTA GITA
A text of Vedanta representing Advaita (q.v.) or non-dualism.

BHAJANS
In Hinduism, devotional songs.

BHAKTI
In Hinduism, the path of devotion.

BODHISATTVA
Enlightened being; in Mahayana Buddhism, the realized spiritual practitioner who had vowed to commit themselves to the liberation of all beings, dedicating their own ultimate realization to that end.

BRAHMAN
In Hinduism, the all-inclusive Absolute.

CONFUCIANISM
The system of ethics, education, and statesmanship taught by Confucius and his disciples stressing love for humanity, ancestor worship, reverence for parents, and harmony in thought and action.

DARSHAN
Being in the presence of a realized being; greeting such a being.

DEPENDENT ARISING
A feature of realization as taught in Buddhism explaining that everything arises in dependence upon causes and conditions and that everything is interdependent.

DHARMA
The Buddha's teachings; the cosmic law or order, truth.

DHARMAKAYA
The absolute aspect of the Buddha and each of us, manifest as formless, luminous, aware emptiness.

DEITIES
The divine awareness beings whose forms and realms are visualized in Tibetan Buddhist Tantric practices.

DZOGCHEN

The Great Perfection or Great Completeness; the teachings of the Nyingma school of Tibetan Buddhism, often called "the view from above," or the Great Consummation; an immediate or direct, non-dual path.

ECKHARDT, MEISTER

A self-realized German mystic and Dominican theologian of the thirteenth and fourteenth centuries.

EIGHTFOLD PATH

The Fourth Noble Truth of Buddha's teachings; the eight principles of enlightened living, the way to the end of suffering.

EMPTINESS

A term used in Buddhism to refer to the insight occurring in realization that all phenomena are interrelated and lack any defining characteristics. (See shunyata)

ENNEAGRAM

A system of nine character fixations or types of ego personalities. It is believed to have been developed by the Sufis.

GARAB DORJE

Recognized as the first human Dzogchen teacher in the Tibetan Buddhist tradition.

GAYATRI MANTRA

The most famous and sacred mantra of Hinduism; it is a prayer to Savitri, the sun, for divine inspiration.

GITA

The Bhagavad Gita, a section of the ancient Hindu epic poem Mahabharata, which recounts a dialogue between Krishna and Arjuna about the nature of Truth and the responsibility to fulfill one's role in life.

GNOSTIC AWARENESS

In western mystical traditions, mystical knowledge, direct experience of the absolute.

HATHA YOGA
A branch of yoga which involves physical movements, postures, and breathing exercises.

HEART SUTRA
A short version of the Prajnaparamita (transcendental wisdom); Sutras recited daily in Buddhist temples and monasteries around the world, which describes and points to the absence of any apparent self-nature in the inextricable interconnectedness of all things appearing as the display of awareness.

I-THOUGHT
In the teachings of Ramana Maharshi (q.v.), the thought "I" is the first thought of the mind; egoity.

JNANA
The universal wisdom of the absolute, non-dual awareness.

JNANI
A Sanscrit term referring to one who has realized the absolute, non-dual awareness, or Self.

KALI YUGA
See Yugas.

KALPA
An eon; a vast period of time during which a world system arises, persists and decays.

KALU RINPOCHE
A twentieth century master of Tibetan Buddhism who died in the 1980s and has been acknowledged to have been reborn in India.

KARMA
The collective results of one's actions; the chain of cause and effect; conditioning; the path of Karma aims to reach enlightenment through virtuous actions.

KASHMIR SHAIVISM
A non-dual spiritual tradition that comes from Kashmir, India which emphasizes the direct realization of its Truth.

KLEIN, JEAN

A musicologist and doctor from Central Europe who is considered one of the greatest teachers of Advaita in the twentieth century. He taught in Europe and the United States for forty years until his death in 1998.

KOAN

A Zen Buddhist practice; an unsolvable riddle designed to take one beyond the conceptual mind.

KRISHNA

An avatar (q.v.) of Vishnu (the Preserver in the Hindu trinity) and hero of the epic poem Mahabharata.

KRISHNAMURTI, J.

A world-renowned Indian spiritual teacher and author of numerous books who taught in India, Europe, and the United States when he was alive.

KRISHNAMURTI, U.G.

A contemporary, iconoclastic "teacher" who simply described his own experience; he authored numerous books.

LAMA

Teacher; the equivalent of the Hindu term guru. A title bestowed by one's teacher.

MADHYMIKA

The Middle Way; Buddhist teaching on emptiness that is beyond extremes.

MAHAMUDRA

Literally, the Great Symbol or Gesture; it refers to the absolute reality itself; how things actually are; it is also the name of a lineage and tradition of teachings in Tibetan Buddhism.

MAHAYANA

Great Vehicle; the majority branch of Buddhism, which emphasizes universal liberation and great compassion.

MANTRA

A sacred syllable or set of syllables, the sound and meaning of which have traditionally been experienced to be evocative of particular states of consciousness.

MAYA
Hindu word for illusion. Literally, "that which is not."

NAMASKAR
A greeting that means the divinity in me recognizes and honors the divinity in you.

NEEM KAROLI BABA
An Indian guru who was also called Maharaji and taught through telling simple stories. He died in 1973.

NEITZCHE, FREDERICK
A nineteenth century German existentialist philosopher and writer.

NIRVANA
Freedom, enlightenment, the transcendence of the ego; a condition that is untouched by space and time.

NISARGADATTA MAHARAJ
A simple, uneducated man who lived in Bombay, India and became a realized master of Advaita (q.v.). He brought Advaita to the West through the book *I Am That*.

PADMASAMBHAVA
The founder of Buddhism in Tibet; Tibetan tradition views him as an emanation of the Buddha of Infinite Light, and refers to him as Guru Rinpoche. His name means "born from a lotus," indicating his miraculous birth from a lotus.

PITH INSTRUCTIONS
The essential teachings or instructions of Tibetan Dzogchen.

POONJA, H.W.L.
A realized Master who lived and taught in Lucknow, India. He is affectionately called Poonjaji and Papaji by his followers. Many Westerners have awakened with him; a powerful force in the awakening of the West. He died in 1997.

PRAJNA
Gnosis, transcendental wisdom.

PRAJNAPARAMITA
The Buddhist teachings of transcendental wisdom and compassion.

PRANAM
Bowing in respect before a teacher or guru.

RAMANA MAHARSHI
A South Indian saint and sage who lived from 1879–1950. He taught primarily through silence and encouraged most seekers to do self-inquiry (q.v.). He is the guru of Poonja.

RAMAKRISHNA
A Bengali Indian saint and visionary mystic who lived from 1836–1886, and was a life-long devotee of the Divine Mother.

RIGPA
Innate wisdom or wakefulness; pure presence; primordial being; a term used in Dzogchen teachings.

SADHANA
Spiritual practice for the purpose of preparing for enlightenment; the way one comes to the Truth.

SADHU
A full-time spiritual seeker, usually one who has given up family life and work in order to pursue enlightenment; they are provided for by the charity of others.

SAHAJA SAMADHI
The natural state of absorption in the Self; permanent realization in which the mind has been irrevocably destroyed.

SAMADHI
An intensely blissful superconscious state or "trance;" the highest condition of human consciousness.

SAMSARA
The finite world of change and illusion. Bondage, delusion; the cycle of suffering, birth conditioning, sickness, death, and rebirth.

SANGHA
A spiritual community of people interested in the Truth.

SAT GURU
True revealer of light; the guru who is real and true.

SATSANG
Fellowship or company with Truth; the conversation and/or company of a realized teacher; association (sangha) with Truth (sat).

SATORI
A term used in Zen Buddhism for sudden enlightenment.

SELF-INQUIRY
A technique utilized in both Advaita and in Buddhism to cut through the mind at its root by asking the question, "Who am I?" Also called Atma Vichara (q.v.).

SHAKTI
The active power of God; the energy that makes the world operate.

SHUNYATA
The teaching of Mahayana Buddhism that everything is empty and open by nature and lacking in inherent, separate self-existence.

SIDDHA YOGA
A school of yoga from the Kashmiri Shaivism tradition brought to the United States by Swami Muktananda (q.v.).

SIDDHI(S)
A supernatural power or faculty; the power to perform miracles.

SIX REALMS OF EXISTENCE
In Buddhist cosmology, the realms through which ignorant sentient beings cycle based on their actions and their principle passions.

SUTRAS
The teachings given by Shakyamuni Buddha, memorized by his disciples, and subsequently written down.

SWAMI MUKTANANDA
A twentieth century Indian guru who wrote many books, came to the West, and started Siddha Yoga Foundation.

TATHAGATA

The Buddha nature that is present in all sentient beings.

THERAVADA

Literally, the tradition of the elders; theravada is the form of Buddhism practiced in Sri Lanka, Thailand, and other south Asian countries; it emphasizes the idea of the Arhat, an individual focused on personal liberation.

TREKCHOD

Cutting through or seeing through; in Dzogchen, the main naked awareness practice of seeing through the apparent forms and recognizing the essence.

TRIPLE GEM OR THE THREE JEWELS

In Buddhism in general, the Buddha, the dharma or teachings of the Buddha and the Sangha are called the Three Jewels; in Dzogchen Rigpa (q.v.), the innate, empty presence of awareness is sometimes referred to as the Three Jewels.

TRUNGPA RINPOCHE

A Tibetan Buddhist master; the eleventh incarnation of the Trungpa Tulka. After leaving Tibet, he established Buddhist study centers in North America and Europe.

UPANISHADS

The most ancient sacred teachings in the Hindu tradition; they form the final part of each Veda (see Vedas).

VAJRA

"Thunderbolt," symbol of immutable power and awareness.

VAJRAYANA BUDDHISM

Vehicle of the Tantra and Dzogchen traditions of Tibetan Buddhism.

VASANAS

Latent tendencies of mind formed by former actions, thoughts, and desires; impressions of anything remaining unconscious in the mind.

VEDAS
Four collections of scriptures dating from 2,000 BC to 500 BC which are the ultimate source of authority for most Hindus.

VEDANTA
The philosophy derived from the Upanishadic (q.v.) texts.

VIDYA
Wisdom; the recognition that one is innately the impersonal awareness in which subject and objects occur.

VIPASSANA
A Buddhist meditation practice; also called Insight Meditation.

YUGAS
In Hindu cosmology, an epic, a cycle or period; a kalpa (q.v.) consists of four yugas which represent four stages of movement away from the Truth and into disharmony. We are now living in the Kali Yuga.

ZAZEN
Zen meditation in a prescribed, crosslegged posture.

ZEN BUDDHISM
A contemplative branch of Mahayana Buddhism developed in Japan from Ch'an Buddhism in China. Zen is the Japanese translation of the Hindu Dhyana, contemplation.

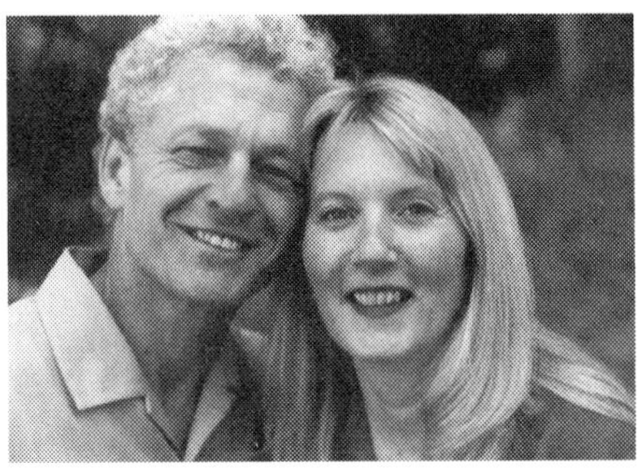

LYNN MARIE LUMIERE is a licensed Marriage, Family Therapist who has a private practice in Oakland, CA. She has fifteen years experience working with individuals and couples. Lynn Marie has been an ardent spiritual seeker for thirty years. This book comes out of her search for Truth and a sincere desire to assist others in this discovery. She is currently writing a book titled *Awareness: The Solution in Which Problems Dissolve* about the integration of non-dual wisdom and psychotherapy. Further information about Lynn Marie's work can be found at conscioustherapy.com

JOHN LUMIERE-WINS is a certified hypnotherapist and counselor who also enjoys writing and working as a carpenter. He has sixteen years experience working in the mental health field and is writing a new book, *The Awakening World: A Journey from Where We Think We Are to Here*. This book addresses the ecological and political climate of our world today and the deepest solution to this condition. John has been on a spiritual path most of his life and initiated *The Awakening West* when he saw that many Westerners were awakening and it wasn't receiving any media attention.